Dysimmune Neuropathies

Dysimmune Neuropathies

Edited by

Yusuf A. Rajabally
Aston Medical School, Aston University, Birmingham, United Kingdom
Regional Neuromuscular Service, Queen Elizabeth Hospital Birmingham,
Birmingham, United Kingdom

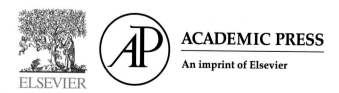

ACADEMIC PRESS

An imprint of Elsevier

Academic Press is an imprint of Elsevier
125 London Wall, London EC2Y 5AS, United Kingdom
525 B Street, Suite 1650, San Diego, CA 92101, United States
50 Hampshire Street, 5th Floor, Cambridge, MA 02139, United States
The Boulevard, Langford Lane, Kidlington, Oxford OX5 1GB, United Kingdom

Notices
Knowledge and best practice in this field are constantly changing. As new research and
experience broaden our understanding, changes in research methods, professional practices, or
medical treatment may become necessary.

Practitioners and researchers must always rely on their own experience and knowledge in
evaluating and using any information, methods, compounds, or experiments described herein.
In using such information or methods they should be mindful of their own safety and the safety
of others, including parties for whom they have a professional responsibility.

To the fullest extent of the law, neither the Publisher nor the authors, contributors, or editors,
assume any liability for any injury and/or damage to persons or property as a matter of products
liability, negligence or otherwise, or from any use or operation of any methods, products,
instructions, or ideas contained in the material herein.

Library of Congress Cataloging-in-Publication Data
A catalog record for this book is available from the Library of Congress

British Library Cataloguing-in-Publication Data
A catalogue record for this book is available from the British Library

ISBN: 978-0-12-814572-2

For information on all Academic Press publications
visit our website at https://www.elsevier.com/books-and-journals

Publisher: Nikky Levy
Acquisitions Editor: Melanie Tucker
Editorial Project Manager: Kristi Anderson
Production Project Manager: Bharatwaj Varatharajan
Cover Designer: Miles Hitchen

Typeset by SPi Global, India

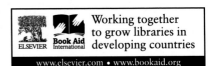

Working together
to grow libraries in
developing countries

www.elsevier.com • www.bookaid.org

Dedication

*To my parents, Mariam and Hanif, who will sadly
not read these lines, for everything they
did for me.*

*To my dearest wife Catherine, for all her continuing
support, help, encouragement
and understanding and all the good and great
happiness she has brought to my life.*

*To my children, Sofia, Hana, Zeinab and Zakariya, who,
each, and in so many ways, have brought and continue
to bring me much joy everyday.*

*To all my patients, who have been my best teachers,
right from the beginning and still today.*

Contents

3.   Chronic inflammatory demyelinating polyneuropathy

Yusuf A. Rajabally, H. Stephan Goedee

4.   Multifocal motor neuropathy

Katie Beadon, Jean-Marc Léger

5. Monoclonal gammopathy associated neuropathy: Focusing on IgM M-protein associated neuropathy

Mariëlle H.J. Pruppers, Ingemar S.J. Merkies, Nicolette C. Notermans,

6. POEMS syndrome

Chiara Briani, Marta Campagnolo, Marco Luigetti, Federica Lessi, Fausto Adami

7. Peripheral nervous system involvement in vasculitis

Stéphane Mathis, Mathilde Duchesne, Laurent Magy,
Jean-Michel Vallat,

8. Paraneoplastic peripheral neuropathies

Jean-Christophe Antoine

9. ## Cervical and lumbosacral radiculoplexus neuropathies

Pariwat Thaisetthawatkul, P. James B. Dyck

10. ## Dysimmune small fiber neuropathies

Anne Louise Oaklander

Contributors

Numbers in parenthesis indicate the pages on which the authors' contributions begin.

Fausto Adami (129), Hematology and Clinical Immunology Unit, Department of Medicine, University of Padova, Padova, Italy

Jean-Christophe Antoine (177), Department of Neurology, University Hospital of Saint-Etienne, Saint-Etienne, France

Katie Beadon (85), National Referral Center for Neuromuscular Diseases, Institut Hospitalo-Universitaire (IHU) de Neurosciences, University Hospital Pitié Salpêtrière, Paris, France

Chiara Briani (129), Department of Neuroscience, University of Padova, Padova, Italy

Marta Campagnolo (129), Department of Neuroscience, University of Padova, Padova, Italy

Pieter A van Doorn (31), Department of Neurology, Erasmus MC, University Medical Center, Rotterdam, Netherlands

Mathilde Duchesne (145), Department of Pathology; Department of Neurology, University Hospital Dupuytren, Limoges, France

P. James B. Dyck (199), Department of Neurology, Mayo Clinic College of Medicine, Rochester, MN, United States

H. Stephan Goedee (31), Brain Center Rudolf Magnus, Department of Neurology and Neurosurgery, University Medical Center Utrecht, Utrecht, The Netherlands

Jean-Marc Léger (85), National Referral Center for Neuromuscular Diseases, Institut Hospitalo-Universitaire (IHU) de Neurosciences, University Hospital Pitié Salpêtrière, Paris, France

Federica Lessi (129), Hematology and Clinical Immunology Unit, Department of Medicine, University of Padova, Padova, Italy

Marco Luigetti (129), Catholic University of the Sacred Heart; Neurology Unit, University Hospital A. Gemelli—IRCCS, Rome, Italy

Laurent Magy (145), Department of Neurology; National Reference Center 'neuropathies périphériques rares', University Hospital Dupuytren, Limoges, France

Stéphane Mathis (145), Department of Neurology, Nerve-Muscle Unit, CHU Bordeaux (Pellegrin University Hospital); National Reference Center 'maladies neuromusculaires du grand sud-ouest', CHU Bordeaux (Pellegrin University Hospital), University of Bordeaux, Bordeaux, France

Ingemar S.J. Merkies (109), Department of Neurology, Maastricht University Medical Center, Maastricht, The Netherlands; Department of Neurology, Sint-Elisabeth Hospital, Willemstad, Curaçao

Nicolette C. Notermans (109), Department of Neurology, University Medical Center Utrecht, Utrecht, The Netherlands

Anne Louise Oaklander (225), Department of Neurology, Massachusetts General Hospital, Harvard Medical School; Department of Pathology (Neuropathology), Massachusetts General Hospital, Boston, MA, United States

Mariëlle H.J. Pruppers (109), Department of Neurology, University Medical Center Utrecht, Utrecht, The Netherlands; Department of Neurology, Maastricht University Medical Center, Maastricht, The Netherlands

Yusuf A. Rajabally (1, 31), Aston Medical School, Aston University; Regional Neuromuscular Service, Queen Elizabeth Hospital Birmingham, Birmingham, United Kingdom

Pariwat Thaisetthawatkul (199), Department of Neurological Sciences, University of Nebraska Medical Center, Omaha, NE, United States

Jean-Michel Vallat (145), Department of Neurology; National Reference Center 'neuropathies périphériques rares', University Hospital Dupuytren, Limoges, France

Chapter 1

Dysimmune neuropathies

Yusuf A. Rajabally

Aston Medical School, Aston University, Birmingham, United Kingdom; Regional Neuromuscular Service, Queen Elizabeth Hospital Birmingham, Birmingham, United Kingdom

Introduction

Dysimmune neuropathies represent an expanding field of a very heterogeneous group of disorders of highly diverse clinical presentations and variable underlying pathophysiology. The diagnostic process is frequently complex and many uncertainties regarding classifications remain, with some of those having very recently appeared as a result of new knowledge. The most exciting aspect of dysimmune neuropathies, within the very wide spectrum of neuromuscular disorders where many are of a genetic basis and unfortunately still mostly untreatable, is certainly their potential for treatment. Recent progress and knowledge indicate that the previous tendencies to clump these disorders in large groups may neither be appropriate nor practical, as treatment modalities vary widely, including in entities with closely related clinical or electrodiagnostic pictures. More splitting appears likely to occur as new data emerge, separating previously grouped disorders. This is not, however, without problems and difficulties with the rarity of the diseases in question and the obvious overlaps that will persist.

In view of the increasing diversity and new developments concerning this group of peripheral nervous system diseases, the need for a dedicated book on the dysimmune neuropathies became apparent. With a primary clinical focus, we have attempted to effectively and comprehensively cover the knowledge base for all main areas, with integration in each chapter of the various epidemiological, diagnostic, and therapeutic elements so as to provide the reader with a readily accessible but as exhaustive as possible clinically directly relevant text.

Starting with Guillain-Barré syndrome, substantial developments have progressively happened in the field over the past century since the initial description of the disorder, including, within the last several years, considerable new knowledge in all areas including diagnostics, pathophysiology, treatment modalities, and potential for novel therapeutic avenues. The chapter offers an up-to-date summary of these important elements of interest. In the chapter on

Dysimmune Neuropathies. **https://doi.org/10.1016/B978-0-12-814572-2.00001-7**

chronic inflammatory demyelinating polyneuropathy (CIDP), the various developments in diagnostic techniques, enhanced by nerve imaging, treatment and use of objective evaluation tools are considered. In the context of the increasing heterogeneity of this entity, with the recent significant discoveries of new antinodal and antiparanodal antibodies in a subset of affected patients, considerable widening the CIDP spectrum has occurred in the last few years. The relative higher prevalence of CIDP compared to other dysimmune neuropathies also led to the need to elaborate on differential diagnosis and mimics as well as the many described associations of CIDP with other diseases. Multifocal motor neuropathy (MMN), which is one of the "newer" dysimmune neuropathies, is also described in its historical, epidemiological, diagnostic, and therapeutic aspects in a chapter that discusses the many important questions that make MMN more than just a single-treatment-responsive disease. A separate chapter focuses on the paraprotein-associated inflammatory neuropathies, particularly the IgM paraproteinaemias. This chapter offers the essential description of a common case scenario in patients with suspected dysimmune neuropathy and highlights the fundamental knowledge required to manage this also heterogeneous, frequently complex and often challenging set of disorders. Polyneuropathy Organomegaly Endocrinopathy M-Protein Skin (POEMS) syndrome is detailed in a dedicated chapter, which was felt essential to elaborate on this rare and previously fatal condition, also associating a neuropathy and a paraprotein, but for which diagnostic modalities and criteria have changed over the years, and importantly, currently available treatments now offer a significantly improved prognosis. An individual chapter covers vasculitic neuropathy. The heterogeneity of this form of dysimmune neuropathy is also wide, ranging from the purely neuropathic nonsystemic forms to those where the neuropathy is part of more diffuse disease. Diagnosis relies on a high index of clinical suspicion and detailed histopathology which is well-illustrated in this chapter which also details the important therapeutic aspects. A dedicated chapter covers the paraneoplastic neuropathies, which although necessarily part of a subsequently unconfirmed differential in many encountered cases of dysimmune neuropathy, represents an area of expanding knowledge both for diagnosis and management. A further separate chapter details cervicobrachial and lumbosacral radiculopexus neuropathies. This is one of the only two anatomically-defined chapters in this volume, the reason being the specific nature of such presentations, which necessitates correct identification of a dysimmune aetiology versus many others, as well as the particular histopathological processes involved, identified in the last few years with important implications for management. The final chapter of this volume elaborates on a new, but substantial clinical problem. Again, this section is necessarily wide, as informs the reader of the dysimmune small fiber neuropathies, to be identified among the many neuropathies of this very specific and separate histopathological subcategory. Identifying those with an immunological basis in this expanding and exciting area is greatly important, as may lead to the need to consider treatments which would otherwise be discounted.

I am extremely grateful to all the recognized major international experts who have kindly contributed to the chapters of this book. All are authorities in the field who have done extensive research, but also and most importantly, they have long and exhaustive direct day-to-day clinical experience in the diagnosis and management of the disorders they describe and detail. We hope this text will cater for the needs of all clinicians in the field and provide readers with a comprehensive, up-to-date and in-depth coverage of the current knowledge-base and thereby ultimately contribute to enhancing the standards of clinical care for the many patients affected by this group of diseases, worldwide.

The timing of the completion of this volume in March/April 2020 is for us all, a moment of profound anxiety and uncertainty due to the COVID-19 pandemic. Undoubtedly, this already has had, for several weeks and will have, for many more to come, substantial consequences on our patients' lives and on the clinical management of their diseases. One hopes that despite the essential focus on the current pandemic, we are capable as healthcare professionals of remaining equally attentive to the needs of our patients with chronic diseases such as dysimmune neuropathies, some of whom will be, themselves or their families, at greater risk, others with less access to care and more still, with many compounded difficulties in their daily lives. Our first challenge at this point will be to ensure they are remembered and continue being looked after in these difficult times.

Chapter 2

Guillain-Barré syndrome

Pieter A van Doorn

Department of Neurology, Erasmus MC, University Medical Center, Rotterdam, Netherlands

Introduction

Guillain-Barré syndrome (GBS) is an immune-mediated polyneuropathy and the most common cause of acute flaccid paralysis.[1] It is characterized by rapidly progressive bilateral weakness of the limbs and hypo- or areflexia.[2, 3] GBS requires early diagnosis, monitoring, and treatment, as it is potentially a life-threatening disorder because respiratory insufficiency and autonomic dysfunction frequently occur. The course is usually progressive, with a monophasic course lasting up to 4 weeks and a more or less stable (plateau) phase for a period of weeks to months, which is followed by a recovery phase that may last months or even years (Fig. 1). GBS typically is preceded by an antecedent event such as an upper respiratory infection, diarrhea, or another immune-stimulating event that induces an aberrant autoimmune response targeting the peripheral nerves and spinal roots.[1] Weakness is often accompanied by sensory symptoms such as paresthesia or numbness that usually start on the distal parts of the extremities. Both cranial nerves and autonomic nerve fibers can be involved.[1, 4] Pain is often present; it can be severe and may even precede the onset of weakness, often causing diagnostic difficulties.[1, 5, 6] GBS has a large clinical spectrum and range of severity.

The clinical presentation of GBS was first described in 1916 in two soldiers by the French neurologists Guillain, Barré, and Strohl.[7] The patients they described had rapidly progressive weakness, mild hypoesthesia, and lowered or absent reflexes. The cerebrospinal fluid (CSF) showed an increased albumin without a cellular reaction, which, at that time, mainly differentiated the disease from poliomyelitis. Treatment consisted of absolute rest, massage of the upper and lower limbs, injections of strychnine, and a soda of phenyl salicylate. Finally, the patients later recovered. Since the 1980s, major progress has been made in the understanding and treatment of GBS.[8–10] Especially in the past 10–15 years, much new evidence has been gathered that has shed light on the immunopathogenesis of GBS, especially concerning the relation between specific infections such as *Campylobacter jejuni*, the presence of antiganglioside antibodies, and

Dysimmune Neuropathies. https://doi.org/10.1016/B978-0-12-814572-2.00002-9

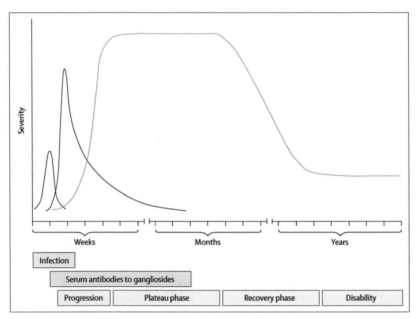

FIG. 1 Course of GBS. *(From Willison HJ, Jacobs BC, van Doorn PA. Guillain-Barré syndrome. Reprinted with permission from Elsevier (The Lancet, 2016, 388(10045): 717–27)).*

the determination of clinical and electrophysiological subgroups. In 2016, a Peripheral Nerve Society meeting was organized in Glasgow. In relation to that meeting, a book celebrating a century of progress in GBS with contributions from more than 100 authors has been published.[11] International collaboration has resulted in large prospective cohort studies such as the International GBS Outcome Study (IGOS) and in the development and publication of a consensus statement on the diagnosis and management of GBS.[12, 13] The first GRADE-based international GBS guideline is currently under construction by members of the European Academy of Neurology (EAN) and the Peripheral Nerve Society (PNS).

Diversity of GBS

The clinical presentation and course of GBS are highly diverse. Usually, GBS is a relatively symmetrical disorder with predominant weakness of the legs. Most patients also have sensory disturbances. Several clinical variants can be distinguished such as the pure motor variant (Fig. 2). A well-known variant characterized by ophthalmoplegia, areflexia, and ataxia is the Miller Fisher syndrome (MFS).[14–16] Some of the other local variants are the pharyngeal-cervical-brachial variant, and paraparetic GBS.[16, 17] Patients with Bickerstaff brainstem encephalitis (BBE) have features of GBS, in particular MFS, but also have disturbance of consciousness that can be so severe that it clinically may even

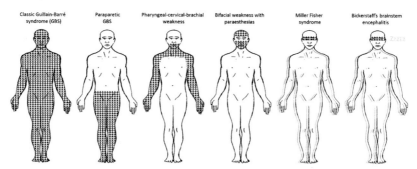

FIG. 2   GBS variants. Patterns of weakness in Guillain-Barré syndrome (GBS), Miller Fisher syndrome, and their subtypes. GBS and Miller Fisher syndrome and their subtypes form a continuum of discrete and overlapping syndromes. Shaded areas indicate weakness. The double outline (blurring the figures) indicates ataxia. "Zzzzz"indicates hypersomnolence. Classic GBS: tetraparesis with or without motor cranial nerve involvement, can be sensory/motor or pure motor; Paraparetic GBS: paresis of lower limbs; Pharyngeal-cervical-brachial weakness: bulbar, neck, and upper limbs; Bifacial weakness with paraesthesias: facial; Miller Fisher syndrome: external ophthalmoplegia; and Bickerstaff's brainstem encephalitis: external ophthalmoplegia. Facial weakness and motor cranial nerve involvement are more frequent in demyelinating-type classic GBS (acute inflammatory demyelinating polyradiculoneuropathy) than in axonal-type (acute motor axonal neuropathy). In Miller Fisher syndrome, there is ataxia and areflexia, and in its central nervous system subtype, Bickerstaff's brainstem encephalitis, there is additional hypersomnolence. *(With permission from Wakerley BR, Yuki N. Mimics and chameleons in Guillain-Barré and Miller Fisher syndromes.* Pract Neurol *2015;15(3):90–9 (Fig. 1)).*

simulate brain death. MRI in BBE can show brainstem and additional white matter involvement. Patients with both MFS and BBE often have serum IgG anti-GQ1b antibodies.[1, 14, 17–19] It is good to realize that there can be overlap between these forms, especially between MFS and the more usual presentation of GBS with limb weakness (MFS-GBS overlap syndrome).

Mainly because the presentation of GBS is highly variable, the diagnosis can be challenging. The diagnosis can be supported by cerebrospinal fluid (CSF) examination and/or nerve conduction studies (NCS). Because NCS may show both signs of demyelination or axonal degeneration, the absence of demyelination does not rule out GBS.[20] This finding and the corresponding pathologic findings were carefully described by the late Professor Griffin et al. This led to the distinction of GBS in the acute inflammatory demyelinating polyneuropathy (AIDP) and the acute motor axonal neuropathy (AMAN).[1, 21, 22] It is important to realize that both CSF protein, but also NCS can be normal, especially in the early phase of disease and thus do not exclude GBS.

The focus of this chapter will be on the diagnostics and management of GBS, but other matters will be discussed. These include the results of recent trials, including with the complement inhibitor eculizumab; future perspectives regarding an intensified IVIg treatment schedule; a study on small volume plasma exchange; and potential other novel therapeutic agents.

Epidemiology and geographical differences

GBS has a reported incidence of 0.81–1.89 cases per 100,000 individuals, and probably is the most common cause of acute flaccid paralysis worldwide.[1] This may indicate that GBS affects about 100,000 people worldwide each year. Based mainly on data from North America and Europe, it has been shown that the GBS incidence increased by 20% for every 10-year increase in age; GBS usually is more frequent in males, with the highest incidence between 50–70 years of age.[23, 24] No major geographical variation has been reported in the incidence of GBS, although there has been a temporary rise in GBS on the Caribbean island of Curacao, likely related to Campylobacter[25] and a rise of Zika-related GBS mainly in South America.[26] The incidence of GBS in children was reported to be relatively high (3.25 cases per 100,000) in Bangladesh[24] (Fig. 3).

However, there is a regional variation in the main subtypes of GBS. It was initially reported that AIDP is the main subtype (60%–80%) of GBS cases in Europe, North America, and Australia, whereas AMAN accounts for 30%–65% of GBS cases in Asia and Central and South America. A recent publication from the International GBS Outcome Study (IGOS) on the first 1000 patients included in this worldwide prospective study shed new light on regional differences.[24] The IGOS study compared three regions based on geography, income, and previous reports: Europe/Americas, Asia (without Bangladesh), and Bangladesh, from which very large numbers of patients were included. The outcome of GBS patients from this lower-income country is different in comparison with the other regions because the majority of GBS patients remain untreated due to a lack of finances. The predominant clinical variant was sensorimotor in Europe/Americas (69%) and Asia (43%), and pure motor in Bangladesh (69%).

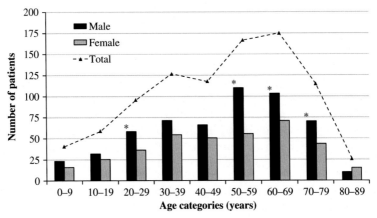

FIG. 3 Age and gender distribution of GBS (Doets Brain 2018 Fig. 1). Age and gender distribution of IGOS cohort. *$P < .05$ for difference in number of males and females per age category. $n = 919$. *(With permission from Doets AY, Verboon C, van den Berg B, et al. Regional variation of Guillain-Barré syndrome. Brain 2018;141(11):2866–77 (Fig. 1)).*

MFS and MFS-GBS overlap syndrome were more common in Asia (22%) than in Europe/Americas (11%) and Bangladesh (1%), ($P < .001$). Pure motor GBS is related to predominant axonal involvement. Rather surprisingly, the predominant electrophysiological subtype was demyelinating in all regions (Europe/Americas: 55%; Asia: 45%; Bangladesh: 40%). However, the axonal subtype occurred more often in Bangladesh (36%) than in Europe/Americas (6%) and other Asian countries (6%) ($P < .001$). This study shows that pure motor GBS is not equivalent to axonal GBS. In all regions, patients with the axonal subtype were younger, had fewer sensory deficits, and showed a trend toward poorer recovery compared to patients with the demyelinating subtype. It is, however, important to realize what criteria have been used to define demyelination and thus classify patients as AIDP, as this may affect the analysis and conclusions. Mortality was higher in Bangladesh (17%) than in Europe/Americas (5%) and Asia (2%) ($P < .001$). This difference, however, is likely due to the fact that the majority of patients in Bangladesh are left untreated with expensive treatments such as intravenous immunoglobulin (IVIg) and plasma exchange (PE). This IGOS study thus showed that factors related to geography have a major influence on clinical phenotype, disease severity, electrophysiological subtype, and outcome of GBS.

Preceding infections

Infections precede GBS in the majority of cases, but other events such as vaccinations have also been reported as preceding GBS.[1, 27] Many different pathogens have been reported in relation with the onset of GBS. Infections that have proven to be associated with GBS in case-control studies are *Campylobacter jejuni* (*C. jejuni*), Cytomegalovirus (CMV), Epstein Barr virus (EBV), *Mycoplasma pneumoniae*, and hepatitis E virus (HEV).[1, 28–33]

Over the past years, large progress has been made in understanding how preceding infections likely result in peripheral nerve damage in GBS, especially in the AMAN subtype. Infections with *Campylobacter jejuni* may trigger cross-reactive antibodies that bind to human peripheral nerve gangliosides (GM1 and GD1a) by a mechanism called "molecular mimicry"[1, 27, 34, 35] (Fig. 4). Identifying the trigger for GBS is important to further understand the underlying pathogenic mechanisms, but also to anticipate a possible rise in incidence following an epidemic or pandemic, as was seen with the recent Zika virus (ZIKV) infection.[26, 36, 37] Interestingly, starting in 2013 an ZIKV outbreak in French Polynesia was followed by a 20-fold increase in GBS cases. A case-control study conducted during the outbreak period found neutralizing antibodies against ZIKV in 100% of GBS cases and 56% of controls.[36] The first confirmed case of ZIKV infection in the Americas was reported in Northeast Brazil in May 2015. Zika rapidly spread across Brazil and to more than 50 other countries and territories on the American continent. Newborns with microcephaly, Zika-related GBS, and other neurological impairments were reported.[38] Since then, multiple studies

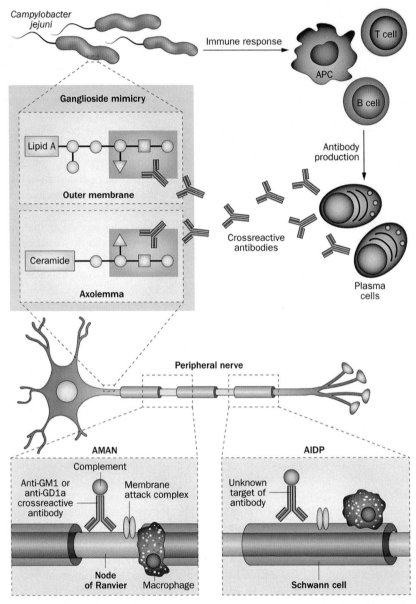

FIG. 4 Immunopathology of GBS. Immunopathogenesis of GBS: molecular mimicry and anti-ganglioside antibodies. Infections with pathogens, such as *Campylobacter jejuni*, can trigger humoral immune and autoimmune responses that result in nerve dysfunction and symptoms of GBS. Lipo-oligosaccharides on the *C. jejuni* outer membrane may elicit the production of antibodies that cross-react with gangliosides, such as GM1 and GD1a on peripheral nerves. The antigens targeted in AMAN are located at or near the node of Ranvier. The anti-GM1 and anti-GD1a antibodies bind to the nodal axolemma, leading to complement activation followed by MAC formation and the disappearance of voltage-gated sodium channels. This damage can lead to the detachment of paranodal

have been performed on the association between ZIKV and GBS, but definitive causality still needs to be established.[26, 39] Although the ZIKV epidemic has now subsided, many unanswered questions remain. A new ZIKV epidemic or other new emerging infections with an increase of GBS cases may occur in South America or in other regions. To act as soon as possible, once a new possibly GBS-related infection comes up, a diagnosis and management consensus statement has been made that supports clinicians, especially in the context of an outbreak wherever it may occur.[12]

Immunopathology

GBS is generally considered to be an immune-mediated disorder in which humoral and likely also cellular immune responses act synergistically in causing nerve damage and subsequently neurological dysfunction.[1, 40] Evidence for the cellular component has mainly originated from experimental allergic neuritis (EAN). Most evidence for a humoral immune response comes from sera of GBS patients, and from studies in mice using monoclonal antibodies that are generated against GM1, other gangliosides, or ganglioside-like structures.[1, 9, 27, 35, 40–42]

A very important finding was that preceding infections with *C. jejuni* are associated with cross-reacting IgG1 and IgG3 antibodies against GM1 or GD1a, and that these antibodies may cause a reversible conduction block in patients with axonal GBS.[41, 43–45] CMV infections were associated with the presence of cross-reactive antibodies against GM2.[46] *M. pneumoniae* infections were recently shown to be associated with the presence of cross-reactive antibodies to galactocerebroside (GalC), a frequent preceding infection, particularly in children with GBS.[47] Anti-GQ1b antibodies are frequently found in patients with MFS.[42, 48] Most infections related to GBS are very common, indicating that host susceptibility factors probably play an additional role in the pathogenesis. For instance, patients with a *C. jejuni*-related GBS have an intrinsic higher dendritic cell response to *C. jejuni* lipo-oligosaccharides than controls.[49] The binding of cross-reactive antibodies (see preceding infections) to peripheral nerves may activate complement and attract macrophages, causing disruption of the axonal membrane.[1, 27]

FIG. 4, CONT'D myelin, and nerve conduction failure. Macrophages then invade from the nodes into the periaxonal space, scavenging the injured axons. The putative antigens targeted in AIDP are, presumably, located on the myelin sheath. The antibodies can activate complement, which leads to the formation of the MAC on the outer surface of Schwann cells, initiation of vesicular degeneration, and invasion of myelin by macrophages. *AIDP*, acute inflammatory demyelinating polyneuropathy; *AMAN*, acute motor axonal neuropathy; *APC*, antigen-presenting cell; *GBS*, Guillain-Barré syndrome; *MAC*, membrane attack complex. *(With permission from van den Berg B, Walgaard C, Drenthen J, Fokke C, Jacobs BC, van Doorn PA. Guillain-Barré syndrome: pathogenesis, diagnosis, treatment and prognosis. Nat Rev Neurol 2014;10(9):469–82 (Fig. 2)).*

Anti-ganglioside antibodies are predominantly found in GBS patients displaying the AMAN variant. The underlying pathogenic mechanism for AIDP seems to be more complex because only in a minority of sera from AIDP patients these antibodies are found. In some patients with AIDP, however, antibodies to individual gangliosides or to ganglioside complexes have been demonstrated, but their exact role in the pathogenesis in these cases is unknown.[1, 4, 50, 51] Fig. 4 shows the immunopathological mechanisms supposed to be involved in AIDP and in AMAN (Fig. 4).

Studies from the Griffin lab showed nodal complement deposition and sub-sarcolemmal macrophage infiltration in peripheral nerves from patients with axonal GBS.[52] Studies from the Willison lab showed strong evidence for complement activation in mice following injections with monoclonal antibodies against various gangliosides.[53] Studies from the lab of Yuki showed that anti-GM1 antibodies caused paresis in Japanese white rabbits.[54] Both human and animal studies have been instrumental for further insight in the immunopathology of GBS.[27, 42, 52, 55-61] These studies, which indicated a very strong protective effect against neuromuscular weakness induced by injections with a monoclonal antibody against GQ1b, subsequently led to both experimental studies and studies in humans using a complement C5 blocker (eculizumab).[53, 62-64]

Diagnosis

Clinical criteria

Currently, the revised criteria for GBS by Asbury and Cornblath are still often used in clinical practice.[2] Updated diagnostic criteria for GBS have recently been proposed[12] (Table 1). The main features of GBS are rapidly progressive weakness of arms and legs (sometimes initially only in the legs), with reduced or absent tendon reflexes in the absence of a CSF cellular reaction ($< 50 \times 10^6$ cells/L) and no symptoms suggesting CNS abnormalities. Mainly for vaccine safety monitoring, the Brighton Collaboration provided new case definitions for GBS and Miller Fisher syndrome (MFS) in 2011.[3] For the Brighton GBS classification, there are four levels of certainty (level 1: highest level of diagnostic certainty; level 4: lowest level of diagnostic certainty) that are based on clinical symptoms, CSF, and nerve conduction study (NCS) findings. The Brighton criteria were subsequently validated in independent cohorts of patients with GBS. It appeared that the Brighton criteria level 1 or 2 was reached in 94%-99% of patients with a complete dataset that were included in cohort studies in the Netherlands and Bangladesh, both in children and in adults.[65-67] To reach level 1 (highest level of certainty) or level 2, abnormal findings of both CSF examination and NCS findings are required. Because these laboratory findings may still be normal or not available at admission or shortly after, these criteria seem less valuable for patients that are just admitted to the hospital. It is usually assumed that the duration of progressive muscle weakness may not extent beyond 4 weeks. In general practice, it was shown that the duration of progression

TABLE 1 Diagnostic criteria for GBS.

Diagnostic criteria for Guillain-Barré syndrome in clinical practice

- Progressive weakness in legs and arms (sometimes initially only in legs)
- Areflexia (or decreased tendon reflexes) in weak limbs

Features that strongly support diagnosis

- Progressive phase lasts days to 4 weeks (usually <2 weeks)
- Relative symmetry
- Mild sensory symptoms or signs (absent in pure motor variant)
- Cranial nerve involvement, especially bilateral facial palsy
- Autonomic dysfunction
- Pain (common) in muscles, radicular or limb pain
- Increased protein in CSF (normal CSF protein does not rule out GBS)
- Electrodiagnostic features of polyneuropathy (can be normal in early stages of GBS)[a]

Features that should raise doubt about the diagnosis of Guillain-Barré syndrome

- Increased numbers of mono- or polymorphonuclear cells in CSF ($>50 \times 10^6$/L)
- Severe respiratory dysfunction with limited limb weakness at onset.
- Severe sensory signs with limited weakness at onset
- Marked, persistent asymmetry of weakness
- Bladder or bowel dysfunction at onset or during course of disease
- Sharp sensory level (suggesting spinal cord injury)
- Fever at onset
- Continued progression for >4 weeks (suggesting a condition such as acute onset CIDP)

[a] *To meet the highest level of the Brighton criteria for Guillain-Barré syndrome, electrodiagnostic abnormalities are required.*[3]
Adapted from diagnostic criteria by the National Institute of Neurological Disorders and Stroke (NINDS), a review paper, and a consensus statement.[1, 2, 12]

usually does not exceed 2 weeks.[24, 67] Due to the rapidly progressive nature of the disease and the absence of a biomarker for GBS, there is a strong wish to have an up-to-date clinical diagnostic guideline for GBS that can also be used as soon as possible after hospital admission. It is important to realize that the presentation of GBS in children may differ from adults, and especially young children can be more difficult to examine, which may cause diagnostic delay. As pain is also a frequent complaint in children with GBS, it should be taken into account when considering the differential diagnosis.[6, 66, 68]

Currently, the European Academy of Neurology (EAN) and the Peripheral Nerve Society (PNS) are in the process of making a diagnostic and treatment guideline for GBS. This new GBS guideline is expected in 2020.

Cerebrospinal fluid (CSF)

Guillain and Barré already described in 1916 the CSF albuminocytological dissociation in patients with GBS.[7] Large cohort studies, however, showed that the CSF protein level is highly dependent on the timing of lumbar puncture.[24] One Dutch study showed that only 49% of patients had an elevated protein level when a lumbar puncture was performed within 1 day from onset of weakness (admission), which increased to 88% of patients after 2 weeks.[67] Therefore, only 64% of GBS patients showed the characteristic albuminocytological dissociation in CSF.[67] In children younger than 6 months, the additional value of CSF total protein determination was considered nil because of large physiological variations in protein levels.[69] In general, if there are no general contraindications, it is suggested to do a diagnostic lumbar puncture in patients suspected of having GBS. An increased CSF protein is not always present, but is compatible with GBS. The determination of the CSF cell count is especially relevant because a clear increased rise of cells ($> 50 \times 10^6$/L) suggests another disorder (see also differential diagnosis).

Nerve conduction studies (NCS): AIDP and AMAN

Two main subtypes of GBS can be distinguished based on NCS: acute inflammatory demyelinating polyradiculoneuropathy (AIDP) and acute motor axonal neuropathy (AMAN).[1] There has been much debate over a long period of time about the most relevant and valid criteria for GBS and its subgroups. Multiple electrophysiological criteria sets have been developed for GBS.[70–72] It has been questioned whether repeated NCS are required for subtyping of GBS.[73, 74] A recent study showed that serial NCS had no effect on GBS subtype proportions.[73] In clinical practice, the main relevance to conduct NCS in patients suspected to have GBS is to confirm the diagnosis, especially if in doubt when patients present with atypical features such as paraparetic GBS. In this case, it could be very helpful to find either signs of demyelination in affected or nonaffected areas suggesting AIDP, or to find electrophysiological abnormalities in regions that are clinically not affected, indicating a more widespread disease, as in GBS. Currently, classification into different subtypes (AIDP or AMAN) has no direct therapeutic implications because it has not been shown that one of these forms requires another treatment. This, however, would become more relevant as soon as more personalized treatment is indicated. Prognostic studies indicate that axonal degeneration is often associated with a poor prognosis, which could indicate that these patients might benefit from additional or more aggressive treatment.[1, 24]

Imaging

There is a need to diagnose GBS as soon as possible in the early phase of the disease. Especially when there is doubt about the diagnosis, new diagnostic techniques that can help diagnose GBS are potentially helpful. Nerve ultrasound (NUS) is a commonly used diagnostic tool in mononeuropathies and currently also gains interest, especially in patients with suspected chronic immune-mediated polyneuropathies when NCS remain inconclusive.[75] NUS could potentially provide a useful painless addition or a potential alternative to NCS, especially in children. Nerve enlargement in GBS is reported to be present already 1–3 days after symptom onset, but it is usually mild and segmentally distributed.[75, 76] Proximal nerve segments and spinal nerve roots seem to be most commonly involved.[75–77] Cervical nerve root enlargement has been described in both AIDP and AMAN, and in MFS.[75, 76] The diagnostic utility of contrast-enhanced spinal MRI in GBS has also been studied.[76, 78–80] Enhancement and thickening of spinal nerve roots and cauda equina were found both in patients with typical GBS, but also with paraparetic GBS.[76, 78–80] Both NUS and MRI therefore potentially could be helpful in some patients, not only to exclude differential diagnostic abnormalities but also to indicate nerve (root) swellings that may add to the diagnosis of GBS. The nature of these nerve swellings is currently not well known. To determine the precise place of both NUS and MRI in patients that may have GBS, additional studies are required.

Differential diagnosis

The acute nature of GBS with rapid progression of weakness rules out a lot of other disorders. The diagnosis, however, can be difficult. Some examples are the clinical situation when there are no sensory disturbances, when there is pain (especially in small children[66]), when there is weakness of the legs and there is doubt about involvement of the arms, when the reflexes are not yet reduced, if there is clear respiratory involvement from the onset of disease, or when there is an increased cell count ($30–50 \times 10^6$/L) in the CSF. It is important to realize that there is often not an increased CSF protein initially.[67] The differential diagnosis is wide. A flowchart is displayed that includes differential diagnostic considerations in specific clinical conditions (Fig. 5).

MFS

MFS itself usually has the three components of ataxia, areflexia, and opthalmoparesis, but one of these can be relatively mild and other cranial nerves may be involved.[14–16] There often is overlap with other features of GBS, as patients may also have weakness of the extremities (MFS-GBS overlap syndrome). Most MFS patients have anti-GQ1b antibodies. Determination of these antiganglioside antibodies especially can be helpful when there is doubt about the diagnosis. Patients with "pure" MFS usually recover well, even without treatment with

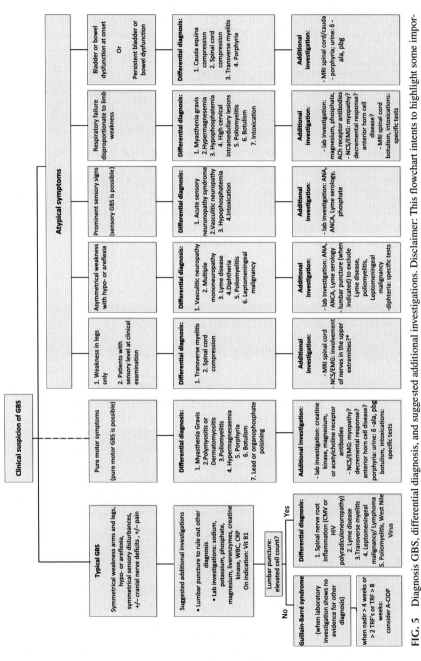

FIG. 5 Diagnosis GBS, differential diagnosis, and suggested additional investigations. Disclaimer: This flowchart intents to highlight some important disorders in the differential diagnosis of GBS. The differential diagnosis, however, is more extended than displayed in this flowchart.

plasma exchange (PE) or intravenous immunoglobulin (IVIg), but opthalmoparesis may persist for many months.

Prognosis of GBS

The course and severity of GBS are highly variable. Therefore, it is often difficult to give a good prognosis. Despite standard treatment, about 25% of patients with GBS require mechanical ventilation.[1] In a recent meta-analysis, an increased risk of intubation was found for patients with a shorter duration from symptom onset to hospital admission, neck or bulbar weakness, and more severe muscle weakness at admission.[81] The Erasmus GBS Respiratory Insufficiency Score (EGRIS) is a prognostic model that predicts the probability of respiratory failure within the first week of admission in individual patients with GBS.[82] Mechanical ventilation appears to be a negative predictive factor for long-term outcome in GBS, and is often accompanied by both local and systemic complications.[83, 84] Several factors have been associated with prolonged mechanical ventilation, including the inability to lift the upper arms from the bed, axonal damage, and unresponsive nerves on NCS. The presence of these features could guide the decision for an early tracheostomy in individual patients in order to prevent tracheal or vocal cord damage.[84] Poor outcome in GBS is often defined as the inability to walk unaided during follow-up. The modified Erasmus GBS Outcome Scale (mEGOS) is a clinical scoring system that predicts the probability of being unable to walk independently during follow-up, based on age, preceding diarrhea, and MRC sum score.[85] Both EGRIS and mEGOS are very easy-to-use clinical prognostic models that can help make clinical decisions and prognosis early in the course of disease.

Treatment

Optimal medical care

Especially because patients with GBS can have a rapidly deteriorating course of disease, it is essential to give optimal medical care as well as regularly monitor the progression of weakness and especially the occurrence of respiratory insufficiency. In addition, it is advised to monitor the occurrence of bulbar dysfunction and the possible presence of autonomic disturbances. Autonomic features such as heart rhythm disturbances (even asystole), abnormal sweating, light-fixed pupils, and bowel and bladder dysfunction may occur in 40%–70% of patients, mainly, but not exclusively, in the first weeks of illness.[86] We usually advise monitoring the patients every 2h in the progressive phase of the disease. As soon as there are symptoms of respiratory insufficiency, swallowing difficulties, or clear autonomic dysfunction, a transfer to the ICU should seriously be considered. It is advised to timely discuss possible deterioration with both the patient and his/her partner, and to try to avoid emergency intubations.

Psychological support is important, especially when the patient is admitted to the ICU and requires artificial ventilation. It is important to ask and to take care for the presence of pain, especially in intubated patients. We offer the possibility to communicate with patient organizations (like the GBS/CIDP Foundation International, or "Spierziekten Nederland"). In our experience, severely affected patients especially appreciate it when they can be visited by dedicated individuals who have had GBS in the past. Physical therapy is important to move the arms and legs, and later to start training. Especially in the recovery phase, rehabilitation is important. A flowchart that can be used to monitor and treat patients can be helpful (Fig. 6).

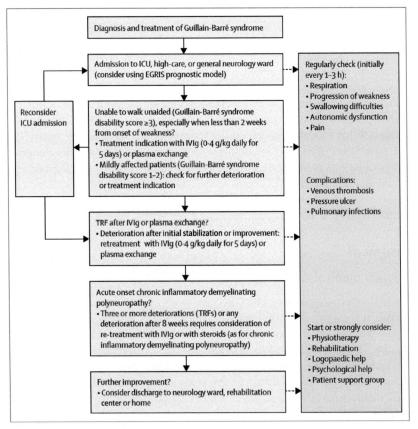

FIG. 6 Flowchart to monitor and treat GBS patients in different phases of the disease. *(From Willison HJ, Jacobs BC, van Doorn PA. Guillain-Barré syndrome. Reprinted with permission from Elsevier (The Lancet, 2016, 388(10045): 717–27)).*

Medical treatment

Almost all trials have been conducted in GBS patients being unable to walk unaided, usually considered to be "severe GBS" compatible with a GBS functional score grade 3 or more. Plasma exchange (PE) started within 4 weeks and IVIg initiated within 2 weeks from the onset of weakness are proven, effective treatments for adult patients with severe GBS.[8, 10, 87–89] If PE was started earlier (within the first weeks after onset), it appeared to be more effective. In severely affected GBS patients, it was shown that despite a standard course of IVIg (2 g/kg bodyweight, usually administered as 0.4 g/kg for 5 consecutive days), or PE treatment (usually 5 treatments administered over 2 weeks, exchanging in total about 5 plasma volumes), GBS remains a life-threatening disorder with substantial morbidity and mortality, emphasizing the need for better treatment. In mildly affected GBS patients still able to walk unaided, it was shown that two PE sessions were better than no exchanges.[90]

Trials that evaluated the effect of corticosteroids surprisingly found no benefit compared to supportive care alone.[91–93] The combination of methylprednisolone (MP) with IVIg was not superior over IVIg alone, though posthoc analysis indicated that the time to recovery seemed somewhat shorter in the IVIg plus MP group after correction for known prognostic factors.[91, 92] No clear benefit was observed when PE was followed by IVIg, compared to PE or IVIg alone.[88, 94] There have been other small randomized controlled trials (RCT) with various drugs that either showed no differences between the treatment arms or were impaired by small numbers of patients.[95]

In some patients, deterioration continues, even after standard treatment with PE or IVIg. These patients might potentially benefit from an additional course of treatment. There is one open prospective study that indicates that a second IVIg course in not effective in GBS patients with a poor prognosis.[96] The definitive results of the Dutch RCT that investigates whether a second course of IVIg is of benefit when administered early in the course of disease (started 2 days after finishing a standard course of IVIg) in GBS patients with a poor prognosis needs to be published.[97]

PE and IVIg are expensive treatments that most patients in low-income countries cannot afford. An open study has been conducted investigating the safety and feasibility of small volume plasma exchange (SVPE). This is a simple procedure where 0.5-L blood is drawn multiple times, the plasma is discharged after sedimentation, and the red blood cells are transfused back to the patient. With this procedure, it was possible to exchange a volume of about 8-L plasma (instead of the usual 10–12 L that is exchanged with standard PE using PE machines) without a high incidence of side effects, especially infections or clotting problems.[98] This potentially is a low-cost alternative for PE. Results of a larger-scale trial are awaited.

Treatment dilemmas in GBS

There are multiple questions related to the use of IVIg or PE (Table 2). This has been addressed in a treatment dilemmas paper.[99] There are several important points to be made. What is the preferred treatment in various clinical conditions (duration from onset, severity, subtype) of GBS? This is sometime difficult, especially when no or insufficient data are available from clinical trials. It is important to realize that there currently is a lack of information on the effect of medical treatment in relatively mildly affected patients with GBS. On the other hand, it is yet unknown what treatment should be given to patients with a poor

TABLE 2 Treatment dilemmas in GBS in daily practice.[99]

Question	Answers
1. Is there a preferred treatment for GBS?	IVIg and PE are about equally effective[10, 100]
	IVIg is readily available and based upon the invasiveness, the preferred treatment in children
2. When should treatment be started?	As soon as possible when a patient is unable to walk unaided. Likely also in patients who rapidly deteriorate while still being able to walk[99]
2. Treatment in patients who can still walk?	Not tested for IVIg. This has been tested for PE: two PE sessions are better than no PE[90]
4. IVIg or PE in patients with MFS?	No trial data. A Cochrane review found no evidence to start with IVIg or PE in MFS[101]
5. What to do if a patient seems unresponsive to IVIg or PE?	No good data. Standard PE followed by IVIg is not superior than either IVIg or PE alone[94]
6. Can the prognosis of GBS be predicted?	Chance to need artificial respiration: use EGRIS[82]
	Prediction walk unaided at 6 months: mEGOS[85]
	Prediction requirement of tracheostomy[84]
7. Repeat IVIg when no improvement or a poor prognosis?[85]	Results from open prognostic study indicate no positive effect of second IVIg course[96]
	Results of RCT (SID-GBS) are awaited[97]
8. Repeat IVIg or PE in patient with TRF?	10% of GBS has a TRF. Although not tested in clinical trials, policy is to retreat with IVIg or PE[99]
9. When to consider A-CIDP?	If there are > 2 TRFs, or when there is deterioration after 2 months[102]
10. Other treatments for GBS available?	Currently not. New treatments are being tested (see novel treatments)

These treatment dilemmas are adapted from Verboon JC, van Doorn PA, Jacobs BC. *J Neurol Neurosurg Psychiatry* 2017;88(4):346–52.

prognosis, or in patients that seem not to respond to a single course of IVIg or PE treatment. PE followed by IVIg doesn't seem to be superior to either IVIg or PE alone, although this was tested in a group of patients irrespective of their initial response to the first treatment.[94] Is a second IVIg course effective early in the disease in patients having a poor prognosis based upon prognostic modelling?[85] The results of an international prospective open study did not suggest a positive effect of a second IVIg course.[96] The definitive results of the second course of IVIg RCT in patients with a predicted poor outcome need to be published.[97] For what period of time is any treatment potentially still effective in GBS? Is there an indication to start IVIg or PE in patients with MFS? This has not been investigated. A Cochrane review found no evidence to start with IVIg or PE.[101]

Is a prognosis good as a patient has symptoms of double vision that last for 3 months or more? It was suggested that IVIg or PE should be considered, especially in patients with MFS-GBS overlap syndrome.

Is there an indication to repeat IVIg or PE in patients who initially improve or stabilize, and subsequently deteriorate again? This clinical condition is known as a treatment-related fluctuation (TRF). Although not tested in clinical trials, it seems current policy often to retreat these patients. If there are more than two TRFs, or if there is a deterioration after 2 months, acute-onset chronic inflammatory demyelinating polyradiculoneuropathy (A-CIDP) needs to be considered.[102] Are there other treatments available for patients with GBS? Not yet, although there are a few new treatments that potentially can be very effective for GBS (see novel treatments). The effect of treatment is often measured by changes (improvement) on the GBS disability scale (ranging from 0–6). However, that scale is focused on ambulation and ventilation, so how about use of the arms, pain, fatigue, or participation in daily life?

Novel treatments

Studies mainly based on mice but also including pathological studies in humans indicated that complement activation plays a role, in particular in anti-ganglioside antibody (mainly GM1 and GQ1b)-induced acute neuropathy (see immunopathology). Therapeutics that prevent the complement-dependent neuronal damage underlying GBS in mice showed a very clear effect.[53, 59] Two randomized, double-blind, placebo-controlled phase 2 trials in patients with GBS showed that eculizumab—a complement factor 5 inhibitor—was deemed safe and well tolerated.[63, 103] The Japanese Eculizumab Trial for GBS (JET-GBS) randomized 23 patients to IVIg with eculizumab, and 12 patients to IVIg with placebo. The primary endpoint was not reached, but a larger proportion of patients in the eculizumab group were able to run at 24 weeks (74%) than in the placebo group (18%).[103] These studies indicate that eculizumab seems safe and well tolerated and might potentially improve outcome in GBS, but larger trials are required. An anti-C1q complement inhibitor was shown to be very effective in mouse models of AMAN and MFS.[59] This drug (ANX005) is currently being tested in a first phase 2 clinical trial and will further be studied in a larger clinical study. Another potentially promising therapeutic agent is the IgG-degrading enzyme that is secreted by *Streptococcus pyogenes* (IdeS). The enzyme cleaves IgG-molecules very rapidly, and is therefore expected to be effective in GBS through the cleavage of pathogenic antibodies.[104] A phase 2 trial using IdeS (a few days later followed by a standard course of IVIg) in GBS is currently being conducted.[105]

Chronic problems

Pain

Pain is a frequently reported symptom at all stages and severity of GBS.[1, 5] The nature of the pain is not always known. In some cases, it may be related to endoneurinal inflammatory edema.[76] In other cases, this could be low back or muscle pain due to immobilization, or neuropathic pain due to distal nerve lesions.

In a subgroup of about one-third of the patients, pain precedes even the onset of weakness, which may induce confusion and diagnostic delay, particularly in children.[1, 5] Pain can be very troublesome, especially when patients are intubated and cannot communicate easily. Therefore, we suggest actively asking about the presence and severity of pain, especially in these patients admitted to the ICU. The management of pain in GBS can be diverse, related to the varying types of pain and unknown underlying pathogenic mechanisms.[1, 5] There currently is no evidence that pain in GBS should be treated differently from other causes of pain.[106] High-quality trials are needed to evaluate the safety and efficacy of therapeutic interventions for various forms of pain in GBS, both in the acute and recovery phases of the disease.

Fatigue

Fatigue is frequently reported in patients with GBS.[107–109] It may persist for years after apparent recovery. It is found in about 80% of patients. The modified FSS was shown to be a good assessment tool for measuring fatigue in inflammatory neuropathies.[110] The nature of fatigue in GBS is not well known, but likely axonal degeneration plays a role.[111]

Attempts to modify the level of fatigue severity, in an analogy to the treatment of fatigue in multiple sclerosis, led to a trial of amantadine in GBS. This RCT, however, did not show any effect of this drug.[112] A physical training study, however, did show that anaerobic exercise could significantly reduce the levels of fatigue.[113, 114]

Quality of life

GBS significantly interferes with the quality of life. Although it was found that the quality of life gradually improved over a 6-month period, longitudinal studies showed that the psychosocial health status was still impaired at 1 year and that this appeared at least partially related with muscle ache and cramps.[115, 116]

Three to six years after onset of GBS, 63% of 122 GBS patients showed one or more changes in their lifestyle, work, or leisure activities, or in the life of their partners. It was concluded that these changes were influenced by an impaired final functional outcome, along with loss of power and poor condition.[117] In a review paper it was stated that GBS impairs function as well as social life beyond 1 year, resulting in work changes in nearly 40% of patients.[118] Most improvement on various aspects of the disease is usually found in the first years after onset. However, as we also were told by patients who have had GBS, it was found that individual patients may experience further slow recovery up to 6 years (or even more) after presentation.[118]

Conclusion and further perspectives

Since GBS was first described over a century ago, knowledge on the pathophysiology and diversity of the clinical syndrome has greatly evolved, and treatment with IVIg or PE has been introduced.[27] The validity of existing electrophysiological criteria for GBS is under debate, and research is being performed on the diagnostic utility of nerve ultrasound and MRI. A new international guideline for the management of GBS is currently being developed by the EAN/PNS. There is increasing evidence that complement activation plays a critical role in the pathophysiology of GBS. Although the first results of small trials with eculizumab are promising, larger studies are required to provide evidence for effectiveness. New studies with different complement inhibitors and with the IgG degrading enzyme IdeS are currently being undertaken. Currently, there is insufficient information that a second course of IVIg is effective in patients with a poor prognosis or who deteriorate despite a standard course of IVIg. Current prognostic models for GBS can be used to personalize treatment. An opportunity to validate these models in an international population of patients and to discover new clinical and biological predictors of outcome will come from IGOS, the world's largest prospective study on GBS.[13]

References

1. Willison HJ, Jacobs BC, van Doorn PA. Guillain-Barré syndrome. *Lancet.* 2016;388(10045): 717–727.
2. Asbury AK, Cornblath DR. Assessment of current diagnostic criteria for Guillain-Barré syndrome. *Ann Neurol.* 1990;27(Suppl):S21–S24.
3. Sejvar JJ, Kohl KS, Gidudu J, et al. Guillain-Barré syndrome and Fisher syndrome: case definitions and guidelines for collection, analysis, and presentation of immunization safety data. *Vaccine.* 2011;29(3):599–612.
4. van den Berg B, Walgaard C, Drenthen J, Fokke C, Jacobs BC, van Doorn PA. Guillain-Barré syndrome: pathogenesis, diagnosis, treatment and prognosis. *Nat Rev Neurol.* 2014;10(8):469–482.
5. Ruts L, Drenthen J, Jongen JL, et al. Pain in Guillain-Barré syndrome: a long-term follow-up study. *Neurology.* 2010;75(16):1439–1447.

6. Roodbol J, de Wit MC, Walgaard C, de Hoog M, Catsman-Berrevoets CE, Jacobs BC. Recognizing Guillain-Barré syndrome in preschool children. *Neurology.* 2011;76(9): 807–810.

7. Guillain G, Barré JA, Strohl A. Sur un syndrome de radiculo-nevrite avec hyperalbuminose du liquide cephalorachidien sans reaction cellulaire. Remarques sur les caracteres cliniques et graphiques des reflexes tendineux. *Bull Soc Med Hop Paris.* 1916;28:1462–1470.

8. The Guillain-Barré syndrome Study Group. Plasmapheresis and acute Guillain-Barré syndrome. *Neurology.* 1985;35(8):1096–1104.

9. Yuki N. Guillain-Barré syndrome and anti-ganglioside antibodies: a clinician-scientist's journey. *Proc Jpn Acad Ser B Phys Biol Sci.* 2012;88(7):299–326.

10. Van Der Meché FG, Schmitz PI. A randomized trial comparing intravenous immune globulin and plasma exchange in Guillain-Barré syndrome. Dutch Guillain-Barré Study Group. *N Engl J Med.* 1992;326(17):1123–1129.

11. Willison HJ, Goodfellow JA. *GBS 100: Celebrating a Century of Progress in Guillain-Barré Syndrome.* San Diego, USA: Peripheral Nerve Society; 2016.

12. Leonhard SE, Mandarakas MR, Gondim FAA, et al. Diagnosis and management of Guillain-Barré syndrome in ten steps. *Nat Rev Neurol.* 2019;15(11):671–683.

13. Jacobs BC, van den Berg B, Verboon C, et al. International Guillain-Barré Syndrome Outcome Study: protocol of a prospective observational cohort study on clinical and biological predictors of disease course and outcome in Guillain-Barré syndrome. *J Peripher Nerv Syst.* 2017;22(2):68–76.

14. Wakerley BR, Yuki N. Mimics and chameleons in Guillain-Barré and Miller Fisher syndromes. *Pract Neurol.* 2015;15(2):90–99.

15. Mori M, Kuwabara S, Yuki N. Fisher syndrome: clinical features, immunopathogenesis and management. *Expert Rev Neurother.* 2012;12(1):39–51.

16. Nagashima T, Koga M, Odaka M, Hirata K, Yuki N. Continuous spectrum of pharyngeal-cervical-brachial variant of Guillain-Barré syndrome. *Arch Neurol.* 2007;64(10):1519–1523.

17. van den Berg B, Fokke C, Drenthen J, van Doorn PA, Jacobs BC. Paraparetic Guillain-Barré syndrome. *Neurology.* 2014;82(22):1984–1989.

18. Odaka M, Yuki N, Yamada M, et al. Bickerstaff's brainstem encephalitis: clinical features of 62 cases and a subgroup associated with Guillain-Barré syndrome. *Brain.* 2003;126:2279–2290.

19. Keisuke Y, Miyuki M, Motoi K, Susumu K. Differences of antibody reactivities against glycolipid complexes among Guillain-Barré syndrome, miller fisher syndrome and bickerstaff brainstem encephalitis. *J Peripher Nerv Syst.* 2017;22(3):313–314.

20. Feasby TE, Gilbert JJ, Brown WF, et al. Acute "axonal" Guillain-Barré polyneuropathy. *Neurology.* 1987;37(2):357.

21. van Doorn PA. Diagnosis, treatment and prognosis of Guillain-Barré syndrome (GBS). *Presse Med.* 2013;42:e193–e201.

22. Griffin JW, Li CY, Macko C, et al. Early nodal changes in the acute motor axonal neuropathy pattern of the Guillain-Barré syndrome. *J Neurocytol.* 1996;25(1):33–51.

23. Sejvar JJ, Baughman AL, Wise M, Morgan OW. Population incidence of Guillain-Barré syndrome: a systematic review and meta-analysis. *Neuroepidemiology.* 2011;36(2):123–133.

24. Doets AY, Verboon C, van den Berg B, et al. Regional variation of Guillain-Barré syndrome. *Brain.* 2018;141(10):2866–2877.

25. van Koningsveld R, Rico R, Gerstenbluth I, et al. Gastroenteritis-associated Guillain-Barré syndrome on the Caribbean island Curacao. *Neurology.* 2001;56(11):1467–1472.

26. Parra B, Lizarazo J, Jimenez-Arango JA, et al. Guillain-Barré syndrome associated with Zika virus infection in Colombia. *N Engl J Med.* 2016;375(16):1513–1523.

27. Goodfellow JA, Willison HJ. Guillain-Barré syndrome: a century of progress. *Nat Rev Neurol.* 2016;12(12):723–731.

28. Jacobs BC, Rothbarth PH, van der Meché FG, et al. The spectrum of antecedent infections in Guillain-Barré syndrome: a case-control study. *Neurology.* 1998;51(4):1110–1115.

29. Geurtsvankessel CH, Islam Z, Mohammad QD, Jacobs BC, Endtz HP, Osterhaus AD. Hepatitis E and Guillain-Barré syndrome. *Clin Infect Dis.* 2013;57(9):1369–1370.

30. van den Berg B, van der Eijk AA, Pas SD, et al. Guillain-Barré syndrome associated with preceding hepatitis E virus infection. *Neurology.* 2014;82(6):491–497.

31. Fukae J, Tsugawa J, Ouma S, Umezu T, Kusunoki S, Tsuboi Y. Guillain-Barré and Miller Fisher syndromes in patients with anti-hepatitis E virus antibody: a hospital-based survey in Japan. *Neurol Sci.* 2016;37(11):1849–1851.

32. Stevens O, Claeys KG, Poesen K, Saegeman V, Van Damme P. Diagnostic challenges and clinical characteristics of hepatitis E virus-associated Guillain-Barré syndrome. *JAMA Neurol.* 2017;74(1):26–33.

33. Dalton HR, Kamar N, van Eijk JJ, et al. Hepatitis E virus and neurological injury. *Nat Rev Neurol.* 2016;12(2):77–85.

34. Ang CW, Jacobs BC, Laman JD. The Guillain-Barré syndrome: a true case of molecular mimicry. *Trends Immunol.* 2004;25(2):61–66.

35. Yuki N. Infectious origins of, and molecular mimicry in, Guillain-Barré and Fisher syndromes. *Lancet Infect Dis.* 2001;1(1):29–37.

36. Cao-Lormeau VM, Blake A, Mons S, et al. Guillain-Barré syndrome outbreak associated with Zika virus infection in French Polynesia: a case-control study. *Lancet.* 2016;387(10027): 1531–1539.

37. Leonhard SE, Amorelli M, Barréira AA, et al. International Zika virus related Guillain-Barré syndrome outcome study (IGOS-Zika): a case-controlled study. *J Peripher Nerv Syst.* 2017;22(3):329–330.

38. Lowe R, Barcellos C, Brasil P, et al. The Zika virus epidemic in Brazil: from discovery to future implications. *Int J Environ Res Public Health.* 2018;15(1).

39. Leonhard SE, Lant S, Jacobs BC, et al. Zika virus infection in the returning traveller: what every neurologist should know. *Pract Neurol.* 2018;18:271–277.

40. Kieseier BC, Mathey EK, Sommer C, Hartung HP. Immune-mediated neuropathies. *Nat Rev Dis Primers.* 2018;4(1):31.

41. Willison HJ, Yuki N. Peripheral neuropathies and anti-glycolipid antibodies. *Brain.* 2002; 125:2591–2625.

42. Willison HJ. The immunobiology of Guillain-Barré syndromes. *J Peripher Nerv Syst.* 2005; 10(2):94–112.

43. Kuwabara S, Yuki N, Koga M, et al. IgG anti-GM1 antibody is associated with reversible conduction failure and axonal degeneration in Guillain-Barré syndrome. *Ann Neurol.* 1998;44(2):202–208.

44. Jacobs BC, Koga M, Van Rijs W, et al. Subclass IgG to motor gangliosides related to infection and clinical course in Guillain-Barré syndrome. *J Neuroimmunol.* 2008;194(1-2): 181–190.

45. Jacobs BC, van Doorn PA, Schmitz PI, et al. Campylobacter jejuni infections and anti-GM1 antibodies in Guillain-Barré syndrome. *Ann Neurol.* 1996;40(2):181–187.

46. Ang CW, Jacobs BC, Brandenburg AH, et al. Cross-reactive antibodies against GM2 and CMV-infected fibroblasts in Guillain-Barré syndrome. *Neurology.* 2000;54(7):1453–1458.

47. Meyer Sauteur PM, Huizinga R, Tio-Gillen AP, et al. Mycoplasma pneumoniae triggering the Guillain-Barré syndrome: a case-control study. *Ann Neurol.* 2016;80(4):566–580.

48. Yuki N. Fisher syndrome and Bickerstaff brainstem encephalitis (Fisher-Bickerstaff syndrome). *J Neuroimmunol*. 2009;215(1-2):1–9.
49. Huizinga R, van den Berg B, van Rijs W, et al. Innate Immunity to Campylobacter jejuni in Guillain-Barré Syndrome. *Ann Neurol*. 2015;78(3):343–354.
50. Rinaldi S, Brennan KM, Kalna G, et al. Antibodies to heteromeric glycolipid complexes in Guillain-Barré syndrome. *PLoS One*. 2013;8(12):e82337.
51. Kusunoki S, Kaida K, Ueda M. Antibodies against gangliosides and ganglioside complexes in Guillain-Barré syndrome: new aspects of research. *Biochim Biophys Acta*. 2008;1780(3):441–444.
52. Griffin JW, Li CY, Ho TW, et al. Pathology of the motor-sensory axonal Guillain-Barré syndrome. *Ann Neurol*. 1996;39(1):17–28.
53. Halstead SK, Zitman FM, Humphreys PD, et al. Eculizumab prevents anti-ganglioside antibody-mediated neuropathy in a murine model. *Brain*. 2008;131(Pt 5):1197–1208.
54. Yuki N, Yamada M, Koga M, et al. Animal model of axonal Guillain-Barré syndrome induced by sensitization with GM1 ganglioside. *Ann Neurol*. 2001;49(6):712–720.
55. Griffin JW, Stoll G, Li CY, Tyor W, Cornblath DR. Macrophage responses in inflammatory demyelinating neuropathies. *Ann Neurol*. 1990;27(Suppl):S64–S68.
56. Hafer-Macko C, Hsieh ST, Li CY, et al. Acute motor axonal neuropathy: an antibody-mediated attack on axolemma. *Ann Neurol*. 1996;40(4):635–644.
57. Hafer-Macko CE, Sheikh KA, Li CY, et al. Immune attack on the Schwann cell surface in acute inflammatory demyelinating polyneuropathy. *Ann Neurol*. 1996;39(5):625–635.
58. Cunningham ME, McGonigal R, Meehan GR, et al. Anti-ganglioside antibodies are removed from circulation in mice by neuronal endocytosis. *Brain*. 2016;139(6):1657–1665.
59. McGonigal R, Cunningham ME, Yao D, et al. C1q-targeted inhibition of the classical complement pathway prevents injury in a novel mouse model of acute motor axonal neuropathy. *Acta Neuropathol Commun*. 2016;2(4):23.
60. McGonigal R, Rowan EG, Greenshields KN, et al. Anti-GD1a antibodies activate complement and calpain to injure distal motor nodes of Ranvier in mice. *Brain*. 2010;133(7):1944–1960.
61. Rupp A, Morrison I, Barrie JA, et al. Motor nerve terminal destruction and regeneration following anti-ganglioside antibody and complement-mediated injury: an in and ex vivo imaging study in the mouse. *Exp Neurol*. 2012;233(2):836–848.
62. Halstead SK, Humphreys PD, Goodfellow JA, Wagner ER, Smith RA, Willison HJ. Complement inhibition abrogates nerve terminal injury in Miller Fisher syndrome. *Ann Neurol*. 2005;58(2):203–210.
63. Davidson AI, Halstead SK, Goodfellow JA, et al. Inhibition of complement in Guillain-Barré syndrome: the ICA-GBS study. *J Peripher Nerv Syst*. 2017;22(1):4–12.
64. Kuwabara S, Misawa S, Sekiguchi Y, Kusunoki S. Japanese eculizumab trial for Guillain-Barré syndrome (JET-GBS). *J Peripher Nerv Syst*. 2017;22(3):323.
65. Islam MB, Islam Z, Farzana KS, et al. Guillain-Barré syndrome in Bangladesh: validation of Brighton criteria. *J Peripher Nerv Syst*. 2016;21(4):345–351.
66. Roodbol J, de Wit MCY, van den Berg B, et al. Diagnosis of Guillain-Barré syndrome in children and validation of the Brighton criteria. *J Neurol*. 2017;264(5):856–861.
67. Fokke C, van den Berg B, Drenthen J, Walgaard C, van Doorn PA, Jacobs BC. Diagnosis of Guillain-Barré syndrome and validation of Brighton criteria. *Brain*. 2014;137(1):33–43.
68. Wu X, Shen D, Li T, et al. Distinct clinical characteristics of pediatric Guillain-Barré syndrome: a comparative study between children and adults in Northeast China. *PLoS One*. 2016;14(11):3.

69. Kahlmann V, Roodbol J, van Leeuwen N, et al. Validated age-specific reference values for CSF total protein levels in children. *Eur J Paediatr Neurol.* 2017;21(4):654–660.

70. Ho TW, Mishu B, Li CY, et al. Guillain-Barré syndrome in northern China. Relationship to Campylobacter jejuni infection and anti-glycolipid antibodies. *Brain.* 1995;118(3): 597–605.

71. Hadden RD, Cornblath DR, Hughes RA, et al. Electrophysiological classification of Guillain-Barré syndrome: clinical associations and outcome. Plasma Exchange/Sandoglobulin Guillain-Barré Syndrome Trial Group. *Ann Neurol.* 1998;44(5):780–788.

72. Rajabally YA, Durand MC, Mitchell J, Orlikowski D, Nicolas G. Electrophysiological diagnosis of Guillain-Barré syndrome subtype: could a single study suffice? *J Neurol Neurosurg Psychiatry.* 2015;86(1):115–119.

73. Van den Bergh PYK, Piéret F, Woodard JL, et al. Guillain-Barré syndrome subtype diagnosis: a prospective multicentric European study. *Muscle Nerve.* 2018;58:23–28.

74. Uncini A, Ippoliti L, Shahrizaila N, Sekiguchi Y, Kuwabara S. Optimizing the electrodiagnostic accuracy in Guillain-Barré syndrome subtypes: criteria sets and sparse linear discriminant analysis. *Clin Neurophysiol.* 2017;128(7):1176–1183.

75. Telleman JA, Grimm A, Goedee S, Visser LH, Zaidman CM. Nerve ultrasound in polyneuropathies. *Muscle Nerve.* 2018;57(5):716–728.

76. Berciano J, Sedano MJ, Pelayo-Negro AL, et al. Proximal nerve lesions in early Guillain-Barré syndrome: implications for pathogenesis and disease classification. *J Neurol.* 2017;264(2):221–236.

77. Mori A, Nodera H, Takamatsu N, et al. Sonographic evaluation of peripheral nerves in subtypes of Guillain-Barré syndrome. *J Neurol Sci.* 2016;364:154–159.

78. Galassi G, Genovese M, Ariatti A, Malagoli M. Early imaging in paraparetic Guillain-Barré syndrome. *Acta Neurol Belg.* 2017;1–2.

79. Resorlu M, Guven M, Aylanc H, Karatag O. Lumbar magnetic resonance imaging findings in Guillain-Barré syndrome. *Spine J.* 2016;16(10):e709–e710.

80. Berciano J, Gallardo E, Orizaola P, et al. Early axonal Guillain-Barré syndrome with normal peripheral conduction: imaging evidence for changes in proximal nerve segments. *J Neurol Neurosurg Psychiatry.* 2016;87(5):563–565.

81. Green C, Baker T, Subramaniam A. Predictors of respiratory failure in patients with Guillain-Barré syndrome: a systematic review and meta-analysis. *Med J Aust.* 2018;208(4):181–188.

82. Walgaard C, Lingsma HF, Ruts L, et al. Prediction of respiratory insufficiency in Guillain-Barré syndrome. *Ann Neurol.* 2010;67(6):781–787.

83. van den Berg B, Storm EF, Garssen MJP, Blomkwist-Markens PH, Jacobs BC. Clinical outcome of Guillain-Barré syndrome after prolonged mechanical ventilation. *J Neurol Neurosurg Psychiatry.* 2018;89(9):949–954.

84. Walgaard C, Lingsma HF, van Doorn PA, van der Jagt M, Steyerberg EW, Jacobs BC. Tracheostomy or not: prediction of prolonged mechanical ventilation in Guillain-Barré syndrome. *Neurocrit Care.* 2017;26(1):6–13.

85. Walgaard C, Lingsma HF, Ruts L, van Doorn PA, Steyerberg EW, Jacobs BC. Early recognition of poor prognosis in Guillain-Barré syndrome. *Neurology.* 2011;76(11):968–975.

86. Anandan C, Khuder SA, Koffman BM. Prevalence of autonomic dysfunction in hospitalized patients with Guillain-Barré syndrome. *Muscle Nerve.* 2017;56(2):331–333.

87. Hughes RA, Swan AV, van Doorn PA. Intravenous immunoglobulin for Guillain-Barré syndrome. *Cochrane Database Syst Rev.* 2014;9:CD002063.

88. Chevret S, Hughes RA, Annane D. Plasma exchange for Guillain-Barré syndrome (Review). *Cochrane Database Syst Rev.* 2017;2:CD001798.

89. Efficiency of plasma exchange in Guillain-Barré syndrome: role of replacement fluids. French Cooperative Group on Plasma Exchange in Guillain-Barré syndrome. *Ann Neurol.* 1987;22(6):753–761.

90. Appropriate number of plasma exchanges in Guillain-Barré syndrome. The French Cooperative Group on Plasma Exchange in Guillain-Barré Syndrome. *Ann Neurol.* 1997;41(3): 298–306.

91. Hughes RA, Brassington R, Gunn AA, van Doorn PA. Corticosteroids for Guillain-Barré syndrome. *Cochrane Database Syst Rev.* 2016;10:CD001446.

92. van Koningsveld R, Schmitz PI, Meché FG, Visser LH, Meulstee J, van Doorn PA. Effect of methylprednisolone when added to standard treatment with intravenous immunoglobulin for Guillain-Barré syndrome: randomised trial. *Lancet.* 2004;363(9404):192–196.

93. Double-blind trial of intravenous methylprednisolone in Guillain-Barré syndrome. Guillain-Barré Syndrome Steroid Trial Group. *Lancet.* 1993;341(8845):586–590.

94. Randomised trial of plasma exchange, intravenous immunoglobulin, and combined treatments in Guillain-Barré syndrome. Plasma Exchange/Sandoglobulin Guillain-Barré Syndrome Trial Group. *Lancet.* 1997;349(9047):225–230.

95. Pritchard J, Hughes RA, Hadden RD, Brassington R. Pharmacological treatment other than corticosteroids, intravenous immunoglobulin and plasma exchange for Guillain-Barré syndrome (Review). *Cochrane Database Syst Rev.* 2016;11:CD008630.

96. Verboon C, Van Den Berg B, Cornblath DR, et al. International second immunoglobulin dose in patients with Guillain-Barré syndrome with poor prognosis (I-SID GBS), a prospective observational study. *J Peripher Nerv Syst.* 2017;22(3):406–407.

97. Walgaard C, Jacobs BC, Lingsma HF, Steyerberg EW, Cornblath DR, van Doorn PA. Second IVIg course in Guillain-Barré syndrome patients with poor prognosis (SID-GBS trial): protocol for a double-blind randomized, placebo-controlled clinical trial. *J Peripher Nerv Syst.* 2018;23(4):210–215.

98. Islam B, Islam Z, Rahman S, et al. Small volume plasma exchange for Guillain-Barré syndrome in low income countries: a safety and feasibility study. *J Peripher Nerv Syst.* 2017;22(3):304.

99. Verboon C, van Doorn PA, Jacobs BC. Treatment dilemmas in Guillain-Barré syndrome. *J Neurol Neurosurg Psychiatry.* 2017;88(4):346–352.

100. Hughes RA, Swan AV, Raphael JC, Annane D, van Koningsveld R, van Doorn PA. Immunotherapy for Guillain-Barré syndrome: a systematic review. *Brain.* 2007;130:2245–2257.

101. Overell JR, Hsieh ST, Odaka M, Yuki N, Willison HJ. Treatment for Fisher syndrome, Bickerstaff's brainstem encephalitis and related disorders. *Cochrane Database Syst Rev.* 2007;1:CD004761.

102. Ruts L, Drenthen J, Jacobs BC, van Doorn PA. Distinguishing acute-onset CIDP from fluctuating Guillain-Barré syndrome: a prospective study. *Neurology.* 2010;74(21):1680–1686.

103. Misawa S, Kuwabara S, Sato Y, et al. Safety and efficacy of eculizumab in Guillain-Barré syndrome: a multicentre, double-blind, randomised phase 2 trial. *Lancet Neurol.* 2018;17(6):519–529.

104. Takahashi R, Yuki N. Streptococcal IdeS: therapeutic potential for Guillain-Barré syndrome. *Sci Rep.* 2015;21(5):10809.

105. Kuwabara S, Misawa S. Future treatment for Guillain-Barré syndrome. *Clin Exp Neuroimmunol.* 2016;7(4):320–323.

106. Liu J, Wang LN, McNicol ED. Pharmacological treatment for pain in Guillain-Barré syndrome. *Cochrane Database Syst Rev.* 2015;4:CD009950.

107. Merkies IS, Faber CG. Fatigue in immune-mediated neuropathies. *Neuromuscul Disord.* 2012;22(Suppl 3):S203–S207.

108. Merkies IS, Schmitz PI, Samijn JP, Van Der Meché FG, van Doorn PA. Fatigue in immune-mediated polyneuropathies. European Inflammatory Neuropathy Cause and Treatment (INCAT) Group. *Neurology.* 1999;53(8):1648–1654.

109. Merkies ISJ, Kieseier BC. Fatigue, pain, anxiety and depression in guillain-barré syndrome and chronic inflammatory demyelinating polyradiculoneuropathy. *Eur Neurol.* 2016;75(3–4): 199–206.

110. van Nes SI, Vanhoutte EK, Faber CG, et al. Improving fatigue assessment in immune-mediated neuropathies: the modified Rasch-built fatigue severity scale. *J Peripher Nerv Syst.* 2009;14(4):268–278.

111. Drenthen J, Jacobs BC, Maathuis EM, van Doorn PA, Visser GH, Blok JH. Residual fatigue in Guillain-Barré syndrome is related to axonal loss. *Neurology.* 2013;81(21):1827–1831.

112. Garssen MP, Schmitz PI, Merkies IS, Jacobs BC, Van Der Meché FG, van Doorn PA. Amantadine for treatment of fatigue in Guillain-Barré syndrome: a randomised, double blind, placebo controlled, crossover trial. *J Neurol Neurosurg Psychiatry.* 2006;77(1):61–65.

113. Garssen MP, Bussmann JB, Schmitz PI, et al. Physical training and fatigue, fitness, and quality of life in Guillain-Barré syndrome and CIDP. *Neurology.* 2004;63(12):2393–2395.

114. White CM, van Doorn PA, Garssen MP, Stockley RC. Interventions for fatigue in peripheral neuropathy. *Cochrane Database Syst Rev.* 2014;12:CD008146.

115. Djordjevic G, Stojanov A, Bozovic I, et al. Six-month prospective study of quality of life in Guillain-Barré syndrome. *Acta Neurol Scand.* 2019. https://doi.org/10.1111/ane.13195.

116. Bernsen RA, de Jager AE, Kuijer W, Van Der Meché FG, Suurmeijer TP. Psychosocial dysfunction in the first year after Guillain-Barré syndrome. *Muscle Nerve.* 2009;41(4):533–539.

117. Bernsen RA, de Jager AE, Schmitz PI, Van Der Meché FG. Residual physical outcome and daily living 3 to 6 years after Guillain-Barré syndrome. *Neurology.* 1999;53(2):409–410.

118. Rajabally YA, Uncini A. Outcome and its predictors in Guillain-Barré syndrome. *J Neurol Neurosurg Psychiatry.* 2012;83:711–718.

Chapter 3

Chronic inflammatory demyelinating polyneuropathy

Yusuf A. Rajabally[a,b], H. Stephan Goedee[c]

[a]Aston Medical School, Aston University, Birmingham, United Kingdom, [b]Regional Neuromuscular Service, Queen Elizabeth Hospital Birmingham, Birmingham, United Kingdom, [c]Brain Center Rudolf Magnus, Department of Neurology and Neurosurgery, University Medical Center Utrecht, Utrecht, The Netherlands

Introduction

Chronic inflammatory demyelinating polyneuropathy (CIDP) is now considered an umbrella term for a spectrum of distinct disorders with pathophysiological differences that all share response to routine immunomodulatory treatment.[1–12] CIDP represents the most common group of inflammatory neuropathies worldwide,[13–19] and was probably first described in the 19th century.[20–22] More recent descriptions date back to those of steroid-responsive relapsing neuropathies in the 1950s by Austin, and the term CIDP was itself coined by the works published in the 1970s, providing the initial characterization of the spectrum of these disorders.[23–28] CIDP occurs more frequently with increasing age, although it is also well recognized in children.[8,15,16,29–32]

The prototypical and most prevalent form of CIDP is characterized by a chronic progressive (monophasic or recurrent) course of symmetric, proximal, and distal weakness of the upper and lower limb muscles and large fiber sensory loss.[1,7,33,34] Less common forms include focal and distal presentations as well as pure motor and pure sensory forms.[1–10,35,36] CIDP may be associated with a number of disorders, although is considered idiopathic. The pathophysiology of CIDP is complex and involves immune mechanisms implicating both cellular and humoral responses.[10,37–40] In recent years, a number of advances, particularly in immunology, have allowed delineating similar but unrelated disorders, such as anti-myelin associated glycoprotein (MAG) neuropathy as well as, more recently still, characterizing new forms of immune-mediated neuropathies related to the presence and presumed pathogenicity of antibodies directed against nodal and paranodal antigens.[41–43]

Dysimmune Neuropathies. https://doi.org/10.1016/B978-0-12-814572-2.00003-0

CIDP treatment relies on three evidence-based treatments from available randomized controlled trials: immunoglobulins, steroids, and plasma exchanges.[34,44] The majority of affected patients respond to these treatments alone or in combination, although incomplete improvement with residual disability as well as refractoriness continue to represent significant problems. Hence, the interest in newer disease-modifying therapies remains and represents an important issue for CIDP management.[34,45] The evaluation of treatment effects and disease monitoring has been the subject of attention in recent years, and the use of different disability scales has been proposed.[46,47] This has become an important area in the management of CIDP in view of cost and availability as well as the side-effect profile of available treatments.[48–53]

Epidemiology

Several epidemiological studies have been conducted worldwide in CIDP, although the majority have been in European populations.[13–19] Reported prevalence rates for CIDP are of 1 to 9 per 100,000. It is likely that these wide differences are related to diagnostic criteria used rather than actual geographical variations.[16,54] CIDP occurs more frequently in men, with reported ratios of 3:2 to nearly 3:1.[13,16] Prevalence increases with age.[13,15–17,54] The incidence of CIDP is also reported as variable, with recent studies suggesting figures around 0.5 to 1.0 per 100,000 per year.[13–18] A recent metaanalysis and systematic review of the epidemiology of CIDP concluded with a pooled prevalence rate of 2.88 per 100,000 and a pooled crude incidence rate of 0.33 per 100,000 person years.[54] Few epidemiological studies have examined the proportions of different CIDP forms. It appears from available limited data that the classic CIDP form is the most common, with focal forms representing a minority and other forms (pure motor, pure sensory, predominantly distal, sensory ataxic) the exception.[1–4,7,8,10,34,55] However, selection bias (e.g., retrospective cohorts with mostly prevalent cases, wide ranges of disease course, and various treatment strategies) and variation in case definition (electrodiagnostic and clinical criteria, lumping/splitting (a)typical forms) all may hamper interpretation from many reported cohorts. Importantly, the lack of systematic studies on the clinical evolution over time may further complicate the accurate definition of CIDP forms.

Diagnosis

Clinical features

The diagnosis of CIDP is a clinical one, based on the presence of symmetrical or asymmetrical muscle weakness and sensory loss to large fiber modalities involving proprioception with accompanying areflexia or hyporeflexia (Fig. 1).[33,34,56] The course is, by definition, over > 8 weeks, progressive or relapsing and remitting, although this can be shorter in a minority of cases.[56]

Clinical criteria for CIDP

≥3 core symptoms
- Subacute, progressive polyneuropathy
- Disease duration ≥ 2 months
- Relapse-remitting/stepwise disease course
- Motor dominant with relative symmetric proximal weakness
- Generalised hyporeflexia or areflexia (*without atrophy*)

Or <3 core symptoms + ≥2 supportive symptoms
- Weakness in 4 extremities
- Proximal weakness ≥ 1 limb
- Focal proximal or distal motor/sensorimotor (*plexus/multiple nerves in upper/lower limb*)
- Reflexes ↓ in affected limbs
- Cranial nerve involvement
- Postural tremor
- Sensory ataxia

Exclusion criteria for CIDP

Other causes for neuropathy
- Diabetic/non-diabetic radiculoplexus neuropathy
- Hereditary demyelinating neuropathy
- IgM MGUS or other paraproteinaemic syndromes (*IgM neuropathy, POEMS, CANOMAD, amyloidosis*)
- Potentially causal drug/toxin exposure
- Renal/hepatic failure, thyroid dysfunction
- Active infections (e.g.,neuroborreliosis, diphteria)
- Diagnosis of multifocal motor neuropathy
- PNS lymphoma

Electrodiagnostic criteria for CIDP

Definite = ≥1 demyelinating feature below in ≥2 nerves
1. DML ↑↑ (*excluding carpal tunnel syndrome*)
2. MCV ↓↓ (*excluding common segments nerve compression*)
3. F-M interval↑↑
4. Definite conduction block (area reduction > 50%, excluding *common segments nerve compression*)
5. Temporal dispersion ↑ (*>30% in arm nerves*)
6. CMAP duration↑
7. Feature from 3-6 in only 1 nerve + ≥1 from 1-6 in other nerve

Probable
- Possible conduction block in ≥ 2 nerves (area reduction > 30%, excluding *common segments nerve compression and leg nerves*)
- Possible conduction block in 1 nerve + ≥1 from 1-6 in other nerve

Possible
- Feature from 1-6 in only 1 nerve

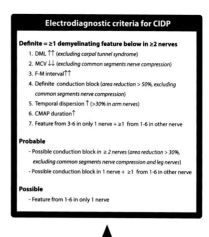

Laboratory investigations in suspected for CIDP

Routine
- Glucose and HbA1c, renal and thyroid function, vitamin B12, folic acid, full blood count, CRP and ESR, M-protein, serum protein immunofixation, antigangliosides and HIV serology.

Additional (*selected cases*)
- Anti-MAG antibodies, VEGF, light chain.
- Screening TTR mutations, PMP22, GJB1, MPZ.
- Antibodies to NF155, NF140, NF186, CNTN1, CASPR1.

Neuroimaging criteria for CIDP

MRI brachial/lumbosacral plexus
- Enlargement nerve roots
- T2-hyperintense signal nerve roots

Nerve ultrasound median nerves + brachial plexus
- Enlargement nerve roots + regional in ≥1 median nerve
- Pronounced enlargement in ≥2 median nerve segments (*excluding carpal tunnel*)

Other supportive criteria for CIDP

CSF
- Protein content ↑ + leukocyte cell count ≤ 10/mm³

Abnormal sensory nerve conduction in ≥1 nerve
- Normal sural with abnormal median/radial SNAP (*excluding carpal tunnel syndrome*)
- Sensory conduction velocity ↓

Nerve biopsy
- Evidence of demyelination and/or remyelination

Objective response to treatment*

Diagnostic categories

Definite CIDP
1. Clinical criteria (≥3 core, or <3 core + ≥2 supportive)
2. No exclusion criteria
3. Electrodiagnostic
   a) Definite;
   b) Probable + abnormal MRI/ultrasound or ≥1 supportive criteria
   c) Possible + abnormal MRI/ultrasound, or ≥2 supportive criteria

Probable CIDP
1. Clinical + no exclusion criteria and
   a) only electrodiagnostic probable, or possible + ≥1 supportive
   b) only abnormal MRI/ultrasound + ≥2 supportive

Possible CIDP
1. Clinical + no exclusion criteria and
   a) only electrodiagnostic possible
   b) only abnormal MRI/ultrasound + 1 supportive
   c) CIDP (definite, probable, possible) associated with concomitant disease

---

FIG. 1 Flowchart in diagnostic workup in patients with suspected CIDP. *HbA1c*, glycosylated hemoglobin; *CRP*, C-reactive protein; *ESR*, erythrocyte sedimentation rate; *MAG*, myelin associated glycoprotein; *VEGF*, vascular endothelial growth factor; *TTR*, transthyretin; *PMP22*, gene for peripheral myelin protein 22 kD; *GJB1*, gene for gap junction protein beta 1; *MPZ*, gene for myelin protein zero; *NF155*, paranodal protein neurofascin 155; *NF140*, nodal protein neurofascin; *NF186*, nodal protein neurofascin 186; *CNTN1*, contactin 1; *CASPR1*, contactin-associated protein 1. *Objective improvement using relevant outcome measures, including handgrip strength. (*Adapted with permission from Wolters Kluwer Health, Inc.:Goedee HS, van der Pol WL, Hendrikse J, van den Berg LH. Nerve ultrasound and magnetic resonance imaging in the diagnosis of neuropathy. Current opinion in neurology 2018;31(5):526–533*).

Acute-onset CIDP may occur in about one case in six and should be suspected in the absence of cranial and respiratory involvement, and particularly in the presence of proprioceptive sensory loss; this was recently suggested as possibly the most helpful distinguishing feature from Guillain-Barré syndrome (GBS).[57–59] Pain may be present, although severe pain is not usual and should suggest alternative diagnoses, as should prominent early atrophy and the presence of autonomic dysfunction, which, despite being present in about 10% of cases, is usually asymptomatic.[1,60–65] Cranial nerve involvement is seen in a minority of patients and respiratory involvement is the exception.[3,7,29,32,66–74]

Central nervous system (CNS) involvement, which should lead to consideration of alternative diagnoses but which may occur as idiopathic CNS demyelination occurring concurrently with the peripheral nerve demyelination of CIDP, has also been the focus of attention despite its rarity.[3,75–82] More recently, CNS involvement has been reported as part of CIDP in the presence on antiparanodal antibodies, specifically antineurofascin 155 (anti-NF155), although this appears to be the case mainly in Japanese populations as it has not been described in European cohorts.[83,84]

There are a number of other, less commonly known clinical manifestations that may occur in CIDP. These include restless leg syndrome, possibly affecting up to 40% of subjects, and fatigue.[85–87] Fatigue may be a prominent symptom in many patients, although the determinants and pathophysiological basis remain poorly understood.[86]

Classic CIDP

In the classic CIDP form (also referred to as "typical" CIDP), as described in the European Federation of Neurological Societies/Peripheral Nerve Society (EFNS/PNS) guidelines in 2006, last updated in 2010, motor weakness affects symmetrically the four limbs in a proximal and distal pattern.[33,56] Sensory loss involves vibratory and proprioceptive modalities. Reflexes are diffusely lost or reduced.[33,56]

Variants of CIDP

In contrast, CIDP variants (also referred to as "atypical" CIDP) concern a heterogeneous group of conditions, each with distinct clinical features and anatomical distribution (Table 1, Fig. 2): focal, predominantly distal, pure sensory including with exclusive small fiber manifestations, pure motor, and sensory ataxic.[2,3,7,10,34,55,91–95] Although several descriptive cohort studies have documented their most distinctive features, small sample sizes and the lack of systematic longitudinal data have hampered accurate definition of their boundaries with regard to presentation and natural disease course. The fact that classic CIDP already has a highly variable time span to evolve into its characteristic features further complicates the distinction, as was illustrated by a recent large Italian study of 460 CIDP patients, among whom up to 20% did not have a debut with typical features.[55] Nevertheless, the prevalence of CIDP variants among the CIDP spectrum may be substantial.[3,55,96]

TABLE 1 Summary of clinical characteristics classic CIDP and variants.

CIDP form	Motor	Sensory	Reflexes	Pain	Tremor	Cranial nerve	Ataxia
						Clinical features	
Classic[3,7,33,55]	++	+	↓/--	+/-	+/-	+/-	+
Focal[7,9,10,35,55,66,88]	++	+	→	+	+/-	+/-	+
Distal predominant[3,55,89,90]	+	++	→	+/-	+	-	+
Pure sensory[2,7,10,55,91]	-	++	↓/--	-	+/-	-	+
Pure motor[6,7,10,55]	++	-	↓/--	-	+/-	-	-
Sensory ataxic[4,7,92a]	-	++	↓/--	-	++	-	++

[a] Two subforms have been observed: (1) chronic immune sensory polyradiculopathy (CISP) with isolated sensory nerve root involvement and normal nerve conduction studies, and (2) ataxic CIDP that has electrophysiological sensory and motor involvement.

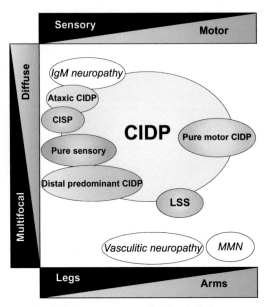

FIG. 2 Summary on the clinical patterns among the chronic inflammatory neuropathies in relation to CIDP as it is known today. *CISP*, chronic immune sensory polyradiculopathy; *LSS*, Lewis-Sumner syndrome; *MMN*, multifocal motor neuropathy.

The most common CIDP variant is focal CIDP, and it was first described by Lewis and Sumner [hence also known as "Lewis-Sumner syndrome" (LSS), MADSAM (multifocal asymmetric demyelinating sensory and motor neuropathy), or MIDN (multifocal inflammatory demyelinating neuropathy)].[5,9,35,66,88] LSS is characterized by multifocal, predominantly distal, and asymmetrical sensorimotor involvement (i.e., patchy multiple nerve distribution, unlike a stocking/glove pattern).[9] Other features may include focal neuropathic pain, tremors, and in some patients, cranial nerve involvement.[9,66] The majority of LSS cases affect exclusively the upper limbs and the disorder needs to be differentiated from multifocal motor neuropathy (MMN), which affects only motor fibers.[9,97] This is important as LSS may be steroid-responsive whereas MMN is not, and may even worsen with steroid treatment.[9,97] There have been reports, however, of deterioration of LSS with steroid therapy, although the literature remains conflicting in this regard, with other reports describing steroid responsiveness.[9]

The distal predominant form [previously referred to as "DADS" (distal acquired demyelinating sensory and motor neuropathy)] is a rare CIDP variant that mainly affects lower limbs and is characterized by distal symmetric sensory involvement with less pronounced weakness and slower progression than classic CIDP.[3,55,89,90] Consequently, it is challenging to recognize this form in routine clinical practice, and especially separate it from more prevalent chronic distal axonopathies or IgM neuropathy.[98] Electrophysiology and exclusion of monoclonal gammopathies are essential for diagnosis.[3,10,42,55,89] A recent Italian retrospective study suggested less frequent treatment effect compared to what may be achieved in typical CIDP,[55] although the validity of traditional CIDP outcome measures for assessment of this variant is debatable, which may cast some uncertainty on these findings.

Pure motor CIDP is another well-recognized variant that needs to be promptly identified as treatable.[6,7,10,55] Pure motor CIDP requires differentiation from other pure motor syndromes, such as MMN (symmetric four-limb involvement at onset as opposed to the asymmetric, predominantly upper limb presentation of MMN), and the lower motor neuron predominant forms of motor neuron disease (progressive muscular atrophy).[6,7,10,55,97,99] Although systematic studies are lacking, the current consensus among experts is that treatment of pure motor CIDP mirrors that of MMN, as it responds to immunoglobulins and may deteriorate with steroid treatment.[100] There are some arguments to include electrophysiology to define pure motor CIDP, as forms with asymptomatic sensory electrophysiological involvement may effectively be treated with steroids, whereas those with normal sensory electrophysiology should lead to the avoidance of steroids.[6,36] As this all comes from small-sized retrospective data, caution is, however, still very much advisable in treating motor CIDP.

Pure sensory CIDP (also described as CISP—chronic immune sensory polyradiculopathy) and sensory ataxic CIDP have also been documented as rare variants.[2–4,7,10,55,91,92,95,101–103] Patients present with distal symmetric or asymmetric, severe proprioceptive loss, areflexia, and sensory ataxia, but with normal muscle strength. There is still a lack of agreement on whether, in the case of clinically exclusive sensory deficits, the electrodiagnostic involvement of motor axons should be viewed as compatible with sensory CIDP. Some prefer lumping cases with electrodiagnostic features compatible with demyelination of motor axons as a pattern potentially evolving into more classic CIDP, whereas others view this as still compatible with pure sensory or even further subcategorize it (sensory dominant, with/without electrodiagnostic involvement of motor axons). Importantly, this form may present with apparently normal electrophysiology, including sensory nerve conduction studies. Such cases are those defined as "CISP." It has been proposed that in those patients, the diagnosis may be supported by delayed somatosensory evoked potentials (SSEPs), which assess preganglionic sensory conduction pathways, and raised cerebrospinal fluid (CSF) protein together with abnormal magnetic resonance[104] imaging of lumbar roots. However, none of these positive test results provides proof of demyelination nor are they specific. More recently, a subset of patients with sensory ataxic CIDP presentations were shown to have antibodies to specific (para)nodal components, illustrating the fact that other diagnostic modalities may further improve diagnosis.[10,37,43,105–108] Some of these CIDP patients with (para)nodal antibodies also have some degree of motor involvement clinically and tremors.[105,106,108] The discovery of these antibodies in a minority of patients has also opened the discussion on CIDP classification, illustrating the need for further improvement of our understanding of specific pathophysiological processes that ultimately lead to such distinctive clinical presentations. In addition, sensory CIDP has also been reported, presenting as a cryptogenic sensory neuropathy with small fiber symptoms, described as responsive to immunotherapy.[95] Great caution is advisable before embarking on immunotherapy in such cases when sensory CIDP with pure small fiber symptoms is suspected, as this is best managed symptomatically.

Electrophysiology

The main diagnostic test for CIDP is electrophysiology, based on motor conduction defects indicating patchy demyelination (Fig. 1). Typically, motor nerve conduction studies demonstrate features compatible with heterogeneously distributed demyelination, such as substantially slowed motor conduction velocities, prolonged distal motor latencies, delayed minimum F-M intervals, motor conduction block, and temporal dispersion (Fig. 3).[56,90,109–114] Distal dispersion of the compound muscle action potential (CMAP) is now of well-established usefulness in the diagnosis of CIDP and may be particularly helpful when nerve conduction studies are poorly tolerated, or reveal little features of demyelination otherwise.[115–118] EMG filter settings are important in the determination of distal CMAP duration as they affect normal values and a recent Japanese-European multicenter study has clarified the respective desirable normative values that may be used with different low-cut filters.[116,119] Also, the chronodispersion of F-waves may be helpful in cases that do not fulfill the electrodiagnostic consensus criteria for CIDP.[114]

Although electrodiagnostic criteria for CIDP are predominantly based on motor conductions, a number of sensory abnormality patterns have been suggested as useful and may help complement the routine motor studies.[120–125] It is important to acknowledge that these sensory patterns merely favor a nonlength dependent origin, rather than providing actual electrodiagnostic proof of demyelination. The "abnormal median normal sural" and "abnormal radial normal sural" sensory conduction patterns have been shown to be diagnostically helpful in different populations, although individually, they are of low sensitivity.[120–122] Slowed sensory conduction velocities may also be of help, again with low sensitivity.[123,124]

Over 15 different sets of electrophysiological criteria have been published for CIDP.[109,111,113,126–131] All rely heavily on the appropriate use of normative values for implementation of demyelinating cut-offs, temperature, and standardization of distances (e.g., fixed distance between stimulus and recording sites).[111,113,128–133] The first documented effort to distinguish demyelinating neuropathy already introduced criteria for conduction slowing that they were based on distribution between groups compared to a scale of normative values (i.e., 60% of median conduction velocity in healthy controls ≈ 38 m/s, still used to classify hereditary (demyelinating) neuropathies).[134] Subsequent proposed electrodiagnostic criteria for CIDP used different sets of normative values and

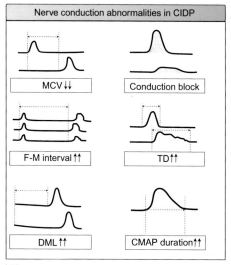

(A)

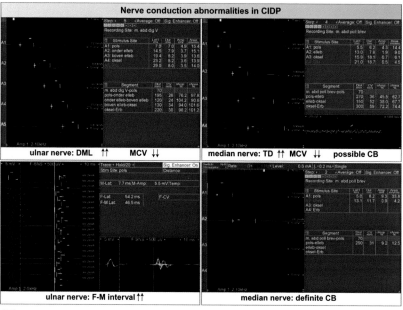

(B)

FIG. 3 Examples of characteristic nerve conduction abnormalities in CIDP. (A) Illustrated summary of nerve conduction abnormalities in CIDP: reduced motor conduction velocity (MCV), prolonged F-M interval and distal motor latency (DML), increased temporal dispersion (TD, and conduction block (CB), and increased compound muscle action potential (CMAP) duration. (B) Examples of nerve conduction abnormalities in found in CIDP patients: reduced MCV and DML, increased TD, prolonged F-M interval, and CB.

required number of affected nerves.[94,111,128–131,135,136] Some investigators evaluated the diagnostic yield of CIDP criteria, based on maximal conduction slowing and other dependent variables in lower motor neuron syndromes.[109] The EFNS/PNS criteria have become the best known and most used in research and in clinical practice, and have demonstrated optimal sensitivity and specificity in multicenter studies of heterogeneous populations.[113,137,138] These criteria are summarized in Table 2. Categorization of levels of electrodiagnostic certainty depend on the fulfillment of the preestablished requirements, leading to three categories: "definite," "probable," and "possible" CIDP. Whereas, the definite and probable subcategories offer high levels of specificity, fulfillment of the possible CIDP subgroup corresponds to a lower level of diagnostic certainty due to its suboptimal specificity.[113]

Multicenter studies in both Europe and North America have shown that motor conductions, performed in forearm and foreleg nerve segments unilaterally, offer > 80% sensitivity in establishing the diagnosis of CIDP as per EFNS/PNS criteria, with high levels of specificity versus other neuropathies, exceeding

TABLE 2 Summary of electrodiagnostic criteria CIDP.

Categories	Criteria for demyelination in electrodiagnostic parameters
Definite	≥ 1 feature(s) of demyelination (below) in at least two nerves[a] - DML ↑↑ - Temporal dispersion ↑↑ - MCV ↓↓ - F-M interval ↑↑ - Distal CMAP duration ↑ - Definite Conduction block (area ↓ > 50%)
Probable	- Possible conduction block in two nerves (area ↓ only > 30%, but < 50%) or with ≥ 1 feature(s) of demyelination in other nerve.
Possible	- Features of demyelination as in definite, but in only 1 nerve

[a] *Although strong evidence is lacking, caution is warranted to rate for these parameters when distal CMAP values are very low. In our experience in patients with suspected CIDP, nerves that have lost the majority of their axons (i.e., CMAP ≤ 1.0 mV) and show conduction slowing meeting EFNS/ PNS criteria, only improve with treatment if they have proximal clinical involvement, in which case the slowing found may indicate a more diffuse presence of inflammatory demyelination. In such cases, it may otherwise be useful to expand the electrodiagnostic protocol to more proximal muscle recordings (i.e., flexor and extensor carpi radialis muscles (respectively, median and radial nerves), biceps brachii muscle (musculocutaneous nerve)) to sample nerves with a sufficient size of the remaining axonal pool. The limitation to this practice for some units may, however, be the absence of available local normative values for these nerves.*

CMAP, compound muscle action potential; DML, distal motor latency; MCV, motor conduction velocity. Criteria for reduction of motor conduction velocity and prolongation of latencies that are compatible with demyelination, may be represented by deviation (in percentages of upper/lower limit of normal values)[94] or based on derivation in disease controls.[109] It is advocated to use area instead of amplitude reduction to define the potential presence of a conduction block, and only evaluate this in nerves with distal CMAP > 1.0 mV.[10,131,139–141]

95%.[111,113,142,143] Proximal upper limb studies, shown to be sensitive and specific for CIDP versus axonal neuropathies, may be helpful to demonstrate proximal conduction blocks and temporal dispersion, and four-limb studies may increase diagnostic sensitivity, both, however, at the expense of specificity.[112,142] Although highly specific, older criteria such as those of the American Academy of Neurology are poorly sensitive, thereby not identifying potentially treatable patients and therefore unsuitable for clinical practice.[128–131,135] It is essential to remember the importance of using adequate normative values and implementing the abnormal cut-offs defined within electrophysiological criteria. This cannot be overemphasized, especially as approximations and general impressions of electrophysiological findings are still unfortunately commonplace in practice worldwide, with major potential implications in depriving or, conversely, inappropriately offering a justification for immunomodulatory treatment, often for long periods.[144–146] Fulfillment of EFNS/PNS criteria in the presence of a compatible clinical picture is both sensitive and specific for a diagnosis of CIDP. Nonfulfillment of electrodiagnostic criteria should, however, not deter from a diagnosis of CIDP in the presence of a strongly suggestive clinical picture, although this is likely to occur in only a minority of patients.[55,113]

Several studies have also addressed the presence and distribution of specific electrophysiological features in CIDP variants compared to the classic presentation. Their main findings are summarized in Table 3. In short, mostly focal conduction blocks and loss of sensory axons are seen in the upper limbs in focal CIDP, whereas sensory ataxic CIDP is characterized by marked sensory loss with preserved or affected motor conductions. In our personal experience with these sensory CIDP variants, motor conduction slowing and conduction blocks are mostly found in proximal nerve segments. Some rare cases may present with completely normal peripheral sensory and motor physiology (CISP).[2,4,7,9,10,35,55,66,91,136,147–149] In contrast, pure motor CIDP has predominantly motor conduction blocks and less slowing, and preserved sensory conduction.[6,10,55,91,149,150] Distal predominant CIDP commonly demonstrates distal loss of sensory more than motor axons and a predominantly distal demyelinating process, with a low terminal latency index,[96] which represents the ratio of distal distance/distal motor latency × motor conduction velocity.[10,55,89,91]

The limitations of electrophysiology in CIDP diagnosis require particular attention. Several other conditions may produce electrophysiological abnormalities that are compatible with parts of the electrodiagnostic criteria for CIDP. These include Guillain-Barré syndrome (GBS), hereditary demyelinating neuropathies, IgM neuropathy with anti-MAG antibodies, familial amyloid neuropathy (FAP), POEMS (polyneuropathy with organomegaly, endocrinopathy, M-protein, and skin rash), and CANOMAD (Chronic Ataxic Neuropathy, Ophthalmoplegia, Monoclonal IgM paraprotein, cold Agglutinins and Disialosyl antibodies). Their clinical and electrodiagnostic features are discussed below in the section on CIDP mimics. Patients suffering from severe diabetic neuropathy or renal failure who present more homogenous severe

TABLE 3 Summary of ancillary investigations in classic CIDP and variants.

CIDP form	EDX	Imaging
		Nerve (root) enlargement
Classic	Symmetric loss sensory and motor axons,[a] multifocal conduction slowing,[b] and blocks	++ (multifocal/regional)
Focal	Focal loss sensory and motor axons, and focal blocks > conduction slowing[c]	+ (multifocal)
Distal predominant	Symmetric loss sensory > motor axons, distal conduction slowing, TLI ↓	+ (multifocal)
Pure sensory with small fiber manifestations	Symmetric loss sensory axons, motor conduction slowing, temporal dispersion, and blocks[d]	++ (multifocal/regional, roots++)
Pure motor	Loss motor axons + normal sensory, multifocal conduction slowing, and blocks[e]	+ (multifocal/regional)
Sensory ataxic		
- ataxic CIDP	Symmetric loss sensory axons, motor conduction slowing, temporal dispersion, and blocks	++ (multifocal/regional, roots++)
- CISP	Normal nerve conduction, abnormal SSEP	++ (multifocal/regional, roots++)

[a] Legs > arms, distally with exception of abnormal median/radial and normal sural in subset.
[b] Motor conduction slowing, prolonged distal latencies or F-M interval, increased temporal dispersion or duration of distal compound muscle action potential (CMAP), all compatible with heterogenous demyelination.
[c] Predominantly upper limb with preserved F-waves and normal distal latencies and CMAP duration; terminal latency index.[96]
[d] Motor studies may be normal and confirmation of sensory conduction block can be challenging, SSEP may be used in selected cases to support nonlength dependent features of sensory involvement.
[e] Preserved sensory conduction, in particularly over segments with motor conduction abnormalities compatible with demyelination.
Two sensory ataxic subforms have been observed: (1) chronic immune sensory polyradiculopathy (CISP) with isolated sensory nerve root involvement and normal nerve conduction studies, yet abnormal somatosensory evoked potential (SSEP), and (2) ataxic CIDP that has electrophysiological sensory and motor involvement.

conduction slowing are the exception. Finally, the issue of axonal loss in CIDP may result in problems identifying electrophysiological features of demyelination. "Axonal" CIDP has long been reported as an immune-mediated and treatment-responsive entity,[151] although it may be argued that greater extensiveness of nerve conductions, including with proximal upper limb studies, may have been diagnostically contributory in such cases, if they had been used. Nevertheless, even extensive and serial electrodiagnostic studies may fail to document any features compatible with demyelination.[152–154] One set of criteria has been proposed that does not require mandatory electrophysiology.[33] Although this may be of help in such clinically typical cases of nonfulfillment of electrodiagnostic requirements, consensus guidelines still advise the support of additional investigations to reach a diagnosis of CIDP.[94] In our experience, such cases remain extremely rare.

Other electrophysiological techniques may help to support a diagnosis of CIDP, although these are neither routinely available nor currently based on strong evidence, to justify advocating widespread implementation. Several reports illustrated the diagnostic potential of SSEPs, specifically the added value of delayed or absent responses in pure sensory CIDP, but this technique only provides support of proximal involvement versus the more common length-dependent origin.[92,101,102,155,156] Needle nerve root stimulation and the triple stimulation technique (TST) have been proposed as complementary techniques to ascertain the presence of a conduction block proximal to Erb's point.[157–161] However, direct nerve root stimulation may be frankly painful for patients, which hampers its use to obtain the supramaximal stimulation needed to reliably distinguish between submaximal and sufficient electrical stimulation. Moreover, cut-offs for a drop in signal amplitude between the cervical and Erb's point are not based on relevant disease controls, resulting in limited specificity as these may also be seen in other disorders.[162–165] Consequently, these techniques require considerable expertise and their use may only be appropriate for highly specialized neuromuscular centers familiar with them.

More recently developed electrophysiological methods have been studied in CIDP, including MUNIX (motor unit index number) and nerve excitability testing.[166] MUNIX was initially developed for motor neuron disease and provides measures that reflect the number and size of functioning motor units.[167–169] Summated values determined from multiple muscles have been shown to correlate with strength, disability scores, and axonal loss in CIDP.[166,170] We have recently studied MUNIX in immunoglobulin-treated subjects with CIDP and have found significant correlations with disability scores as well as significant improvement 2 weeks after treatment, suggesting that this novel technique may provide an objective marker of response to immunoglobulin therapy.[171] Nerve excitability testing was introduced by Bostock and colleagues, and mainly designed to test membrane properties from which ion-channel dysfunction may be inferred, and subsequently verified by modeling.[172–177] Elevated thresholds for several excitability parameters have been found in CIDP, including threshold electrotonus and activity-dependent hyperpolarization, indicating paranodal involvement and activity-dependent conduction block.[178–180] Subsequent studies have also documented amelioration of these effects after immunoglobulin therapy.[181,182] Interestingly, another study illustrated the potential diagnostic profiles that may aid in the distinction between GBS and CIDP of acute onset.[183] The fact that nerve excitability testing is mainly suited to sample distal nerve segments while also requiring specific hardware and software as well as extensive knowledge of normal nerve physiology, limit its widespread implementation. Temperature control is also of importance as well as further development of test protocols.[184–186]

Cerebrospinal fluid studies

An elevated cerebrospinal fluid (CSF) protein level without pleiocytosis is a helpful finding in suspected CIDP, occurring in 80%–90% of cases (Fig. 1).[127,187–189] However, the frequently used cut-off value of >45 mg/dL suffers from poor diagnostic performance as such levels may be encountered in a substantial number of healthy controls and as substantial variations exist between different laboratories.[190,191] New data on age-based cut-offs for CSF protein elevation require consideration in the diagnosis of CIDP, as does awareness of the poor specificity of elevated levels, particularly versus subjects with diabetes or demyelinating genetic neuropathy.[144,192] Furthermore, the clinical phenotype is of major importance, as illustrated by the low sensitivity of CSF protein elevation in CIDP variants.[9,66,193] This reduces the value of systematic CSF protein level measurement in suspected cases. Although studies on CSF cell count in CIDP are lacking, they are normal in most cases and exceed the current consensus limit of <10/mm^3 only exceptionally.[94,194,195] Consequently, lumbar punctures may be justifiably avoided nowadays in the majority of patients whose clinical and electrophysiological picture are unequivocal. In subjects for whom a malignant process or infectious basis may be suspected, or the history relatively short, CSF study remains, however, mandatory.

Imaging

Neuroimaging of the peripheral nervous system has in recent years been described as a valuable complement for the diagnostic process in CIDP (Fig. 1).[196] Magnetic resonance imaging (MRI) and nerve ultrasound (US) are the most commonly used modalities to study various morphological aspects of nerves and nerve roots, each with their own advantages and limitations. Dedicated MRI protocols have been developed, often referred to as MR neurography (MRN), to study cervical and lumbosacral roots and plexuses in CIDP.[197–201] In routine practice, the most essential sequences to evaluate the plexuses are based on T2 images in the coronal plane, such as advanced short tau inversion recovery (STIR) and maximal intensity projection (MIP), that can be complemented by imaging in the sagittal plane to correlate the anatomy and T1 sequences.[196] This allows the evaluation of the presence of nerve root hypertrophy, increased signal intensity, and gadolinium contrast enhancement (Fig. 4).[202] High-resolution ultrasound, using probes with frequencies between 15 and 18 MHz, can be used to evaluate nerves and cervical plexus for the presence of nerve enlargement (Fig. 4).[196] Nerve US has superior spatial resolution, but MRI compensates this with excellent tissue contrast and the ability to document signal intensity and

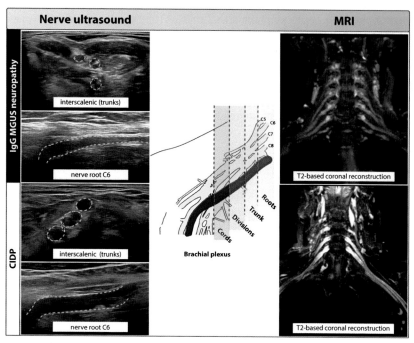

FIG. 4   Examples of characteristic MRI and nerve US findings in CIDP. Nerve root enlargement in patient with CIDP *(lower panels)* compared to patient with IgM MGUS (monoclonal gammopathy of unknown significance) neuropathy *(upper panels)* on nerve ultrasound *(left panels)* and MRI *(right panels)*. *(From Bunschoten C, Jacobs BC, Van den Bergh PYK, Cornblath DR, van Doorn PA. Progress in diagnosis and treatment of chronic inflammatory demyelinating polyradiculoneuropathy. Lancet neurology Reprinted with permission from Elsevier (The Lancet, 2019, 18(8), 784–794)).*

contrast enhancement. Early case reports and case series on these techniques suggested that inflammation and myelin dysfunction led to a thickening of nerves in patients with CIDP, which could be detected by both MRI and nerve US.[203–209] Subsequent MRI studies explored the frequency of abnormalities in spinal nerve roots, but suffered from a lack of objective cut-off values for abnormality and used different protocols in heterogenous groups with small sample sizes, resulting in considerable variation in the detected abnormalities.[196] In contrast, ultrasound studies focused more on large arm and leg nerves but used various cut-off values and protocols, and have resulted in several scoring systems that still need to be validated.[196] In short, MRI may reveal a hyperintense signal in 44%–72% of CIDP patients, enlargement in 13%–88%, and postgadolinium enhancement in 10%–89%.[196,197,204,206,210] MRI abnormalities are more often symmetrical in typical CIDP, the reverse being true in LSS, in line with what may be expected clinically and electrophysiologically.[197,211,212] The available data from nerve US in CIDP and the few comparative studies with MRI indicate that its diagnostic performance to detect nerve root enlargement is considerably higher than that of MRI.[152,213–216] However, similar changes have been described in CMT1A, IgM neuropathy, vasculitic neuropathy, idiopathic or diabetic cervical and lumbosacral radiculoplexus neuropathies, neuralgic amyotrophy, and neurolymphomatosis, making the specificity of MR imaging for CIDP versus clinically relevant controls uncertain (also see section on CIDP mimics).[104,197,202,217–222] Consequently, results from nerve imaging should be weighed carefully in the appropriate clinical context. Furthermore, some studies have suggested US as a helpful way to separate acute-onset CIDP from GBS.[223–225] Nevertheless, this needs to be validated in independent large cohorts and should merely lead to an increase in clinical vigilance for such a presentation of CIDP with simple and routine but careful serial clinical evaluations after onset of an acute polyradiculoneuropathy. It may clearly be argued, therefore, that clinical monitoring only overrides any potential utility of nerve US in this setting. Taken together, the routine use of MRN and US may be helpful in some cases, particularly when electrophysiology does not provide the answer.[93,152,226,227] The interrater reliability for nerve imaging techniques remains uncertain, with a limited number of reports on various nerve US protocols [228–231] and a recent study raising some concerns.[232] However, it is important to remember that this issue applies to all operator-dependent tests, including electrophysiology, for which data are also similarly very scarce. Further prospective studies addressing the diagnostic value of MRI and nerve US are needed to improve our understanding of their diagnostic performance in patients with suspected CIDP. Adequate, well-conducted clinical phenotyping and electrophysiology remain the essential priority to identify inflammatory neuropathies and therefore effectively contribute to the ultimate therapeutic decision-making process.

Routine blood investigations

Routine blood investigations are essential when a diagnosis of CIDP is under consideration. Evaluation of the glycosylated hemoglobin (HbA1c) level is mandatory as CIDP may occur in diabetics (see below) and as measures are desirable in patients with newly identified impaired glucose metabolism, with the additional neuropathic consequences possible as a result. Excluding a monoclonal gammopathy by immunofixation is essential, as is early detection of an inflammatory syndrome that may suggest an etiology, in particular, malignant. Testing for antimyelin associated antibody (MAG) positivity is required in the presence of an IgM paraprotein, as is measurement of the vascular endothelial growth factor (VEGF) level in the presence of an IgA or IgG, or even IgM paraprotein, with a lambda light chain, to investigate for POEMS syndrome. It has to be kept in mind, however, that CIDP may coexist with low-level anti-MAG antibodies and benefit from usual CIDP treatment.[233] Similarly, IgG, IgA, and IgM monoclonal gammopathies of uncertain significance (MGUS) may be present in otherwise typical CIDP, with no proven link, and do not alter usual CIDP treatment modalities. The issue of IgM monoclonal proteins requires special attention with consideration of anti-MAG (myelin associated glycoprotein) antibody status being desirable, as discussed in the dedicated chapter on the subject in this volume. In subjects with pain and suggestion of autonomic dysfunction, genetic screening for transthyretin (TTR) mutations is mandatory, whereas in those with exclusive or predominant distal and motor dominant involvement, consideration should be given for screening for Charcot-Marie-Tooth disease type 1A, followed by screening of other demyelinating CMT subtypes and eventual gene panel testing. More recently, and as will be subsequently detailed, new antibodies to nodal and paranodal proteins have been identified in a small proportion of patients with CIDP, with, for the majority, suggestive phenotypes and frequent refractoriness to conventional therapies.

Nerve pathology

In the early descriptions and diagnostic criteria for CIDP, nerve histology was considered the gold standard.[1,23,128,189] As electrodiagnostic testing became more widely accepted to be proficient for CIDP diagnosis, and it became apparent that the important limitations of a nerve biopsy outweighed its added diagnostic value, the routine use of nerve histology dissipated. Although characteristic, the visualization of macrophage-induced demyelination is very rare, and other histopathological findings are frequently of low sensitivity and poor specificity.[38,234–236] The fact that consensus is lacking on optimal techniques and that these are considerably operator- and sampling-dependent further complicates the interpretation of results.[237,238] Consequently, a sural nerve biopsy is not recommended in the setting of typical CIDP presentations, and may only be helpful if and when a specific alternative diagnosis, particularly amyloid or vasculitic neuropathy, as well as malignant infiltration, particularly lymphomatous, are under concurrent consideration. Despite these reservations, histology may, in the research setting, improve our understanding of the underlying pathophysiological processes in the spectrum of CIDP.[10,37,239] For example, it has been demonstrated recently that cases with antiparanodal antibodies display histopathological paranodal dissection from IgG4 attachment at the paranodal junctions, this in absence of macrophage-induced demyelination. The process of macrophage-induced demyelination itself appears to occur at different sites, nodal or internodal, and this may relate the CIDP clinical subtype.[37]

CIDP mimics

Several mimics may initially be misdiagnosed as CIDP; their clinical features and characteristics of ancillary investigation are summarized in Table 4.[64] A more detailed discussion is provided below.

GBS

Although GBS is typically a postinfectious neuropathy, with acute onset and a clinically well-delineated short disease course of progression, some cases may

TABLE 4 Summary of characteristics of common CIDP mimics.

Mimics	Clinical	EDX	Imaging Nerve (root) enlargement	CSF Protein content ↑	Lab
CMT1	Childhood onset affected family members slowly progressive distal motor predominant pes cavus hammer toes diffuse atrophy lower legs	Homogeneous motor conduction slowing[a]	++	+	PMP22, GJB1, MPZ
GBS (with TRF)	Acute onset submaximal improvement on treatment with subsequent deterioration sensorimotor cranial nerve involvement	Loss sensory and motor axons, multifocal conduction slowing, and/ or conduction block[a]	+/−	+	
IgM neuropathy	Indolent progression distal sensory ataxia	Predominant loss longer and sensory axons, distal conduction slowing, TLI ↓ (<0.26)	++	+	IgM protein anti-MAG
Amyloid neuropathy	Slowly progressive distal sensory predominant pain, CTS, autonomic involvement	Loss sensory > motor axons, may have multifocal conduction slowing[a]	+/++	+	TTR
POEMS	Subacute, progressive distal motor predominant pain	Loss sensory and motor axons, conduction slowing in intermediate nerve segments[a] TLI 0.35–0.6	+	+/−	IgG/IgA protein Lambda light chain + VEGF ↑ thrombocytes ↑
CANOMAD	Slowly progressive distal sensory predominant ataxia ophthalmoplegia	Predominant loss sensory axons, multifocal conduction slowing[a]	+	+/−	Disialosyl antibodies: IgM protein anti-GD1b/GQ1b Cold Agglutinins

[a] Compatible with demyelination.

IgM, monoclonal immunogobulin M protein (of unknown significance IgM MGUS); CMT1, Charcot-Mary-Tooth type 1; CBS, Guillain-Barré-Syndrome index; TRF, treatment-related fluctuation; POEMS, polyneuropathy with organomegaly, endocrinopathy, M-protein, and skin rash; CANOMAD, chronic ataxic neuropathy, ophthalmoplegia, monoclonal IgM protein, cold agglutinins and disialosyl antibodies; CTS, carpal tunnel syndrome; TLI, terminal latency; anti-MAC, antibodies to myelin associated glycoprotein; TTR, transthyretin; IgG, monoclonal immunoglobulin protein G; IgA, monoclonal immunoglobulin protein A; VEGF, vascular endothelial growth factor; anti-GD1b, antibodies to ganglioside GD1b; anti-GQ1b, antibodies to ganglioside GQ1b.

remain challenging, especially when deficits and disability continue progressing beyond 4 weeks.[240] Treatment-related fluctuations (TRF) that can be seen in at least a subset of GBS patients should be distinguished from CIDP with acute onset.[57,59,241,242] Cranial and respiratory involvement favor GBS, whereas their absence combined with prominent proprioceptive sensory loss and sensory ataxia are more compatible with CIDP.[57,59] CSF and blood investigations will not aid in this distinction.[57,59] Differentiating electrophysiologically acute-onset CIDP (AO-CIDP) from GBS is most frequently difficult, although we have found in practice that severe reduction of motor conduction velocities (< 30 m/s in the upper limbs and < 20 m/s in the lower limbs) is highly uncommon in GBS and may, as a result, suggest AO-CIDP. Nerve imaging may show nerve root enlargement in both conditions,[204,206,213,243,244] whereas the extension of such a process in large arm nerves may favor CIDP.[223,224,245] Ultimately, given the poor diagnostic performance of most of these tests, only close serial clinical monitoring will allow accurate distinction.

Demyelinating Charcot-Marie-Tooth disease

Distinguishing CIDP from demyelinating Charcot-Marie-Tooth (CMT) disease is usually straightforward due to the expected distinct clinical and electrodiagnostic features.[64,246] Although both may present as a motor dominant neuropathy with areflexia, the distal predominance in the presence of foot deformities and indolent progression are usually sufficient to indicate CMT, whereas CIDP is characterized by prominent proximal weakness, proprioceptive sensory loss, and relapses. Electrodiagnostically, the heterogeneous slowing in CIDP as opposed to the homogeneous slowing in CMT as well as the detection of conduction block and excessive temporal dispersion, which are characteristics of CIDP but the exception in CMT, further aid their distinction.[247–254] Similarly, diffuse nerve enlargement is a typical ultrasound characteristic of CMT1, as opposed to more regional in CIDP, but extension into these patterns can be seen in both, rendering uncertain the discriminating value in less straightforward cases.[255–257] In contrast to adults, the prevalence of demyelinating CMT in children is higher than CIDP, complicating the diagnosis of CIDP in children and misdiagnosis of late onset forms of demyelinating CMT as CIDP.[29–32,144,246] Improved descriptions of CMT forms that may unexpectedly present with electrodiagnostic features of CIDP, the search for Myelin Protein Zero and GJB1 mutations, and gene panel testing in addition to PMP22 duplication have improved their identification to avoid misdiagnosis and unnecessary treatments. It is, however, likely from observation in clinical practice that this may still be of common occurrence today, for the partly understandable reason of willingness to attempt treating an undiagnosed although suspected CMT. Active avoidance of unproven treatments is, however, of paramount importance in this setting to avoid exposure to toxic drugs in these children.

IgM neuropathy (with anti-MAG antibodies)

Although IgM neuropathy is mainly a clinical-laboratory diagnosis, several clinical and electrodiagnostic features are shared with CIDP.[258–261] Typically, IgM neuropathy has an indolent disease progression and sensory predominance, but some have considerable weakness and the reduced or absent tendon reflexes combined with prominent ataxia and tremor that can also be seen in certain CIDP presentations.[41] As a substantial portion of patients with IgM neuropathy—particularly in the presence of anti-MAG antibodies—fulfill the electrodiagnostic criteria of CIDP, the recognition of a characteristic distal predominant slowing combined with decreased terminal latency indices (TLIs) helps to redirect clinicians to complete appropriate laboratory testing on paraprotein presence.[42,218,258] Similarly, the widespread enlargement of nerve(root)s can be seen in both CIDP and IgM neuropathy, merely indicating the extent of the disease processes, albeit possibly more prominent in proximal segments of median nerves in the case of IgM neuropathy.[217,218,262,263] Nevertheless, a plexus MRI is not helpful in this distinction and the results from nerve ultrasound studies need to be replicated in independent cohorts, but will certainly not remove the need for the required blood testing. Also, main CIDP treatment modalities have failed to produce significant clinical improvement in IgM neuropathy with anti-MAG antibodies, but this simply cannot be considered diagnostic.[264]

Amyloid neuropathy

Another genetic neuropathy causing similar electrophysiological difficulties in mimicking CIDP and that has been the focus of recent attention is familial amyloid polyneuropathy (FAP).[265] Although suggestive clinical features, namely pain and autonomic dysfunction, are expected to help question a CIDP diagnosis, it appears from recent studies that misdiagnosis due to electrophysiology is not uncommon.[98,247,266,267] Enlargement of peripheral nerves, similar to CIDP, has also been documented in FAP with nerve ultrasound and MRI.[268,269] Consequently, FAP remains primarily a genetic diagnosis and transthyretin (TTR) gene sequencing should be considered early when appropriate in the diagnostic work-up. The advent of new effective treatments for FAP makes it imperative to be aware of this to avoid diagnostic and therapeutic delays in treating this fatal condition.[270]

POEMS

POEMS is a rare but important CIDP mimic that can be suspected clinically based on distal predominant neuropathy with prominent pain and signs of multisystem involvement.[271] This disorder is described in detail in a dedicated chapter. Its motor predominance and heterogeneity clinically, combined with subacute onset and progressive course, are very similar to CIDP. Increased levels of vascular endothelial growth factor (VEGF), thrombocytosis, and the presence of a lambda light chain are indicative of a diagnosis of POEMS, whereas IgA and IgG monoclonal gammopathies can also be seen in CIDP without concomitant hematologic disease [IgA/IgG monoclonal gammopathy of unknown significance (MGUS)].[98,271,272] Considerable conduction slowing is also frequent in the electrodiagnostic testing of POEMS, but appears predominantly to involve the intermediate nerve segments with less distal slowing than in CIDP.[273,274] Therefore, nerve conduction studies (NCS) that reveal motor conduction slowing of intermediate nerve segments and increased TLI combined with lack of temporal dispersion and conduction blocks may facilitate an early focus on other causes of neuropathy when associated with IgA/IgG paraproteins.[273,274] Systematic nerve imaging studies comparing POEMS and CIDP are lacking. A single case description noted widespread enlargements of arm nerves on ultrasound in POEMS, which was also documented in a more recent study but not corroborated by another case series.[275–277] It remains unclear how this pattern of sonographic nerve involvement compares to that seen in CIDP, and therefore should not be used diagnostically in this setting. Taken together, POEMS is primarily a clinical and laboratory diagnosis in which electrophysiology may help to redirect the diagnostic path when some of these elements were not sufficiently appreciated or atypical.

CANOMAD

CANOMAD (chronic ataxic neuropathy, ophthalmoplegia, monoclonal IgM protein, cold agglutinins and disialosyl antibodies) is an extremely rare, slowly progressive sensory predominant ataxic neuropathy that classically presents with ophthalmoplegia, although the extraocular involvement may be absent/delayed or even misinterpreted as focal cranial nerve involvement of CIDP, as relapses may also occur.[278, 279] The laboratory features of CANOMAD include the presence of IgM paraprotein and antiganglioside antibodies (anti-GD1b/GQ1b), and of cold agglutinins.[278] The fact that the electrophysiological features of CANOMAD may be compatible with demyelination and even fulfill the criteria for CIDP further complicates their distinction.[278] A recent retrospective study documented regional enlargement of arm nerves on US.[280] However, systematic studies comparing the electrophysiological and nerve US patterns are lacking. Therefore, clinicians should primarily rely on the clinical phenotype and laboratory features for correct identification of these patients. Finally, these patients may also show partial response to IVIg, plasmapheresis, or steroids.[278]

Pathophysiology

Despite several different approaches that have been deployed to unravel the causes of CIDP, much of the pathophysiological mechanisms involved are still unknown. Most of the research on the pathophysiology has been populated predominantly by observations in the most typical presentations of CIDP.

The early studies described pathological changes exclusively in the sensory nerves of the distal lower leg,[1,188] but systematic histologic studies of multiple nerve segments and mixed nerves in lower and upper limbs are still lacking. Electrodiagnostic studies have revealed the loss of longer axons and multifocal demyelination noninvasively.[90] Subsequently, more detailed electrophysiological studies, predominantly in distal segments or large arm nerves, have indicated that the paranode may constitute one of the primary nerve targets in CIDP, and can evolve to sites of axonal injury as well.[180] Also, nerve imaging has revealed widespread nerve involvement, even when nerve function is still retained.[196,281] More recent reports sparked the interest in blood and CSF markers, identifying different traces of inflammatory processes predominantly distant from the blood-nerve barrier and diseased nerves. A detailed synthesis of all these findings can be found elsewhere.[39] Below, we summarize the most relevant insights of immunopathophysiology in CIDP.

An immune basis is indicated in CIDP by the evidence of inflammatory phenomena in peripheral nerves and blood as well as the response to immunomodulatory therapies including immunoglobulins, steroids, and plasma exchanges. The pathophysiological mechanisms involved include the synergistic action of both humoral and cellular immunity. The implication of cellular mechanisms is illustrated by the presence of inflammatory infiltrates in diseased nerves, altered cytokine expression in blood, and CSF.[10,37,38,235,282–285] The migration of activated T cells across a disrupted blood nerve barrier, which then produce inflammatory mediators, results in further increased permeability of the barrier, thereby allowing entry of soluble factors including pathogenic antibodies.[38,107,194,286] The release of cytokines and chemokines results in macrophage activation and upregulation of vascular cell adhesion molecules.[37,194,283,287] The infiltration of inflammatory cells occurs within affected nerves, predominantly by macrophages, which then play a major role, by antigen presentation, the release of proinflammatory cytokines, demyelination, and phagocytosis (Figs. 5 and 6).[37,282,287] CD8[+] T cells are believed to drive cell-mediated attack on nerves, and it is possible that immunoglobulin therapy may reduce CD8[+] cells as well as ameliorate the activation of proinflammatory cytokine pathways.[38,194,286,288] On the other hand, regulatory T cell dysfunction may also contribute to the inappropriate immune response.[22,288] Although the specific autoantibody response is still unknown in the majority of patients, humoral mechanism implication is suggested in CIDP by response to plasma exchange therapy as well as immunohistological studies.[1,10,37,107,108] The responsibility of a role for the major myelin antigens P0, P2, PMP22, and connexin is not established. The focus in more recent years has been on antigens located in nodal, paranodal, and juxtaparanodal regions, vital for normal saltatory conduction (Fig. 5). IgG4 subclass antibodies against neurofascin 155 and contactin 1 as well as CASPR1 have been associated with a rare CIDP subtype with characteristic clinical features and poor immunoglobulin response.[10,37,43,105–108] These CIDP subtypes are further detailed later in this chapter.

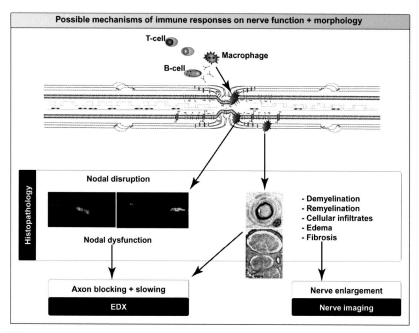

FIG. 5 Summary of possible mechanisms related to the involvement of the immune system in CIDP as it is known today. Schematic overview on only the partially elucidated balance of both humoral and cellular immununologic processes that are known to be involved in CIDP, and ultimately result in disruption of the peripheral nerve myelin, nodal structure, and function. Also, part of their downstream effects may be detected with routine electrodiagnostic studies (EDX) and nerve imaging. *(Adapted with permission from Wolters Kluwer Health, Inc.:Goedee HS, van der Pol WL, Hendrikse J, van den Berg LH. Nerve ultrasound and magnetic resonance imaging in the diagnosis of neuropathy. Current opinion in neurology 2018;31(5):526–533).*

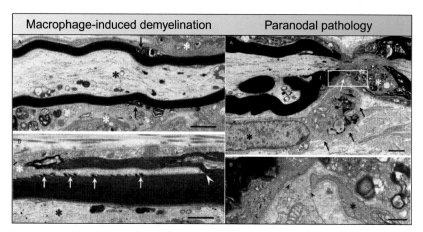

FIG. 6 Examples of macrophage-induced demyelination and (para)nodal involvement. A high-powered view of the region of macrophage-induced demyelination and paranodal pathology. Focal unraveling and swelling of myelin apposed to the cytoplasm of a macrophage is observed adjacent to the Schmidt-Lanterman incisures *(left upper panel)*. The surface of myelin adjacent to the cytoplasm of macrophages becomes fuzzy as a result of the disruption of myelin lamellae *(left lower panel)*. The *arrowhead* indicates the top of the macrophage process lifting layers of myelin. The cytoplasm of the macrophage extends to the node of Ranvier and enters into the tube of the basement membrane and phagocytoses the right paranode *(right upper panel)*. The nucleus and cytoplasm located outside the tube of the basement membrane are indicated by a *black asterisk* and *black arrows*, respectively. A point where the macrophage invades into the basement membrane is shown by *arrows*.

Associations of CIDP with other diseases

CIDP may be associated with a number of disorders.[94] This may be problematic as it may make the diagnostic process more difficult as well as complicate management decisions. Knowledge of these potential associations and of the issues that may result is important in clinical practice. Some drugs used for non-neurological indications have also been associated with CIDP, raising important questions regarding the continuation of these implicated treatments in affected subjects.

Diabetes

Although it is known that CIDP may occur in diabetics in addition to a diabetic polyneuropathy, whether diabetics are more susceptible to developing CIDP has been the subject of debate. A higher risk of CIDP, reaching up to nine-fold, had been suggested by earlier nonpopulation-based studies.[16,289,290] This was not, however, subsequently supported by two epidemiological studies conducted in the United States and Italy, neither of which found a higher CIDP prevalence in diabetics.[8,291] More recently, this has again been the subject of attention with a study of a large insurance healthcare database from North America, indicating a nine-fold increased CIDP prevalence in diabetics compared to nondiabetics, with reported figures of 54 per 100,000 versus 6 per 100,000.[292] These results have proved controversial, particularly in relation to the important issue of CIDP misdiagnosis, as illustrated by recent studies.[144] The prevalence figure in nondiabetics appears compatible with that of the other North American study performed and also consistent with worldwide figures, although an excess diagnostic rate in diabetics due, among other reasons, to the overinterpretation of clinical and especially electrophysiological findings appears quite possible.[290] Although the issue of frequency of association remains currently unresolved, CIDP does clearly occur in some patients with diabetes and prompt identification and treatment are highly desirable. The diagnosis of CIDP in such cases is in our experience, however, unfortunately often delayed due to symptoms being erroneously attributed to diabetic neuropathy, resulting in late treatment that may, in turn, contribute to suboptimal improvement as a result of continuing irreversible axonal loss. Adequate clinical evaluation is paramount as the principal clinical features of symmetrical proximal weakness and proprioceptive sensory loss, with gait imbalance, are unexpected in diabetic polyneuropathy and should raise suspicion of CIDP. In practice, as patients with diabetes are seldom systematically referred for neurology opinions for their diabetic neuropathy, delays in recognizing these features may occur commonly. The diagnostic process is also complicated from the electrophysiological point of view. Although only mild degrees of electrophysiological demyelination can be expected in diabetic polyneuropathy, these should not reach demyelinating cut-offs of current EFNS/PNS criteria for CIDP.[56,117,290] However, both electrophysiological under- and overdiagnosis is not uncommon.[131,144,293] In the first case, lack of attention given to the presence of excessive demyelination for diabetic poly-neuropathy, particularly in an appropriate clinical setting suggestive of CIDP, may be encountered. In the latter, misplaced emphasis on minimal slowing not meeting requirements for CIDP, in the presence of a clinically purely diabetic polyneuropathy, may unfortunately similarly occur. CSF protein elevation is often unhelpful as elevated protein levels occurs commonly in diabetes. Levels in excess of 1 g/L may, however, be diagnostically useful.[294] Imaging both with MR neurography and ultrasonography is currently of uncertain value in identi-fying CIDP in patients with diabetes, as the detected structural abnormalities, although well described in CIDP, have also been recently reported in diabetic neuropathy.[104,196,295,296] The usefulness of nerve pathology in this setting is also highly uncertain due to the low sensitivity in CIDP as well as the technical ex-pertise required, which is unavailable in many centers.[236,297] Treatment response to immunoglobulins has importantly been found as frequently in diabetics as in nondiabetics.[290] However, the degree of amelioration has been described as less in diabetics, possibly due to accompanying axonal loss from the associated diabetic polyneuropathy.

Monoclonal gammopathy of uncertain significance (MGUS)

MGUS are monoclonal proteins secreted in excess by plasma cells, with-out associated sign of hematological disease. It is important to recognize that the prevalence of MGUS increases with age, as does that of CIDP.[17,298] Coincidental coexistence of the two disorders is therefore not unexpected. MGUS can be of IgG, IgM, or IgA heavy chain subtypes. Light chains can be of the kappa or lambda subtype. The case of IgM deserves special atten-tion, as it may be of heterogeneous presentation in the setting of neuropathy; this is detailed in another chapter. Lambda light chains should, despite a low paraprotein level, raise the possibility of POEMS syndrome. The presence of antimyelin-associated-glycoprotein (MAG) antibodies needs to be excluded, as this would lead to a diagnosis of anti-MAG neuropathy, distinct clinically and electrophysiologically from CIDP, and require a very different therapeu-tic approach.[98] Recent data suggest that the search for high-titer anti-MAG antibodies should be performed, even in the absence of a detectable IgM monoclonal protein on immunofixation.[299] However, when the appropriate he-matological investigations have confirmed MGUS (IgG, IgM or IgA heavy chain subtype, kappa or lambda light chain) instead of an alternative malignant disorder, the management of a concurrent CIDP diagnosed on clinical and elec-trophysiological grounds does not differ from that of CIDP without MGUS.[98] Hematological input is highly advisable, as is the collaborative interaction be-tween the specialities in this setting and monitoring of the monoclonal protein level, necessary on a 6- to 12-month basis.

Charcot-Marie-Tooth disease (CMT)

The coexistence of inflammatory and genetic neuropathy has been reported widely.[247] CIDP occurring in a context of CMT has been described in a few cases, although this needs to be recognized promptly for adequate management. In patients attending routine follow-up for CMT, recent unexpected rapid decline in function, with new motor deficits, particularly in proximal limb regions as well as proprioceptive sensory loss, should serve as red flags to suggest the possibility of associated CIDP. The association has been reported in a number of CMT subtypes, as expected more frequently with the commoner CMT1A, but also with X-linked CMT and CMT due to MPZ mutations. Rare case reports describe possible similar associations with CMT 4C, CMT 4J, HNPP (hereditary neuropathy with liability to pressure palsies), and HSAN I (hereditary sensory and autonomic neuropathy). However, in some of these cases, it is possible that the genetic neuropathy itself had a CIDP-like phenotype rather than there being a true association with an inflammatory neuropathic component. The electrophysiology in the presence of associated CIDP may reveal heterogeneous slowing, conduction block, and excessive temporal dispersion, all uncharacteristic of genetic neuropathy, although the existence of these features in some pure genetic neuropathy subtypes such as those with GJB1 mutations needs to be recognized.[247–254] CSF studies may be helpful, particularly when protein levels > exceed 1 g/L, as this is infrequent in CMT. Nerve pathology, although previously described as diagnostic, is unlikely to be helpful in the majority of cases.[300] In our experience, CIDP associated with genetic neuropathy is rare but responds well to existing treatments that may substantially improve the function and quality of life of affected patients, who may easily miss out on such effective therapies in view of their known underlying CMT, hence the need to promptly identify the association by adequate clinical evaluation.

Other autoimmune disorders

The association of CIDP with a number of other autoimmune conditions is described in the literature.[301] It is possible that a susceptibility to immune disorders may be present in some individuals, hence a frequent association of two or more dysimmune diseases. Systemic Lupus Erythematosus (SLE) has been reported in association with CIDP in multiple reports.[301,302] The nonneurological literature reporting this does not, however, adequately detail the neuropathic presentations or electrophysiology for a confident CIDP diagnosis, as per current criteria, in some of these cases. Furthermore, there are no described features to indicate a specific CIDP phenotype occurring in association with SLE, suggesting that the two disorders may occur coincidentally. Associations of CIDP have also been reported with Hashimoto's thyroiditis, Sjögren's syndrome, rheumatoid arthritis, and inflammatory bowel disease.[301] The possibility of coincidental association cannot be excluded in these cases either, particularly in view of the small numbers involved. A large population study from Sweden otherwise showed an association of coeliac disease with CIDP.[303] Also, in sarcoidosis, a CIDP phenotype has been reported to precede systemic involvement.[304] However, this is the exception, with small-fiber neuropathy being far more common together with multifocal sensory predominant neuropathy.[305] It is, of course, imperative to take a systematic detailed general medical history from patients with suspected CIDP and to perform, in the case of suggestive features, the appropriate screening investigations for some or all of the above. Rare cases of myasthenia gravis and CIDP have also been reported.[306–309]

How concurrent autoimmune diagnoses should affect CIDP management strategies is uncertain. In patients responding to standard first-line CIDP treatment, concurrent diagnoses are unlikely to represent a reason to alter effective therapy. However, the question may be raised either in case of refractoriness or when the need arises for immunotherapy of the associated disorder. In such cases, potential effects on both conditions need to be sought to minimize the treatments attempted and the side-effect risks.

Malignancy

Several cases of CIDP occurring concurrently with cancer have been reported. In a recent literature review on the subject, we found that hematological malignancies were by far the most frequent, with non-Hodgkin's lymphomas (NHLs) four times more common than Hodgkin lymphomas (HLs).[310] Of note, as many as a quarter of patients with NHL and a paraneoplastic syndrome may have CIDP and the same may be true for up to a fifth of those with Waldenström's macroglobulinaemia[311] and neuropathy. Melanoma has also been described in association with CIDP, importantly commonly with the presence of antiganglioside antibodies. CIDP is often diagnosed before the malignancy and suggestive features may include ataxia, distal or upper limb predominance, and cranial, respiratory, or autonomic involvement. Early awareness of the possibility of an associated malignancy and consideration of a suggestive clinical picture and of appropriate further investigations is essential. Cancer treatment alone may be effective for CIDP, although the concurrent use of immunomodulatory agents including steroids, immunoglobulins, and plasma exchange appears of potential benefit if cancer therapy is insufficient or in the case of severe and disabling or progressive neuropathic disease.[310]

Infection

Although CIDP, as opposed to GBS, is considered to be preceded by infection in only a small percentage of cases (10% versus 70%), an infective or postinfective etiology has been described in the literature for many years.[58,301] HIV infection has been well known to be a trigger of CIDP, and systematic HIV serology is appropriate in de novo cases.[312] Affected patients appear to respond to standard

CIDP therapy in addition to antiretroviral treatment, and the prognosis appears good. Hepatitis B and C infections have also been described in the setting of CIDP.[313–318] One study suggested that chronic Epstein Barr virus (EBV) infection may be implicated in CIDP, although this has not to our knowledge been replicated.[319] Rare cases of acute-onset post-*Mycoplasma pneumoniae* infection CIDP have also been described.[320,321]

Drug-induced CIDP

A number of drugs have been described as triggering inflammatory neuropathies, both acute and chronic in onset.[70,322–324] CIDP has been described after short- and long-term use of antitumor necrosis factor alpha (TNF-alpha) agents.[322] Such presentations may occur weeks to years after initiation of the treatment and may be in the typical and atypical forms of the disease. Anti-TNF-alpha drug withdrawal is usually performed, although standard CIDP immunomodulatory therapy may be required in the longer term. Reintroduction of the presumed responsible drug has been described without further relapse in some cases, although it would appear appropriate to cautiously consider other therapeutic options. Bortezomib, a proteasome inhibitor drug used in myeloma, has also been described as causing a demyelinating neuropathy resembling CIDP with good response to immunomodulatory therapy.[325] Coincidentally, bortezomib has also been attempted in the treatment of refractory CIDP in a few cases.[326] Tacrolimus, used to prevent graft rejection, has similarly rarely been described as causing a CIDP-like illness.[327–329] In drug-triggered cases, the pathophysiological processes involved remain uncertain, and may involve differences with idiopathic CIDP.

CIDP with antibodies to nodal and paranodal proteins

Since 2013, new autoantibodies to nodal and paranodal proteins have been reported in a small proportion of patients with CIDP.[43] This area has generated considerable interest in the field, at the current time, disproportionate to the numbers of patients implicated. This is in part due to the potential for new immunological biomarkers to be discovered in the future related to more common forms of the disease, as up to one-third of patients with CIDP have serum reactivity to dorsal root ganglion neurons, Schwann cells, or motor neurons in vitro.[330,331] These new antibodies, suggested as pathogenic by pathological studies of paranodal destruction in nerve and skin biopsy-obtained fibers and by animal studies, have been found in subjects with atypical clinical presentations and frequent unresponsiveness to first-line CIDP therapies.[10,37,43,105–107] The method used for detection appears of importance, with ELISA using human antigens offering optimal sensitivity and specificity.[43] The newly discovered antibodies include those to the paranodal proteins neurofascin 155 (NF155), contactin 1 (CNTN1), and contactin-associated protein 1 (CASPR1) as well as the nodal proteins neurofascin 140 (NF140) and neurofascin 186 (NF186).[43]

Paranodal antibodies are mostly of the IgG4 isotype. The presence of these antibodies has been found to have direct clinical associations. CNTN1 antibody-positive patients have aggressive disease with poor IVIg response and nephrotic syndrome, whereas NF155-antibody positive subjects have been described with distal-predominant weakness, tremor of the cerebellar type, and poor IVIg response.[43,105-108] Despite the cerebellar features, the majority of patients with anti-NF155 reactivity have no CNS MRI abnormality, although this has been reported in a proportion of Japanese patients.[83] Of note, a small number of cases have to date been reported with reactivity to the CNTN1/CASPR1 complex.[332,333] Such patients have an aggressive neuropathy.[334,335] As the experience with these new CIDP subtypes is very small so far, it is difficult to be confident of a clinical phenotype indicating the presence of a specific antibody at this stage. Indeed, these cases may present quite heterogeneously, with some that have an initial IVIg response.[108] Whether all CIDP patients need testing is currently a matter of debate, although it appears clear that this should be the case, when possible, in patients with poor or incomplete IVIg response.

These new entities are important to recognize as they are most often poorly responsive to conventional CIDP treatments. IVIg is frequently ineffective, whereas steroids have proved beneficial in some reported cases. Both in subjects with anti-NF155 and anti-CNTN1 antibodies, B-cell depleting agents, in particular rituximab, have been described as effective in producing substantial amelioration.[43,105,107,108,336] This needs to be kept in mind at an early stage, particularly in aggressive disease, so as to attempt to reduce the deleterious effects of progressive axonal loss and minimize the time and risks of exposure to unhelpful drugs.

It is argued that the nodo-paranodopathies should not constitute part of the CIDP spectrum, as they are neither strictly pathologically demyelinating nor pathophysiologically inflammatory.[34] This may be challenged as unhelpful and confusing, as a chronic neuropathy presenting with electrophysiological features of demyelination with not only conduction blocks (i.e., also severe motor conduction slowing, prolonged latencies and F-waves, with albumino-cytological dissociation and hyperintensity and hypertrophy or MR neurography) will be considered as part of the CIDP spectrum, in clinical practice. In addition, it may be considered that an extension of the CIDP spectrum itself to include such new entities may now require further thought through reconsideration of the very definition of CIDP. We propose it may be useful in the future to consider the words "*chronic immune-determined polyneuropathy*" as defining *CIDP* instead of the terms "inflammatory" and "demyelinating," as well as the notion of "radiculopathy" as these clearly do not apply to all cases.

Treatment of CIDP

CIDP is a treatable but chronic disorder with a current evidence base for three main first-line therapies (Table 5): corticosteroids, immunoglobulins, and plasma exchange.[34,44]

TABLE 5 Summary of treatment of CIDP.

Modality	Dosing	Level of evidence
Immunogobulins		
- IVIg	Induction 2 g/kg in 3–5 days, maintenance 0.4–1.0 g/kg/2–4 weeks	1a
- SCIg	0.2–0.4 g/kg/week	1b
Steroids		
- Prednisone	1 mg/kg	1b
- Dexamethasone	40 mg/day on 4 days/month	1b
- Methylprednisolone	500 mg/day on 4 days/month or 1000 mg/month	1b
Plasma exchange	Induction 5 sessions/2–3 weeks maintenance 1 session/2–4 weeks	1a

IVIg, intravenous immunoglobulins; *SCIg*, subcutaneous immunoglobulins.

The justification to use corticosteroids is based on a single randomized controlled trial (RCT), with additional studies having demonstrated a comparable effect on disability to that of intravenous immunoglobulins.[11,44,337] There is no significant difference of efficacy between pulsed oral or intravenous steroid therapy and daily oral steroids.[44,338] However, pulsed therapy has been shown to be effective more quickly and to offer a better side-effect profile, particularly as regards moon-like facies and sleeplessness.[339] In addition, pulsed therapy may offer an advantage with regards to glycemic control and weight gain.[337] Pulsed therapy is commonly used at a dose of 500 mg or 1000 mg daily, with 4 weekly administrations of 2 g, or using oral dexamethasone at a dose of 40 mg daily for 4 days every month.[337,339,340] Up to six courses are usually administered. Daily prednisolone regimens may be given on a daily or alternate day basis, with an initial dose of 1 mg/kg with subsequent gradual reductions to the minimum effective dose allowing stabilization. Gastric protection as well as bone protection are mandatory with both regimens.

Intravenous immunoglobulins have been demonstrated as effective in CIDP in five different RCTs versus a placebo over the short term.[44] Importantly, a variety of different outcome measures were used. All trials used an initial dose of 2 g/kg of actual body weight, with one single longer-term trial subsequently, after one loading dose, using a maintenance dose of 1 g/kg every 3 weeks and a crossover, response-conditional design. This regimen is currently used in clinical practice widely. However, dose reductions to the minimal effective and trials off treatment have been advocated and shown to be appropriate in a few studies and dose-reducing protocols have been proposed.[341,342] In a recent retrospective analysis, we demonstrated the clinical and economic benefits of individualized dosing versus standard dosing as well as that of "dosing weight" rather than actual body weight in initial treatment stages in patients with a raised body mass index (BMI).[52] That intravenous immunoglobulins are effective in CIDP is very clear from the evidence base and clinical practice. However, how to optimally use this therapy remains to a degree uncertain, although this is important given the availability and cost issues as well as the high remission rate described in several different cohorts and the high-rate of continuing overtreatment found in research settings.[52] Furthermore, although serious thromboembolic complications of intravenous immunoglobulin therapy are very rare, they are non-negligible, particularly in patients with high cardiovascular risk, and caution is therefore required.[53] In recent years, subcutaneous immunoglobulin (SCIg) therapy has become the focus of attention as a more convenient alternative to the intravenous route of administration.[53] Few studies showed the effectiveness of SCIg in comparison to IVIg and a placebo.[343–345] A recent large, international, multicenter RCT has demonstrated the effectiveness of both a low dose (0.2 g/kg/week) and a high dose (0.4 g/kg/week) of SCIg versus a placebo.[346] No difference was ascertained between the two doses.

Plasma exchanges (PE) are advised in CIDP refractory to corticosteroids and intravenous immunoglobulins.[44] The effect of PE was demonstrated versus sham exchange in studies performed in the late 1980s and 1990s.[347] Despite methodological issues, PE have been found to be of equivalent efficacy to intravenous immunoglobulins for CIDP, although they are often impractical and of transient benefit, implying the need for repeated treatment. The use of peripheral venous access has facilitated the use of PE and made this option far more attractive than with central venous access. PE are generally well tolerated and most side effects described are relatively mild. The number of exchange sessions used per treatment course is variable across centers, with four or five being the most frequent. Other regimes, used in some centers, include biweekly ongoing exchanges for several consecutive weeks until clinical amelioration.

There is currently no evidence for the use of immunosuppressant therapy in CIDP. However, many clinicians still use this in an attempt to reduce the reliance on first-line treatments or in refractory disease. RCTs have shown no benefit of azathioprine, methotrexate, or interferon beta-1a, and the most recent trial of fingolimod was prematurely interrupted because interim analysis showed futility.[45,348] Some other agents found helpful in case reports or case series have been cyclophosphamide, rituximab, cyclosporine, and mycophenolate mofetil. In the absence of evidence, considering the side-effect risk and given the availability of three proven effective therapies, the justification for use of immunosuppressants requires careful consideration on a case-by-case basis.[34,349] We consider immunosuppressants exclusively in severely disabling refractory disease. Also, we and others have found cyclophosphamide and rituximab of benefit, sometimes remarkably so, in this setting in individual patients.

The choice of first-line treatment is an important issue in CIDP. Steroids and immunoglobulins are preferred to PE, as they are more practical. Steroids are obviously cheaper whereas both the availability and cost are of concern with immunoglobulins. The side-effect profile of steroids, on the other hand, are a concern while immunoglobulins pose generally few issues except in patients with high vascular risk. Immunoglobulins appear to have a quicker effect and are particularly useful in severely disabled individuals, whereas steroids have a slower action, which appears to be particularly the case with daily oral regimens. Importantly, long-term follow-up studies have shown longer remission periods after steroid treatment in comparison to immunoglobulin therapy.[337,339] Steroids and immunoglobulins used in combination may hence represent an interesting option and this is currently being investigated in an RCT, the OPTIC trial.[350] All these factors need consideration in the decision-making process, which ideally needs to be tailored to each subject, considering age, gender, co-morbidities, and concurrent treatments.[351,352] In case of unresponsiveness to the first agent attempted, the second should be considered followed by PE, which itself may also be combined effectively with steroids.

Outcome measures for CIDP

Several scoring systems have been introduced in research practice to determine the outcome in CIDP, including heterogenous sets of items of motor and sensory functions. The issue of outcome measures is of fundamental importance in CIDP, as on them should solely rely therapeutic decisions for initiation, tailoring, and continuation of therapy.

Early research studies have used different primary outcomes, including the Neuropathy Impairment Score (NIS), later known as the Neuropathy Disability Score (NDS), the Hughes Disability Scale or the Hammersmith Motor Ability Scale (HMAS), with the Medical Research Council (MRC) sum score utilized as a frequent secondary outcome. Over the past two decades, other scales were used in the research arena, including the Inflammatory Neuropathy Cause and Treatment (INCAT) scale and the Overall Neuropathy Limitation Score (ONLS).[46,353–355] In recent years, attention has focused on the Rasch-built scales, which have been advocated to overcome limitations and the variable item importance on older scales as well as differential weighing. An inflammatory neuropathy Rasch-built Overall Disability Scale (I-RODS) for CIDP and GBS was proposed in 2011, and a new Rasch-built MRC scoring system was also proposed in 2012.[46,47,356] Neither has been implemented in research practice in CIDP, as a primary outcome measure, to date.

Handgrip strength as measured by a Martin vigorimeter or Jamar dynamometer has also been found to be a useful measure in CIDP, correlating well with global disability; it is frequently used in centers with neuromuscular expertise.[356] However, even in patients that are clinically considered stable, there may be day-to-day variability up to 10% in this handgrip strength,[357,358] illustrating the importance of timing and the accurate definition of clinically relevant changes. The ability to walk may appear an attractive measure for routine clinical practice, but lacks important responsiveness to general functionality.[47] Although quantification of the walking capacity may improve responsiveness, it should only be used to complement other measures rather than replace them.[359,360]

A key issue with outcome measures is the concept of minimal clinically important difference (MCID), which is essential in interpreting changes on scales used.[361] These can be determined by different methods and provide meaningful cut-offs to be used. This notion is currently not widely applied in clinical practice but requires attention and consideration, as in addition to proper regular use of available scales, the valuation of genuine patient-relevant changes is of obvious utmost importance.

Clinical practice currently uses highly variable outcome measures, which is clearly very inadequate. These may vary from subjective descriptions of improvement and binary partially objective single outcomes to MRC scores in limited muscles or the more extensive use of one or more of the above-mentioned scales and methods. There is currently no consensus on what would be the most practical measures to evaluate treatment in clinical practice, although regulating bodies and insurance companies may request one or several to justify continuing treatment.[362]

Regardless, it appears imperative that monitoring measures are used, particularly given the implications of ineffective, inappropriate, and potentially harmful treatment. The more recently described scales, including INCAT, ONLS, and I-RODS as well as grip strength, despite obvious limitations for each, represent very useful ways of ensuring therapeutic decisions are being made as objectively as possible.

Conclusion

Although a relatively recently described disorder, CIDP has been the subject of considerable research and now represents a spectrum of immune-mediated neuropathies with heterogeneous clinical presentations, diagnostic modalities, and differing treatment options. CIDP as a whole remains rare and the subtypes described to date still rarer, but all have the potential to respond to treatment.

Early diagnosis of CIDP relies on the accurate recognition of suggestive clinical features as well as the adequate use of diagnostic techniques, particularly electrophysiology, maybe imaging, and immunology. The issue of misdiagnosis is clear and while it is imperative to tackle inappropriate overdiagnosis, it is similarly important to avoid underdiagnosis and its long-term effects. The lack of a valid and practical biomarker for CIDP contributes to diagnostic difficulties, with the recent progress in immunology bringing hope that more pathogenic antibodies concerning larger proportions of affected subjects may be identified in the coming years.

Despite several decades of research on CIDP management, treatment is still predominantly confined to classic modalities: steroids, immunoglobulins, and plasmapheresis. Although these are effective treatments for CIDP, they often do not offer a cure. Many affected patients show incomplete response and are left with long-term disability. This contrasts with what occurs in a proportion of subjects for whom full remission is, on the other hand, achieved with the same treatments. More research is therefore needed, focusing specifically on unraveling the underlying pathophysiology and development of biomarkers such as pathogenic antibodies that may offer better targets for treatment, which could further improve the outcome and help to reduce the individual treatment load. Also, research to enhance tailored treatments may also include a combination of different therapeutic modalities, particularly in groups of patients with poorer prognosis. It may be important to recognize that the quest for new treatments may not be appropriate for all types of CIDP, although low prevalence often unfortunately leads to the temptation to widen the eligibility criteria for study inclusion. This poses, in our opinion, important although most often unrecognized ethical questions relating to what may clearly be the inappropriate inclusion of subjects with a potential excellent prognosis in studies using novel agents of possible high toxicity. The evaluation of treatment effects is closely linked to all the above-mentioned issues. Contrary to other disorders where objective, patient, and observer-independent outcomes are available, the assessment of CIDP is conditioned by the evaluation tool itself, with compounded difficulties relating to patient and examiner bias. The impact of the inaccurate evaluation of treatment effects clearly remains a fundamental issue that will necessarily impact the relevance of future research. Despite these many challenges, future exciting developments are awaited and expected in the field, with hopefully better outcomes for affected patients worldwide.

References

1. McCombe PA, Pollard JD, McLeod JG. Chronic inflammatory demyelinating polyradiculoneuropathy. A clinical and electrophysiological study of 92 cases. *Brain.* 1987;110(Pt 6): 1617–1630.
2. Oh SJ, Joy JL, Kuruoglu R. "Chronic sensory demyelinating neuropathy": chronic inflammatory demyelinating polyneuropathy presenting as a pure sensory neuropathy. *J Neurol Neurosurg Psychiatry.* 1992;55(8):677–680.
3. Rotta FT, Sussman AT, Bradley WG, Ram Ayyar D, Sharma KR, Shebert RT. The spectrum of chronic inflammatory demyelinating polyneuropathy. *J Neurol Sci.* 2000;173(2):129–139.
4. Yato M, Ohkoshi N, Sato A, Shoji S, Kusunoki S. Ataxic form of chronic inflammatory demyelinating polyradiculoneuropathy (CIDP). *Eur J Neurol.* 2000;7(2):227–230.
5. Van den Berg-Vos RM, Van den Berg LH, Franssen H, et al. Multifocal inflammatory demyelinating neuropathy: a distinct clinical entity? *Neurology.* 2000;54(1):26–32.
6. Sabatelli M, Madia F, Mignogna T, Lippi G, Quaranta L, Tonali P. Pure motor chronic inflammatory demyelinating polyneuropathy. *J Neurol.* 2001;248(9):772–777.
7. Busby M, Donaghy M. Chronic dysimmune neuropathy. A subclassification based upon the clinical features of 102 patients. *J Neurol.* 2003;250(6):714–724.

8. Chio A, Cocito D, Bottacchi E, et al. Idiopathic chronic inflammatory demyelinating polyneuropathy: an epidemiological study in Italy. *J Neurol Neurosurg Psychiatry*. 2007;78(12):1349–1353.

9. Rajabally YA, Chavada G. Lewis-Sumner syndrome of pure upper-limb onset: diagnostic, prognostic, and therapeutic features. *Muscle Nerve*. 2009;39(2):206–220.

10. Ikeda S, Koike H, Nishi R, et al. Clinicopathological characteristics of subtypes of chronic inflammatory demyelinating polyradiculoneuropathy. *J Neurol Neurosurg Psychiatry*. 2019;90(9):988–996.

11. Dyck PJ, O'Brien PC, Oviatt KF, et al. Prednisone improves chronic inflammatory demyelinating polyradiculoneuropathy more than no treatment. *Ann Neurol*. 1982;11(2):136–141.

12. Iijima M, Yamamoto M, Hirayama M, et al. Clinical and electrophysiologic correlates of IVIg responsiveness in CIDP. *Neurology*. 2005;64(8):1471–1475.

13. Lunn MP, Manji H, Choudhary PP, Hughes RA, Thomas PK. Chronic inflammatory demyelinating polyradiculoneuropathy: a prevalence study in south East England. *J Neurol Neurosurg Psychiatry*. 1999;66(5):677–680.

14. Mygland A, Monstad P. Chronic polyneuropathies in Vest-Agder, Norway. *Eur J Neurol*. 2001;8(2):157–165.

15. Iijima M, Koike H, Hattori N, et al. Prevalence and incidence rates of chronic inflammatory demyelinating polyneuropathy in the Japanese population. *J Neurol Neurosurg Psychiatry*. 2008;79(9):1040–1043.

16. Rajabally YA, Simpson BS, Beri S, Bankart J, Gosalakkal JA. Epidemiologic variability of chronic inflammatory demyelinating polyneuropathy with different diagnostic criteria: study of a UK population. *Muscle Nerve*. 2009;39(4):432–438.

17. Mahdi-Rogers M, Hughes RA. Epidemiology of chronic inflammatory neuropathies in Southeast England. *Eur J Neurol*. 2014;21(1):28–33.

18. Visser NA, Notermans NC, Linssen RS, van den Berg LH, Vrancken AF. Incidence of polyneuropathy in Utrecht, the Netherlands. *Neurology*. 2015;84(3):259–264.

19. Mendell JR, Barohn RJ, Freimer ML, et al. Randomized controlled trial of IVIg in untreated chronic inflammatory demyelinating polyradiculoneuropathy. *Neurology*. 2001;56(4):445–449.

20. Thomas HM. Recurrent polyneuritis: a clinical lecture. *Phil Med J*. 1898;1:885–889.

21. Hoestermann E. Über rekurrierende polyneuritis. *Dtsch Z Nervenheilkunde*. 1914;51:116–123.

22. Burns TM. Chronic inflammatory demyelinating polyradiculoneuropathy. *Arch Neurol*. 2004;61(6):973–975.

23. Austin JH. Recurrent polyneuropathies and their corticosteroid treatment; with five-year observations of a placebo-controlled case treated with corticotrophin, cortisone, and prednisone. *Brain*. 1958;81(2):157–192.

24. Thomas PK, Lascelles RG, Hallpike JF, Hewer RL. Recurrent and chronic relapsing Guillain-Barre polyneuritis. *Brain*. 1969;92(3):589–606.

25. Matthews WB, Howell DA, Hughes RD. Relapsing corticosteroid-dependent polyneuritis. *J Neurol Neurosurg Psychiatry*. 1970;33(3):330–337.

26. Bonnaud E, Vital C, Cohere G, Castaing R, Loiseau P. Recurrent and relapsing polyneuritis. Four cases with ultrastructural studies of the peripheral nerves. *Pathol Eur*. 1974;9(2):109–118.

27. Prineas JW, McLeod JG. Chronic relapsing polyneuritis. *J Neurol Sci*. 1976;27(4):427–458.

28. Abramsky O, Webb C, Teitelbaum D, Arnon R. Cell-mediated immunity to neural antigens in idiopathic polyneuritis and myeloradiculitis. Clinical-immunologic classification of several autoimmune demyelinating disorders. *Neurology*. 1975;25(12):1154–1159.

29. Simmons Z, Wald JJ, Albers JW. Chronic inflammatory demyelinating polyradiculoneuropathy in children: I. Presentation, electrodiagnostic studies, and initial clinical course, with comparison to adults. *Muscle Nerve*. 1997;20(8):1008–1015.

30. McMillan HJ, Kang PB, Jones HR, Darras BT. Childhood chronic inflammatory demyelinating polyradiculoneuropathy: combined analysis of a large cohort and eleven published series. *Neuromuscul Disord*. 2013;23(2):103–111.

31. Haliloglu G, Yuksel D, Temocin CM, Topaloglu H. Challenges in pediatric chronic inflammatory demyelinating polyneuropathy. *Neuromuscul Disord*. 2016;26(12):817–824.

32. Cabasson S, Tardieu M, Meunier A, Rouanet-Larriviere MF, Boulay C, Pedespan JM. Childhood CIDP: study of 31 patients and comparison between slow and rapid-onset groups. *Brain Dev*. 2015;37(10):943–951.

33. Koski CL, Baumgarten M, Magder LS, et al. Derivation and validation of diagnostic criteria for chronic inflammatory demyelinating polyneuropathy. *J Neurol Sci*. 2009;277(1–2):1–8.

34. Bunschoten C, Jacobs BC, Van den Bergh PYK, Cornblath DR, van Doorn PA. Progress in diagnosis and treatment of chronic inflammatory demyelinating polyradiculoneuropathy. *Lancet Neurol*. 2019;18(8):784–794.

35. Lewis RA, Sumner AJ, Brown MJ, Asbury AK. Multifocal demyelinating neuropathy with persistent conduction block. *Neurology*. 1982;32(9):958–964.

36. Kimura A, Sakurai T, Koumura A, et al. Motor-dominant chronic inflammatory demyelinating polyneuropathy. *J Neurol*. 2010;257(4):621–629.

37. Koike H, Nishi R, Ikeda S, et al. Ultrastructural mechanisms of macrophage-induced demyelination in CIDP. *Neurology*. 2018;91(23):1051–1060.

38. Van Rhijn I, Van den Berg LH, Bosboom WM, Otten HG, Logtenberg T. Expression of accessory molecules for T-cell activation in peripheral nerve of patients with CIDP and vasculitic neuropathy. *Brain*. 2000;123(Pt 10):2020–2029.

39. Mathey EK, Park SB, Hughes RA, et al. Chronic inflammatory demyelinating polyradiculoneuropathy: from pathology to phenotype. *J Neurol Neurosurg Psychiatry*. 2015;86(9):973–985.

40. Franssen H, Straver DC. Pathophysiology of immune-mediated demyelinating neuropathies—part II: neurology. *Muscle Nerve*. 2014;49(1):4–20.

41. Notermans NC, Franssen H, Eurelings M, Van der Graaf Y, Wokke JH. Diagnostic criteria for demyelinating polyneuropathy associated with monoclonal gammopathy. *Muscle Nerve*. 2000;23(1):73–79.

42. Franssen H, Notermans NC. Length dependence in polyneuropathy associated with IgM gammopathy. *Ann Neurol*. 2006;59(2):365–371.

43. Querol L, Devaux J, Rojas-Garcia R, Illa I. Autoantibodies in chronic inflammatory neuropathies: diagnostic and therapeutic implications. *Nat Rev Neurol*. 2017;13(9):533–547.

44. Oaklander AL, Lunn MP, Hughes RA, van Schaik IN, Frost C, Chalk CH. Treatments for chronic inflammatory demyelinating polyradiculoneuropathy (CIDP): an overview of systematic reviews. *Cochrane Database Syst Rev*. 2017;1:CD010369. https://doi.org/10.1002/14651858.CD010369.pub2.

45. Mahdi-Rogers M, Brassington R, Gunn AA, van Doorn PA, Hughes RA. Immunomodulatory treatment other than corticosteroids, immunoglobulin and plasma exchange for chronic inflammatory demyelinating polyradiculoneuropathy. *Cochrane Database Syst Rev*. 2017;5:CD003280. https://doi.org/10.1002/14651858.CD003280.pub5.

46. Merkies IS, Schmitz PI, van der Meche FG, et al. Clinimetric evaluation of a new overall disability scale in immune mediated polyneuropathies. *J Neurol Neurosurg Psychiatry*. 2002;72(5):596–601.

47. Draak TH, Gorson KC, Vanhoutte EK, et al. Does ability to walk reflect general functionality in inflammatory neuropathies? *J Peripher Nerv Syst*. 2016;21(2):74–81.

48. Divino V, Mallick R, DeKoven M, Krishnarajah G. The economic burden of CIDP in the United States: a case-control study. *PLoS One*. 2018;13(10):e0206205.

49. Guptill JT, Bromberg MB, Zhu L, et al. Patient demographics and health plan paid costs in chronic inflammatory demyelinating polyneuropathy. *Muscle Nerve.* 2014;50(1):47–51.

50. Owens GM. The economic burden and managed care implications of chronic inflammatory demyelinating polyneuropathy. *Am J Manag Care.* 2018;24(17 Suppl):S380–S384.

51. Rajabally YA. Cost of illness, cost of immunoglobulin therapy and their determinants in chronic inflammatory demyelinating polyneuropathy. *Muscle Nerve.* 2019;59(3):E22.

52. Rajabally YA, Afzal S. Clinical and economic comparison of an individualised immunoglobulin protocol vs. standard dosing for chronic inflammatory demyelinating polyneuropathy. *J Neurol.* 2019;266(2):461–467.

53. Abbas A, Rajabally YA. Complications of immunoglobulin therapy and implications for treatment of inflammatory neuropathy: a review. *Curr Drug Saf.* 2019;14(1):3–13.

54. Broers MC, Bunschoten C, Nieboer D, Lingsma HF, Jacobs BC. Incidence and prevalence of chronic inflammatory demyelinating polyradiculoneuropathy: a systematic review and meta-analysis. *Neuroepidemiology.* 2019;52(3–4):161–172.

55. Doneddu PE, Cocito D, Manganelli F, et al. Atypical CIDP: diagnostic criteria, progression and treatment response. Data from the Italian CIDP database. *J Neurol Neurosurg Psychiatry.* 2019;90(2):125–132.

56. Van den Bergh PY, Hadden RD, Bouche P, et al. European Federation of Neurological Societies/Peripheral Nerve Society guideline on management of chronic inflammatory demyelinating polyradiculoneuropathy: report of a joint task force of the European Federation of Neurological Societies and the Peripheral Nerve Society—first revision. *Eur J Neurol.* 2010;17(3):356–363.

57. Ruts L, Drenthen J, Jacobs BC, van Doorn PA, Dutch GBSSG. Distinguishing acute-onset CIDP from fluctuating Guillain-Barre syndrome: a prospective study. *Neurology.* 2010;74(21):1680–1686.

58. Dionne A, Nicolle MW, Hahn AF. Clinical and electrophysiological parameters distinguishing acute-onset chronic inflammatory demyelinating polyneuropathy from acute inflammatory demyelinating polyneuropathy. *Muscle Nerve.* 2010;41(2):202–207.

59. Alessandro L, Pastor Rueda JM, Wilken M, et al. Differences between acute-onset chronic inflammatory demyelinating polyneuropathy and acute inflammatory demyelinating polyneuropathy in adult patients. *J Peripher Nerv Syst.* 2018;23(3):154–158.

60. Boukhris S, Magy L, Khalil M, Sindou P, Vallat JM. Pain as the presenting symptom of chronic inflammatory demyelinating polyradiculoneuropathy (CIDP). *J Neurol Sci.* 2007;254(1–2):33–38.

61. Bjelica B, Peric S, Bozovic I, et al. One-year follow-up study of neuropathic pain in chronic inflammatory demyelinating polyradiculoneuropathy. *J Peripher Nerv Syst.* 2019;24(2):180–186.

62. Stamboulis E, Katsaros N, Koutsis G, Iakovidou H, Giannakopoulou A, Simintzi I. Clinical and subclinical autonomic dysfunction in chronic inflammatory demyelinating polyradiculoneuropathy. *Muscle Nerve.* 2006;33(1):78–84.

63. Figueroa JJ, Dyck PJ, Laughlin RS, et al. Autonomic dysfunction in chronic inflammatory demyelinating polyradiculoneuropathy. *Neurology.* 2012;78(10):702–708.

64. Neligan A, Reilly MM, Lunn MP. CIDP: mimics and chameleons. *Pract Neurol.* 2014;14(6):399–408.

65. Lozeron P, Mariani LL, Dodet P, et al. Transthyretin amyloid polyneuropathies mimicking a demyelinating polyneuropathy. *Neurology.* 2018;91(2):e143–e152.

66. Viala K, Renie L, Maisonobe T, et al. Follow-up study and response to treatment in 23 patients with Lewis-Sumner syndrome. *Brain.* 2004;127(Pt 9):2010–2017.

67. Alwan AA, Mejico LJ. Ophthalmoplegia, proptosis, and lid retraction caused by cranial nerve hypertrophy in chronic inflammatory demyelinating polyradiculoneuropathy. *J Neuroophthalmol.* 2007;27(2):99–103.

68. Hickman SJ, Allen JA, Baisre A, et al. Neuro-ophthalmological complications of chronic inflammatory demyelinating polyradiculoneuropathy. *Neuroophthalmology.* 2013;37(4):146–156.

69. Al-Bustani N, Weiss MD. Recurrent isolated sixth nerve palsy in relapsing-remitting chronic inflammatory demyelinating polyneuropathy. *J Clin Neuromuscul Dis.* 2015;17(1):18–21.

70. Yao A, Chan H, Macdonell RAL, Shuey N, Khong JJ. Bilateral facial nerve palsies secondary to chronic inflammatory demyelinating polyneuropathy following adalimumab treatment. *Clin Neurol Neurosurg.* 2018;164:64–66.

71. Mehndiratta MM. Trigeminal motor neuropathy with tongue fasciculations in a patient with chronic inflammatory demyelinating polyradiculoneuropathy. *J Clin Neurosci.* 2010;17(10):1355–1356.

72. Hemmi S, Kutoku Y, Inoue K, Murakami T, Sunada Y. Tongue fasciculations in chronic inflammatory demyelinating polyradiculoneuropathy. *Muscle Nerve.* 2008;38(4):1341–1343.

73. Escorcio-Bezerra ML, Manzano GM, Bichuetti DB, et al. Tonic pupils: an unusual autonomic involvement in chronic inflammatory demyelinating polyneuropathy (CIDP). *Neurol Sci.* 2019;40(8):1725–1727.

74. Zivkovic SA, Peltier AC, Iacob T, Lacomis D. Chronic inflammatory demyelinating polyneuropathy and ventilatory failure: report of seven new cases and review of the literature. *Acta Neurol Scand.* 2011;124(1):59–63.

75. Mendell JR, Kolkin S, Kissel JT, Weiss KL, Chakeres DW, Rammohan KW. Evidence for central nervous system demyelination in chronic inflammatory demyelinating polyradiculoneuropathy. *Neurology.* 1987;37(8):1291–1294.

76. Ohtake T, Komori T, Hirose K, Tanabe H. CNS involvement in Japanese patients with chronic inflammatory demyelinating polyradiculoneuropathy. *Acta Neurol Scand.* 1990;81(2):108–112.

77. Feasby TE, Hahn AF, Koopman WJ, Lee DH. Central lesions in chronic inflammatory demyelinating polyneuropathy: an MRI study. *Neurology.* 1990;40(3 Pt 1):476–478.

78. Uncini A, Gallucci M, Lugaresi A, Porrini AM, Onofrj M, Gambi D. CNS involvement in chronic inflammatory demyelinating polyneuropathy: an electrophysiological and MRI study. *Electromyogr Clin Neurophysiol.* 1991;31(6):365–371.

79. Zephir H, Stojkovic T, Latour P, et al. Relapsing demyelinating disease affecting both the central and peripheral nervous systems. *J Neurol Neurosurg Psychiatry.* 2008;79(9):1032–1039.

80. Ioannidis P, Parissis D, Karapanayiotides T, Maiovis P, Karacostas D, Grigoriadis N. Spinal cord involvement in chronic inflammatory demyelinating polyradiculoneuropathy: a clinical and MRI study. *Acta Neurol Belg.* 2015;115(2):141–145.

81. Cortese A, Franciotta D, Alfonsi E, et al. Combined central and peripheral demyelination: clinical features, diagnostic findings, and treatment. *J Neurol Sci.* 2016;363:182–187.

82. Wang YQ, Chen H, Zhuang WP, Li HL. The clinical features of combined central and peripheral demyelination in Chinese patients. *J Neuroimmunol.* 2018;317:32–36.

83. Kawamura N, Yamasaki R, Yonekawa T, et al. Anti-neurofascin antibody in patients with combined central and peripheral demyelination. *Neurology.* 2013;81(8):714–722.

84. Ogata H, Matsuse D, Yamasaki R, et al. A nationwide survey of combined central and peripheral demyelination in Japan. *J Neurol Neurosurg Psychiatry.* 2016;87(1):29–36.

85. Rajabally YA, Shah RS. Restless legs syndrome in chronic inflammatory demyelinating polyneuropathy. *Muscle Nerve.* 2010;42(2):252–256.

86. Boukhris S, Magy L, Gallouedec G, et al. Fatigue as the main presenting symptom of chronic inflammatory demyelinating polyradiculoneuropathy: a study of 11 cases. *J Peripher Nerv Syst.* 2005;10(3):329–337.

87. Merkies IS, Kieseier BC. Fatigue, pain, anxiety and depression in Guillain-Barre syndrome and chronic inflammatory demyelinating polyradiculoneuropathy. *Eur Neurol.* 2016;75(3–4): 199–206.

88. Saperstein DS, Amato AA, Wolfe GI, et al. Multifocal acquired demyelinating sensory and motor neuropathy: the Lewis-Sumner syndrome. *Muscle Nerve.* 1999;22(5):560–566.

89. Katz JS, Saperstein DS, Gronseth G, Amato AA, Barohn RJ. Distal acquired demyelinating symmetric neuropathy. *Neurology.* 2000;54(3):615–620.

90. Rajabally YA, Narasimhan M. Distribution, clinical correlates and significance of axonal loss and demyelination in chronic inflammatory demyelinating polyneuropathy. *Eur J Neurol.* 2011;18(2):293–299.

91. Kuwabara S, Isose S, Mori M, et al. Different electrophysiological profiles and treatment response in 'typical' and 'atypical' chronic inflammatory demyelinating polyneuropathy. *J Neurol Neurosurg Psychiatry.* 2015;86(10):1054–1059.

92. Sinnreich M, Klein CJ, Daube JR, Engelstad J, Spinner RJ, Dyck PJ. Chronic immune sensory polyradiculopathy: a possibly treatable sensory ataxia. *Neurology.* 2004;63(9):1662–1669.

93. Viala K. Diagnosis of atypical forms of chronic inflammatory demyelinating polyradiculoneuropathy: a practical overview based on some case studies. *Int J Neurosci.* 2016;126(9):777–785.

94. Joint Task Force of the E, the PNS. European Federation of Neurological Societies/Peripheral Nerve Society guideline on management of chronic inflammatory demyelinating polyradiculoneuropathy: report of a joint task force of the European Federation of Neurological Societies and the Peripheral Nerve Society—first revision. *J Peripher Nerv Syst.* 2010;15(1):1–9.

95. Chin RL, Latov N, Sander HW, et al. Sensory CIDP presenting as cryptogenic sensory polyneuropathy. *J Peripher Nerv Syst.* 2004;9(3):132–137.

96. Viala K, Maisonobe T, Stojkovic T, et al. A current view of the diagnosis, clinical variants, response to treatment and prognosis of chronic inflammatory demyelinating polyradiculoneuropathy. *J Peripher Nerv Syst.* 2010;15(1):50–56.

97. Vlam L, van der Pol WL, Cats EA, et al. Multifocal motor neuropathy: diagnosis, pathogenesis and treatment strategies. *Nat Rev Neurol.* 2011;8(1):48–58.

98. Rajabally YA. Neuropathy and paraproteins: review of a complex association. *Eur J Neurol.* 2011;18(11):1291–1298.

99. Garg N, Park SB, Vucic S, et al. Differentiating lower motor neuron syndromes. *J Neurol Neurosurg Psychiatry.* 2017;88(6):474–483.

100. Eftimov F, Liesdek MH, Verhamme C, van Schaik IN, Group Ps. Deterioration after corticosteroids in CIDP may be associated with pure focal demyelination pattern. *BMC Neurol.* 2014;14:72.

101. Ayrignac X, Viala K, Koutlidis RM, et al. Sensory chronic inflammatory demyelinating polyneuropathy: an under-recognized entity? *Muscle Nerve.* 2013;48(5):727–732.

102. Devic P, Petiot P, Mauguiere F. Diagnostic utility of somatosensory evoked potentials in chronic polyradiculopathy without electrodiagnostic signs of peripheral demyelination. *Muscle Nerve.* 2016;53(1):78–83.

103. Rubin M, Mackenzie CR. Clinically and electrodiagnostically pure sensory demyelinating polyneuropathy. *Electromyogr Clin Neurophysiol.* 1996;36(3):145–149.

104. Massie R, Mauermann ML, Staff NP, et al. Diabetic cervical radiculoplexus neuropathy: a distinct syndrome expanding the spectrum of diabetic radiculoplexus neuropathies. *Brain.* 2012;135(Pt 10):3074–3088.

105. Querol L, Nogales-Gadea G, Rojas-Garcia R, et al. Neurofascin IgG4 antibodies in CIDP associate with disabling tremor and poor response to IVIg. *Neurology.* 2014;82(10):879–886.

106. Devaux JJ, Miura Y, Fukami Y, et al. Neurofascin-155 IgG4 in chronic inflammatory demyelinating polyneuropathy. *Neurology.* 2016;86(9):800–807.

107. Delmont E, Manso C, Querol L, et al. Autoantibodies to nodal isoforms of neurofascin in chronic inflammatory demyelinating polyneuropathy. *Brain*. 2017;140(7):1851–1858.

108. Doppler K, Stengel H, Appeltshauser L, et al. Neurofascin-155 IgM autoantibodies in patients with inflammatory neuropathies. *J Neurol Neurosurg Psychiatry*. 2018;89(11):1145–1151.

109. Van Asseldonk JT, Van den Berg LH, Kalmijn S, Wokke JH, Franssen H. Criteria for demyelination based on the maximum slowing due to axonal degeneration, determined after warming in water at 37 degrees C: diagnostic yield in chronic inflammatory demyelinating polyneuropathy. *Brain*. 2005;128(Pt 4):880–891.

110. Van Asseldonk JT, Van den Berg LH, Wieneke GH, Wokke JH, Franssen H. Criteria for conduction block based on computer simulation studies of nerve conduction with human data obtained in the forearm segment of the median nerve. *Brain*. 2006;129(Pt 9):2447–2460.

111. Bromberg MB. Review of the evolution of electrodiagnostic criteria for chronic inflammatory demyelinating polyradicoloneuropathy. *Muscle Nerve*. 2011;43(6):780–794.

112. Rajabally YA, Jacob S. Proximal nerve conduction studies in chronic inflammatory demyelinating polyneuropathy. *Clin Neurophysiol*. 2006;117(9):2079–2084.

113. Rajabally YA, Nicolas G, Pieret F, Bouche P, Van den Bergh PY. Validity of diagnostic criteria for chronic inflammatory demyelinating polyneuropathy: a multicenter European study. *J Neurol Neurosurg Psychiatry*. 2009;80(12):1364–1368.

114. Rajabally YA, Varanasi S. Practical electrodiagnostic value of F-wave studies in chronic inflammatory demyelinating polyneuropathy. *Clin Neurophysiol*. 2013;124(1):171–175.

115. Rajabally YA, Nicolas G. Value of distal compound muscle action potential duration prolongation in acute inflammatory demyelinating polyneuropathy: a European perspective. *Muscle Nerve*. 2011;43(5):751–755.

116. Rajabally YA, Lagarde J, Cassereau J, Viala K, Fournier E, Nicolas G. A European multicenter reappraisal of distal compound muscle action potential duration in chronic inflammatory demyelinating polyneuropathy. *Eur J Neurol*. 2012;19(4):638–642.

117. Thaisetthawatkul P, Logigian EL, Herrmann DN. Dispersion of the distal compound muscle action potential as a diagnostic criterion for chronic inflammatory demyelinating polyneuropathy. *Neurology*. 2002;59(10):1526–1532.

118. Isose S, Kuwabara S, Kokubun N, et al. Utility of the distal compound muscle action potential duration for diagnosis of demyelinating neuropathies. *J Peripher Nerv Syst*. 2009;14(3):151–158.

119. Mitsuma S, Van den Bergh P, Rajabally YA, et al. Effects of low frequency filtering on distal compound muscle action potential duration for diagnosis of CIDP: a Japanese-European multicenter prospective study. *Clin Neurophysiol*. 2015;126(9):1805–1810.

120. Bromberg MB, Albers JW. Patterns of sensory nerve conduction abnormalities in demyelinating and axonal peripheral nerve disorders. *Muscle Nerve*. 1993;16(3):262–266.

121. Tamura N, Kuwabara S, Misawa S, Mori M, Nakata M, Hattori T. Superficial radial sensory nerve potentials in immune-mediated and diabetic neuropathies. *Clin Neurophysiol*. 2005;116(10):2330–2333.

122. Rajabally YA, Narasimhan M. The value of sensory electrophysiology in chronic inflammatory demyelinating polyneuropathy. *Clin Neurophysiol*. 2007;118(9):1999–2004.

123. Bragg JA, Benatar MG. Sensory nerve conduction slowing is a specific marker for CIDP. *Muscle Nerve*. 2008;38(6):1599–1603.

124. Rajabally YA, Samarasekera S. Electrophysiological sensory demyelination in typical chronic inflammatory demyelinating polyneuropathy. *Eur J Neurol*. 2010;17(7):939–944.

125. Rajabally YA, Narasimhan M. Characteristics and correlates of sensory function in chronic inflammatory demyelinating polyneuropathy. *J Neurol Sci*. 2010;297(1–2):11–14.

126. Albers JW, Kelly Jr. JJ. Acquired inflammatory demyelinating polyneuropathies: clinical and electrodiagnostic features. *Muscle Nerve*. 1989;12(6):435–451.

127. Barohn RJ, Kissel JT, Warmolts JR, Mendell JR. Chronic inflammatory demyelinating polyradiculoneuropathy. Clinical characteristics, course, and recommendations for diagnostic criteria. *Arch Neurol*. 1989;46(8):878–884.

128. Cornblath DR, Asbury AK, Albers JW, et al. Research criteria for diagnosis of chronic inflammatory demyelinating polyneuropathy (CIDP). Report from an ad hoc Subcommittee of the American Academy of Neurology AIDS Task Force. *Neurology*. 1991;41(5):617–618.

129. Bromberg MB. Comparison of electrodiagnostic criteria for primary demyelination in chronic polyneuropathy. *Muscle Nerve*. 1991;14(10):968–976.

130. Molenaar DS, Vermeulen M, de Haan RJ. Comparison of electrodiagnostic criteria for demyelination in patients with chronic inflammatory demyelinating polyneuropathy (CIDP). *J Neurol*. 2002;249(4):400–403.

131. Wilson J, Chawla J, Fisher M. Sensitivity and specificity of electrodiagnostic criteria for CIDP using ROC curves: comparison to patients with diabetic and MGUS associated neuropathies. *J Neurol Sci*. 2005;231(1–2):19–28.

132. Franssen H, Wieneke GH. Nerve conduction and temperature: necessary warming time. *Muscle Nerve*. 1994;17(3):336–344.

133. Franssen H, Wieneke GH, Wokke JH. The influence of temperature on conduction block. *Muscle Nerve*. 1999;22(2):166–173.

134. Buchthal F, Behse F. Peroneal muscular atrophy (PMA) and related disorders. I. Clinical manifestations as related to biopsy findings, nerve conduction and electromyography. *Brain*. 1977;100(Pt 1):41–66.

135. Sander HW, Latov N. Research criteria for defining patients with CIDP. *Neurology*. 2003; 60(8 Suppl 3):S8–15.

136. De Sousa EA, Chin RL, Sander HW, Latov N, Brannagan 3rd. TH. Demyelinating findings in typical and atypical chronic inflammatory demyelinating polyneuropathy: sensitivity and specificity. *J Clin Neuromuscul Dis*. 2009;10(4):163–169.

137. Breiner A, Brannagan 3rd. TH. Comparison of sensitivity and specificity among 15 criteria for chronic inflammatory demyelinating polyneuropathy. *Muscle Nerve*. 2014;50(1):40–46.

138. Rajabally YA, Fowle AJ, Van den Bergh PY. Which criteria for research in chronic inflammatory demyelinating polyradiculoneuropathy? An analysis of current practice. *Muscle Nerve*. 2015;51(6):932–933.

139. Bromberg MB, Franssen H. Practical rules for electrodiagnosis in suspected multifocal motor neuropathy. *J Clin Neuromuscul Dis*. 2015;16(3):141–152.

140. Rhee EK, England JD, Sumner AJ. A computer simulation of conduction block: effects produced by actual block versus interphase cancellation. *Ann Neurol*. 1990;28(2):146–156.

141. Oh SJ, Kim DE, Kuruoglu HR. What is the best diagnostic index of conduction block and temporal dispersion? *Muscle Nerve*. 1994;17(5):489–493.

142. Vo ML, Hanineva A, Chin RL, Carey BT, Latov N, Langsdorf JA. Comparison of 2-limb versus 3-limb electrodiagnostic studies in the evaluation of chronic inflammatory demyelinating polyneuropathy. *Muscle Nerve*. 2015;51(4):549–553.

143. Rajabally YA, Jacob S, Hbahbih M. Optimizing the use of electrophysiology in the diagnosis of chronic inflammatory demyelinating polyneuropathy: a study of 20 cases. *J Peripher Nerv Syst*. 2005;10(3):282–292.

144. Allen JA, Lewis RA. CIDP diagnostic pitfalls and perception of treatment benefit. *Neurology*. 2015;85(6):498–504.

145. Allen JA, Ney J, Lewis RA. Electrodiagnostic errors contribute to chronic inflammatory demyelinating polyneuropathy misdiagnosis. *Muscle Nerve*. 2018;57(4):542–549.

146. Rajabally YA. Chronic inflammatory demyelinating polyneuropathy misdiagnosis: a clinical more than electrophysiogical problem? *Muscle Nerve*. 2018;57(5):E131–E132.

147. Simmons Z, Tivakaran S. Acquired demyelinating polyneuropathy presenting as a pure clinical sensory syndrome. *Muscle Nerve*. 1996;19(9):1174–1176.

148. Rajabally YA, Wong SL. Chronic inflammatory pure sensory polyradiculoneuropathy: a rare CIDP variant with unusual electrophysiology. *J Clin Neuromuscul Dis*. 2012;13(3):149–152.

149. Herraets I, Goedee HS, Telleman JA, et al. Nerve ultrasound improves detection of treatment-responsive chronic inflammatory neuropathies. *Neurology*. 2020; pii: 10.1212/WNL.0000000000008978. http://dx.doi.org/ 10.1212/WNL.0000000000008978.

150. Donaghy M, Mills KR, Boniface SJ, et al. Pure motor demyelinating neuropathy: deterioration after steroid treatment and improvement with intravenous immunoglobulin. *J Neurol Neurosurg Psychiatry*. 1994;57(7):778–783.

151. Uncini A, Sabatelli M, Mignogna T, Lugaresi A, Liguori R, Montagna P. Chronic progressive steroid responsive axonal polyneuropathy: a CIDP vaariant or a primary axonal disorder? *Muscle Nerve*. 1996;19(3):365–371.

152. Goedee S, Herraets I, Visser L, et al. Nerve ultrasound for the identification of treatment-responsive chronic neuropathies without nerve conduction abnormalities. *J Peripher Nerv Syst*. 2018;23(4):275–276.

153. Goedee HS, Herraets IJT, Visser LH, et al. Nerve ultrasound can identify treatment-responsive chronic neuropathies without electrodiagnostic features of demyelination. *Muscle Nerve*. 2019;60(4):415–419.

154. Lucke IM, Adrichem ME, Wieske L, et al. Intravenous immunoglobulins in patients with clinically suspected chronic immune-mediated neuropathy. *J Neurol Sci*. 2019;397:141–145.

155. Yiannikas C, Vucic S. Utility of somatosensory evoked potentials in chronic acquired demyelinating neuropathy. *Muscle Nerve*. 2008;38(5):1447–1454.

156. Tsukamoto H, Sonoo M, Shimizu T. Segmental evaluation of the peripheral nerve using tibial nerve SEPs for the diagnosis of CIDP. *Clin Neurophysiol*. 2010;121(1):77–84.

157. Vucic S, Cairns KD, Black KR, Chong PS, Cros D. Cervical nerve root stimulation. Part I: technical aspects and normal data. *Clin Neurophysiol*. 2006;117(2):392–397.

158. Vucic S, Black K, Siao Tick Chong P, Cros D. Cervical nerve root stimulation. Part II: findings in primary demyelinating neuropathies and motor neuron disease. *Clin Neurophysiol*. 2006;117(2):398–404.

159. Takada H, Ravnborg M. Magnetically evoked motor potentials in demyelinating and axonal polyneuropathy: a comparative study. *Eur J Neurol*. 2000;7(1):63–69.

160. Attarian S, Franques J, Elisabeth J, et al. Triple-stimulation technique improves the diagnosis of chronic inflammatory demyelinating polyradiculoneuropathy. *Muscle Neurol*. 2015;51(4):541–548.

161. Cao D, Guo X, Yuan T, Hao J. Diagnosing chronic inflammatory demyelinating polyradiculoneuropathy with triple stimulation technique. *J Neurol*. 2018;265(8):1916–1921.

162. Magistris MR, Rosler KM, Truffert A, Myers JP. Transcranial stimulation excites virtually all motor neurons supplying the target muscle. A demonstration and a method improving the study of motor evoked potentials. *Brain*. 1998;121(Pt 3):437–450.

163. Magistris MR, Rosler KM, Truffert A, Landis T, Hess CW. A clinical study of motor evoked potentials using a triple stimulation technique. *Brain*. 1999;122(Pt 2):265–279.

164. Rosler KM, Magistris MR. Triple stimulation technique (TST) in amyotrophic lateral sclerosis. *Clin Neurophysiol*. 2004;115(7):1715.

165. Deroide N, Uzenot D, Verschueren A, Azulay JP, Pouget J, Attarian S. Triple-stimulation technique in multifocal neuropathy with conduction block. *Muscle Nerve.* 2007;35(5):632–636.

166. Delmont E, Benvenutto A, Grimaldi S, et al. Motor unit number index (MUNIX): is it relevant in chronic inflammatory demyelinating polyradiculoneuropathy (CIDP)? *Clin Neurophysiol.* 2016;127(3):1891–1894.

167. Nandedkar SD, Nandedkar DS, Barkhaus PE, Stalberg EV. Motor unit number index (MUNIX). *IEEE Trans Biomed Eng.* 2004;51(12):2209–2211.

168. Neuwirth C, Nandedkar S, Stalberg E, Weber M. Motor unit number index (MUNIX): a novel neurophysiological technique to follow disease progression in amyotrophic lateral sclerosis. *Muscle Nerve.* 2010;42(3):379–384.

169. Neuwirth C, Braun N, Claeys KG, et al. Implementing motor unit number index (MUNIX) in a large clinical trial: real world experience from 27 centres. *Clin Neurophysiol.* 2018;129(8):1756–1762.

170. Paramanathan S, Tankisi H, Andersen H, Fuglsang-Frederiksen A. Axonal loss in patients with inflammatory demyelinating polyneuropathy as determined by motor unit number estimation and MUNIX. *Clin Neurophysiol.* 2016;127(1):898–904.

171. Lawley A, Seri S, Rajabally YA. Motor unit number index (MUNIX) in chronic inflammatory demyelinating polyneuropathy: a potential role in monitoring response to intravenous immunoglobulins. *Clin Neurophysiol.* 2019;130(10):1743–1749.

172. Bostock H, Cikurel K, Burke D. Threshold tracking techniques in the study of human peripheral nerve. *Muscle Nerve.* 1998;21(2):137–158.

173. Kuwabara S, Cappelen-Smith C, Lin CS, Mogyoros I, Bostock H, Burke D. Excitability properties of median and peroneal motor axons. *Muscle Nerve.* 2000;23(9):1365–1373.

174. Burke D, Kiernan MC, Bostock H. Excitability of human axons. *Clin Neurophysiol.* 2001;112(9):1575–1585.

175. Sleutjes B, Kovalchuk MO, Durmus N, et al. Simulating perinodal changes observed in immune-mediated neuropathies – impact on conduction in a model of myelinated motor and sensory axons. *J Neurophysiol.* 2019;.

176. Stephanova DI, Alexandrov AS. Simulating mild systematic and focal demyelinating neuropathies: membrane property abnormalities. *J Integr Neurosci.* 2006;5(4):595–623.

177. Stephanova DI, Krustev SM, Negrev N, Daskalova M. The myelin sheath aqueous layers improve the membrane properties of simulated chronic demyelinating neuropathies. *J Integr Neurosci.* 2011;10(1):105–120.

178. Cappelen-Smith C, Kuwabara S, Lin CS, Mogyoros I, Burke D. Activity-dependent hyperpolarization and conduction block in chronic inflammatory demyelinating polyneuropathy. *Ann Neurol.* 2000;48(6):826–832.

179. Cappelen-Smith C, Kuwabara S, Lin CS, Mogyoros I, Burke D. Membrane properties in chronic inflammatory demyelinating polyneuropathy. *Brain.* 2001;124(Pt 12):2439–2447.

180. Garg N, Park SB, Howells J, et al. Conduction block in immune-mediated neuropathy: paranodopathy versus axonopathy. *Eur J Neurol.* 2019;26(8):1121–1129.

181. Boerio D, Creange A, Hogrel JY, Gueguen A, Bertrand D, Lefaucheur JP. Nerve excitability changes after intravenous immunoglobulin infusions in multifocal motor neuropathy and chronic inflammatory demyelinating neuropathy. *J Neurol Sci.* 2010;292(1–2):63–71.

182. Lin CS, Krishnan AV, Park SB, Kiernan MC. Modulatory effects on axonal function after intravenous immunoglobulin therapy in chronic inflammatory demyelinating polyneuropathy. *Arch Neurol.* 2011;68(7):862–869.

183. Sung JY, Tani J, Park SB, Kiernan MC, Lin CS. Early identification of 'acute-onset' chronic inflammatory demyelinating polyneuropathy. *Brain.* 2014;137(Pt 8):2155–2163.

184. Kovalchuk MO, Franssen H, Van Schelven LJ, Sleutjes B. Comparing excitability at 37 degrees C versus at 20 degrees C: differences between motor and sensory axons. *Muscle Nerve.* 2018;57(4):574–580.

185. Kovalchuk MO, Franssen H, FEV S, Van Schelven LJ, Van Den Berg LH, Sleutjes B. Warming nerves for excitability testing. *Muscle Nerve.* 2019;60(3):279–285.

186. Hageman S, Kovalchuk MO, Sleutjes B, van Schelven LJ, van den Berg LH, Franssen H. Sodium-potassium pump assessment by submaximal electrical nerve stimulation. *Clin Neurophysiol.* 2018;129(4):809–814.

187. Said G. Chronic inflammatory demyelinative polyneuropathy. *J Neurol.* 2002;249(3):245–253.

188. Bouchard C, Lacroix C, Plante V, et al. Clinicopathologic findings and prognosis of chronic inflammatory demyelinating polyneuropathy. *Neurology.* 1999;52(3):498–503.

189. Dyck PJ, Lais AC, Ohta M, Bastron JA, Okazaki H, Groover RV. Chronic inflammatory polyradiculoneuropathy. *Mayo Clinic Proc.* 1975;50(11):621–637.

190. Hegen H, Auer M, Zeileis A, Deisenhammer F. Upper reference limits for cerebrospinal fluid total protein and albumin quotient based on a large cohort of control patients: implications for increased clinical specificity. *Clin Chem Lab Med.* 2016;54(2):285–292.

191. Bourque PR, Breiner A, Moher D, et al. Adult CSF total protein: higher upper reference limits should be considered worldwide. A web-based survey. *J Neurol Sci.* 2019;396:48–51.

192. Breiner A, Bourque PR, Allen JA. Updated cerebrospinal fluid total protein reference values improve chronic inflammatory demyelinating polyneuropathy diagnosis. *Muscle Nerve.* 2019;60(2):180–183.

193. Tackenberg B, Lunemann JD, Steinbrecher A, et al. Classifications and treatment responses in chronic immune-mediated demyelinating polyneuropathy. *Neurology.* 2007;68(19):1622–1629.

194. Press R, Pashenkov M, Jin JP, Link H. Aberrated levels of cerebrospinal fluid chemokines in Guillain-Barre syndrome and chronic inflammatory demyelinating polyradiculoneuropathy. *J Clin Immunol.* 2003;23(4):259–267.

195. Lucke IM, Peric S, van Lieverloo GGA, et al. Elevated leukocyte count in cerebrospinal fluid of patients with chronic inflammatory demyelinating polyneuropathy. *J Peripher Nerv Syst.* 2018;23(1):49–54.

196. Goedee HS, van der Pol WL, Hendrikse J, van den Berg LH. Nerve ultrasound and magnetic resonance imaging in the diagnosis of neuropathy. *Curr Opin Neurol.* 2018;31(5):526–533.

197. Shibuya K, Sugiyama A, Ito S, et al. Reconstruction magnetic resonance neurography in chronic inflammatory demyelinating polyneuropathy. *Ann Neurol.* 2015;77(2):333–337.

198. Fargeot G, Viala K, Theaudin M, et al. Diagnostic usefulness of plexus magnetic resonance imaging in chronic inflammatory demyelinating polyradiculopathy without electrodiagnostic criteria of demyelination. *Eur J Neurol.* 2019;26(4):631–638.

199. Hiwatashi A, Togao O, Yamashita K, et al. Lumbar plexus in patients with chronic inflammatory demyelinating polyradiculoneuropathy: evaluation with simultaneous T2 mapping and neurography method with SHINKEI. *Br J Radiol.* 2018;91(1092):20180501. https://doi.org/10.1259/bjr.20180501.

200. Hiwatashi A, Togao O, Yamashita K, et al. Evaluation of chronic inflammatory demyelinating polyneuropathy: 3D nerve-sheath signal increased with inked rest-tissue rapid acquisition of relaxation enhancement imaging (3D SHINKEI). *Eur Radiol.* 2017;27(2):447–453.

201. Ishikawa T, Asakura K, Mizutani Y, et al. MR neurography for the evaluation of CIDP. *Muscle Nerve.* 2017;55(4):483–489.

202. van Es HW. MRI of the brachial plexus. *Eur Radiol.* 2001;11(2):325–336.

203. Schady W, Goulding PJ, Lecky BR, King RH, Smith CM. Massive nerve root enlargement in chronic inflammatory demyelinating polyneuropathy. *J Neurol Neurosurg Psychiatry.* 1996;61(6):636–640.

204. Kuwabara S, Nakajima M, Matsuda S, Hattori T. Magnetic resonance imaging at the demyelinative foci in chronic inflammatory demyelinating polyneuropathy. *Neurology*. 1997;48(4):874–877.
205. Midroni G, de Tilly LN, Gray B, Vajsar J. MRI of the cauda equina in CIDP: clinical correlations. *J Neurol Sci*. 1999;170(1):36–44.
206. Duggins AJ, McLeod JG, Pollard JD, et al. Spinal root and plexus hypertrophy in chronic inflammatory demyelinating polyneuropathy. *Brain*. 1999;122(Pt 7):1383–1390.
207. Matsuoka N, Kohriyama T, Ochi K, et al. Detection of cervical nerve root hypertrophy by ultrasonography in chronic inflammatory demyelinating polyradiculoneuropathy. *J Neurol Sci*. 2004;219(1–2):15–21.
208. Zaidman CM, Al-Lozi M, Pestronk A. Peripheral nerve size in normals and patients with polyneuropathy: an ultrasound study. *Muscle Nerve*. 2009;40(6):960–966.
209. Goedee HS, Brekelmans GJ, Visser LH. Multifocal enlargement and increased vascularization of peripheral nerves detected by sonography in CIDP: a pilot study. *Clin Neurophysiol*. 2014;125(1):154–159.
210. Tanaka K, Mori N, Yokota Y, Suenaga T. MRI of the cervical nerve roots in the diagnosis of chronic inflammatory demyelinating polyradiculoneuropathy: a single-institution, retrospective case-control study. *BMJ Open*. 2013;3(8):e003443.
211. Jongbloed BA, Bos JW, Rutgers D, van der Pol WL, van den Berg LH. Brachial plexus magnetic resonance imaging differentiates between inflammatory neuropathies and does not predict disease course. *Brain Behav*. 2017;7(5):e00632.
212. Rajabally YA, Knopp MJ, Martin-Lamb D, Morlese J. Diagnostic value of MR imaging in the Lewis-Sumner syndrome: a case series. *J Neurol Sci*. 2014;342(1–2):182–185.
213. Goedee HS, van der Pol WL, van Asseldonk JH, et al. Diagnostic value of sonography in treatment-naive chronic inflammatory neuropathies. *Neurology*. 2017;88(2):143–151.
214. Goedee HS, Jongbloed BA, van Asseldonk JH, et al. A comparative study of brachial plexus sonography and magnetic resonance imaging in chronic inflammatory demyelinating neuropathy and multifocal motor neuropathy. *Eur J Neurol*. 2017;24(10):1307–1313.
215. Grimm A, Heiling B, Schumacher U, Witte OW, Axer H. Ultrasound differentiation of axonal and demyelinating neuropathies. *Muscle Nerve*. 2014;50(6):976–983.
216. Grimm A, Rattay TW, Winter N, Axer H. Peripheral nerve ultrasound scoring systems: benchmarking and comparative analysis. *J Neurol*. 2017;264(2):243–253.
217. Eurelings M, Notermans NC, Franssen H, et al. MRI of the brachial plexus in polyneuropathy associated with monoclonal gammopathy. *Muscle Nerve*. 2001;24(10):1312–1318.
218. Goedee HS, Notermans NC, Visser LH, et al. Neuropathy associated with immunoglobulin M monoclonal gammopathy: a combined sonographic and nerve conduction study. *Muscle Nerve*. 2019.
219. Goedee SH, Brekelmans GJ, van den Berg LH, Visser LH. Distinctive patterns of sonographic nerve enlargement in Charcot-Marie-Tooth type 1A and hereditary neuropathy with pressure palsies. *Clin Neurophysiol*. 2015;126(7):1413–1420.
220. Goedee HS, van der Pol WL, van Asseldonk JH, et al. Nerve sonography to detect peripheral nerve involvement in vasculitis syndromes. *Neurol Clin Pract*. 2016;6(4):293–303.
221. van Rosmalen M, Lieba-Samal D, Pillen S, van Alfen N. Ultrasound of peripheral nerves in neuralgic amyotrophy. *Muscle Nerve*. 2019;59(1):55–59.
222. Bourque PR, Warman Chardon J, Bryanton M, Toupin M, Burns BF, Torres C. Neurolymphomatosis of the brachial plexus and its branches: case series and literature review. *Can J Neurol Sci*. 2018;45(2):137–143.
223. Grimm A, Decard BF, Axer H, Fuhr P. The ultrasound pattern sum score-UPSS. A new method to differentiate acute and subacute neuropathies using ultrasound of the peripheral nerves. *Clin Neurophysiol*. 2015;126(11):2216–2225.

224. Grimm A, Oertl H, Auffenberg E, et al. Differentiation between Guillain-Barre syndrome and acute-onset chronic inflammatory demyelinating polyradiculoneuritis – a prospective follow-up study using ultrasound and neurophysiological measurements. *Neurotherapeutics.* 2019;16(3):838–847.

225. Kerasnoudis A, Pitarokoili K, Behrendt V, Gold R, Yoon MS. Nerve ultrasound score in distinguishing chronic from acute inflammatory demyelinating polyneuropathy. *Clin Neurophysiol.* 2014;125(3):635–641.

226. Gasparotti R, Lucchetta M, Cacciavillani M, et al. Neuroimaging in diagnosis of atypical polyradiculoneuropathies: report of three cases and review of the literature. *J Neurol.* 2015;262(7):1714–1723.

227. Lozeron P, Lacour MC, Vandendries C, et al. Contribution of plexus MRI in the diagnosis of atypical chronic inflammatory demyelinating polyneuropathies. *J Neurol Sci.* 2016;360:170–175.

228. Tagliafico A, Cadoni A, Fisci E, Bignotti B, Padua L, Martinoli C. Reliability of side-to-side ultrasound cross-sectional area measurements of lower extremity nerves in healthy subjects. *Muscle Nerve.* 2012;46(5):717–722.

229. Boehm J, Scheidl E, Bereczki D, Schelle T, Aranyi Z. High-resolution ultrasonography of peripheral nerves: measurements on 14 nerve segments in 56 healthy subjects and reliability assessments. *Ultraschall Med.* 2014;35(5):459–467.

230. Garcia-Santibanez R, Dietz AR, Bucelli RC, Zaidman CM. Nerve ultrasound reliability of upper limbs: effects of examiner training. *Muscle Nerve.* 2018;57(2):189–192.

231. Telleman JA, Herraets IJT, Goedee HS, et al. Nerve ultrasound: a reproducible diagnostic tool in peripheral neuropathy. *Neurology.* 2018;.

232. Oudeman J, Eftimov F, Strijkers GJ, et al. Diagnostic accuracy of MRI and ultrasoundin chronic immune-mediated neuropathies. *Neurology.* 2020;94(1):e62–e74.

233. Magy L, Kabore R, Mathis S, et al. Heterogeneity of polyneuropathy associated with anti-MAG antibodies. *J Immunol Res.* 2015;2015:450391.

234. Molenaar DS, Vermeulen M, de Haan R. Diagnostic value of sural nerve biopsy in chronic inflammatory demyelinating polyneuropathy. *J Neurol Neurosurg Psychiatry.* 1998;64(1):84–89.

235. Bosboom WM, Van den Berg LH, Dieks HJ, et al. Unmyelinated nerve fiber degeneration in chronic inflammatory demyelinating polyneuropathy. *Acta Neuropathol.* 2000;99(5):571–578.

236. Bosboom WM, van den Berg LH, Franssen H, et al. Diagnostic value of sural nerve demyelination in chronic inflammatory demyelinating polyneuropathy. *Brain.* 2001;124(Pt 12):2427–2438.

237. England JD, Gronseth GS, Franklin G, et al. Practice parameter: evaluation of distal symmetric polyneuropathy: role of autonomic testing, nerve biopsy, and skin biopsy (an evidence-based review). Report of the American Academy of Neurology, American Association of Neuromuscular and Electrodiagnostic Medicine, and American Academy of Physical Medicine and Rehabilitation. *Neurology.* 2009;72(2):177–184.

238. Sommer C, Toyka K. Nerve biopsy in chronic inflammatory neuropathies: in situ biomarkers. *J Peripher Nerv Syst.* 2011;16(Suppl 1):24–29.

239. Dalakas MC. Medscape. Advances in the diagnosis, pathogenesis and treatment of CIDP. *Nat Rev Neurol.* 2011;7(9):507–517.

240. van den Berg B, Walgaard C, Drenthen J, Fokke C, Jacobs BC, van Doorn PA. Guillain-Barre syndrome: pathogenesis, diagnosis, treatment and prognosis. *Nat Rev Neurol.* 2014;10(8):469–482.

241. Ruts L, van Koningsveld R, van Doorn PA. Distinguishing acute-onset CIDP from Guillain-Barre syndrome with treatment related fluctuations. *Neurology.* 2005;65(1):138–140.

242. Odaka M, Yuki N, Hirata K. Patients with chronic inflammatory demyelinating polyneuropathy initially diagnosed as Guillain-Barre syndrome. *J Neurol.* 2003;250(8):913–916.

243. Perry JR, Fung A, Poon P, Bayer N. Magnetic resonance imaging of nerve root inflammation in the Guillain-Barre syndrome. *Neuroradiology.* 1994;36(2):139–140.

244. Gorson KC, Ropper AH, Muriello MA, Blair R. Prospective evaluation of MRI lumbosacral nerve root enhancement in acute Guillain-Barre syndrome. *Neurology.* 1996;47(3):813–817.

245. Kerasnoudis A, Pitarokoili K, Behrendt V, Gold R, Yoon MS. Bochum ultrasound score versus clinical and electrophysiological parameters in distinguishing acute-onset chronic from acute inflammatory demyelinating polyneuropathy. *Muscle Nerve.* 2015;51(6):846–852.

246. Laura M, Pipis M, Rossor AM, Reilly MM. Charcot-Marie-tooth disease and related disorders: an evolving landscape. *Curr Opin Neurol.* 2019;.

247. Rajabally YA, Adams D, Latour P, Attarian S. Hereditary and inflammatory neuropathies: a review of reported associations, mimics and misdiagnoses. *J Neurol Neurosurg Psychiatry.* 2016;87(10):1051–1060.

248. Lewis RA, Sumner AJ. The electrodiagnostic distinctions between chronic familial and acquired demyelinative neuropathies. *Neurology.* 1982;32(6):592–596.

249. Kaku DA, Parry GJ, Malamut R, Lupski JR, Garcia CA. Uniform slowing of conduction velocities in Charcot-Marie-Tooth polyneuropathy type 1. *Neurology.* 1993;43(12):2664–2667.

250. Stanton M, Pannoni V, Lewis RA, et al. Dispersion of compound muscle action potential in hereditary neuropathies and chronic inflammatory demyelinating polyneuropathy. *Muscle Nerve.* 2006;34(4):417–422.

251. Uncini A, Parano E, Lange DJ, De Vivo DC, Lovelace RE. Chronic inflammatory demyelinating polyneuropathy in childhood: clinical and electrophysiological features. *Childs Nerv Syst.* 1991;7(4):191–196.

252. Benstead TJ, Kuntz NL, Miller RG, Daube JR. The electrophysiologic profile of Dejerine-Sottas disease (HMSN III). *Muscle Nerve.* 1990;13(7):586–592.

253. Hoogendijk JE, de Visser M, Bour LJ, Jennekens FG, Ongerboer BW. Conduction block in hereditary motor and sensory neuropathy type I. *Muscle Nerve.* 1992;15(4):520–521 [author reply 523].

254. Lewis RA, Sumner AJ, Shy ME. Electrophysiological features of inherited demyelinating neuropathies: a reappraisal in the era of molecular diagnosis. *Muscle Nerve.* 2000;23(10):1472–1487.

255. Zaidman CM, Harms MB, Pestronk A. Ultrasound of inherited vs. acquired demyelinating polyneuropathies. *J Neurol.* 2013;260(12):3115–3121.

256. Grimm A, Vittore D, Schubert V, et al. Ultrasound pattern sum score, homogeneity score and regional nerve enlargement index for differentiation of demyelinating inflammatory and hereditary neuropathies. *Clin Neurophysiol.* 2016;127(7):2618–2624.

257. Niu J, Cui L, Liu M. Multiple sites ultrasonography of peripheral nerves in differentiating Charcot-Marie-tooth type 1A from chronic inflammatory demyelinating polyradiculoneuropathy. *Front Neurol.* 2017;8:181.

258. Joint Task Force of the E, the PNS. European Federation of Neurological Societies/Peripheral Nerve Society Guideline on management of paraproteinemic demyelinating neuropathies. Report of a joint task force of the European Federation of Neurological Societies and the peripheral nerve society—first revision. *J Peripher Nerv Syst.* 2010;15(3):185–195.

259. Stork AC, van der Pol WL, Franssen H, Jacobs BC, Notermans NC. Clinical phenotype of patients with neuropathy associated with monoclonal gammopathy: a comparative study and a review of the literature. *J Neurol.* 2014;261(7):1398–1404.

260. Eurelings M, Ang CW, Notermans NC, Van Doorn PA, Jacobs BC, Van den Berg LH. Antiganglioside antibodies in polyneuropathy associated with monoclonal gammopathy. *Neurology.* 2001;57(10):1909–1912.

261. Stork AC, Jacobs BC, Tio-Gillen AP, et al. Prevalence, specificity and functionality of anti-ganglioside antibodies in neuropathy associated with IgM monoclonal gammopathy. *J Neuroimmunol*. 2014;268(1–2):89–94.

262. Lucchetta M, Padua L, Granata G, et al. Nerve ultrasound findings in neuropathy associated with anti-myelin-associated glycoprotein antibodies. *Eur J Neurol*. 2015;22(1):193–202.

263. Athanasopoulou IM, Rasenack M, Grimm C, et al. Ultrasound of the nerves—an appropriate addition to nerve conduction studies to differentiate paraproteinemic neuropathies. *J Neurol Sci*. 2016;362:188–195.

264. Lunn MP, Nobile-Orazio E. Immunotherapy for IgM anti-myelin-associated glycoprotein paraprotein-associated peripheral neuropathies. *Cochrane Database Syst Rev*. 2012;5(5): CD002827.

265. Adams D, Cauquil C, Labeyrie C. Familial amyloid polyneuropathy. *Curr Opin Neurol*. 2017;30(5):481–489.

266. Mariani LL, Lozeron P, Theaudin M, et al. Genotype-phenotype correlation and course of transthyretin familial amyloid polyneuropathies in France. *Ann Neurol*. 2015;78(6):901–916.

267. Cortese A, Vegezzi E, Lozza A, et al. Diagnostic challenges in hereditary transthyretin amyloidosis with polyneuropathy: avoiding misdiagnosis of a treatable hereditary neuropathy. *J Neurol Neurosurg Psychiatry*. 2017;88(5):457–458.

268. Capek S, Amrami KK, Dyck PJ, Spinner RJ. Targeted fascicular biopsy of the sciatic nerve and its major branches: rationale and operative technique. *Neurosurg Focus*. 2015;39(3):E12.

269. McKenzie GA, Broski SM, Howe BM, et al. MRI of pathology-proven peripheral nerve amyloidosis. *Skeletal Radiol*. 2017;46(1):65–73.

270. Plante-Bordeneuve V. Transthyretin familial amyloid polyneuropathy: an update. *J Neurol*. 2018;265(4):976–983.

271. Keddie S, D'Sa S, Foldes D, Carr AS, Reilly MM, Lunn MPT. POEMS neuropathy: optimising diagnosis and management. *Pract Neurol*. 2018;18(4):278–290.

272. Joint Task Force of the E, the PNS. European Federation of Neurological Societies/Peripheral Nerve Society guideline on management of multifocal motor neuropathy. Report of a joint task force of the European Federation of Neurological Societies and the Peripheral Nerve Society—first revision. *J Peripher Nerv Syst*. 2010;15(4):295–301.

273. Nasu S, Misawa S, Sekiguchi Y, et al. Different neurological and physiological profiles in POEMS syndrome and chronic inflammatory demyelinating polyneuropathy. *J Neurol Neurosurg Psychiatry*. 2012;83(5):476–479.

274. Mauermann ML, Sorenson EJ, Dispenzieri A, et al. Uniform demyelination and more severe axonal loss distinguish POEMS syndrome from CIDP. *J Neurol Neurosurg Psychiatry*. 2012;83(5):480–486.

275. Yanik B, Conkbayir I, Keyik B, Yoldas TK. Sonographic findings in a case of polyneuropathy associated with POEMS syndrome. *J Clin Ultrasound*. 2011;39(8):473–476.

276. Mitsuma S, Misawa S, Shibuya K, et al. Altered axonal excitability properties and nerve edema in POEMS syndrome. *Clin Neurophysiol*. 2015;126(10):2014–2018.

277. Lucchetta M, Pazzaglia C, Granata G, Briani C, Padua L. Ultrasound evaluation of peripheral neuropathy in POEMS syndrome. *Muscle Nerve*. 2011;44(6):868–872.

278. Willison HJ, O'Leary CP, Veitch J, et al. The clinical and laboratory features of chronic sensory ataxic neuropathy with anti-disialosyl IgM antibodies. *Brain*. 2001;124(Pt 10):1968–1977.

279. Kam C, Balaratnam MS, Purves A, et al. Canomad presenting without ophthalmoplegia and responding to intravenous immunoglobulin. *Muscle Nerve*. 2011;44(5):829–833.

280. Garcia-Santibanez R, Zaidman CM, Sommerville RB, et al. CANOMAD and other chronic ataxic neuropathies with disialosyl antibodies (CANDA). *J Neurol*. 2018;265(6):1402–1409.

281. Goedee HS, van der Pol WL, Herraets IJT, van Asseldonk JTH, Visser LH, van den Berg LH. *Functional and morphological consequences of cellular and humoral responses in treatment-naive chronic inflammatory demyelinating polyneuropathy: a combined sonographic and nerve conduction study.* In: *Paper Presented at: Peripheral Nerve Society Meeting 2017, Sitges, Barcelona, Spain*; 2017.

282. Sommer C, Koch S, Lammens M, Gabreels-Festen A, Stoll G, Toyka KV. Macrophage clustering as a diagnostic marker in sural nerve biopsies of patients with CIDP. *Neurology.* 2005;65(12):1924–1929.

283. Sainaghi PP, Collimedaglia L, Alciato F, et al. The expression pattern of inflammatory mediators in cerebrospinal fluid differentiates Guillain-Barre syndrome from chronic inflammatory demyelinating polyneuropathy. *Cytokine.* 2010;51(2):138–143.

284. Beppu M, Sawai S, Misawa S, et al. Serum cytokine and chemokine profiles in patients with chronic inflammatory demyelinating polyneuropathy. *J Neuroimmunol.* 2015;279:7–10.

285. Bonin S, Zanotta N, Sartori A, et al. Cerebrospinal fluid cytokine expression profile in multiple sclerosis and chronic inflammatory demyelinating polyneuropathy. *Immunol Invest.* 2018;47(2):135–145.

286. Yang M, Peyret C, Shi XQ, et al. Evidence from human and animal studies: pathological roles of CD8(+) T cells in autoimmune peripheral neuropathies. *Front Immunol.* 2015;6:532.

287. Vital C, Vital A, Lagueny A, et al. Chronic inflammatory demyelinating polyneuropathy: immunopathological and ultrastructural study of peripheral nerve biopsy in 42 cases. *Ultrastruct Pathol.* 2000;24(6):363–369.

288. Meyer Zu Horste G, Cordes S, Pfaff J, et al. Predicting the response to intravenous immunoglobulins in an animal model of chronic neuritis. *PLoS One.* 2016;11(10):e0164099.

289. Haq RU, Pendlebury WW, Fries TJ, Tandan R. Chronic inflammatory demyelinating polyradiculoneuropathy in diabetic patients. *Muscle Nerve.* 2003;27(4):465–470.

290. Rajabally YA, Stettner M, Kieseier BC, Hartung HP, Malik RA. CIDP and other inflammatory neuropathies in diabetes—diagnosis and management. *Nat Rev Neurol.* 2017;13(10):599–611.

291. Laughlin RS, Dyck PJ, Melton 3rd LJ, Leibson C, Ransom J, Dyck PJ. Incidence and prevalence of CIDP and the association of diabetes mellitus. *Neurology.* 2009;73(1):39–45.

292. Bril V, Blanchette CM, Noone JM, Runken MC, Gelinas D, Russell JW. The dilemma of diabetes in chronic inflammatory demyelinating polyneuropathy. *J Diabetes Complications.* 2016;30(7):1401–1407.

293. Wilson JR, Park Y, Fisher MA. Electrodiagnostic criteria in CIDP: comparison with diabetic neuropathy. *Electromyogr Clin Neurophysiol.* 2000;40(3):181–185.

294. Lozeron P, Nahum L, Lacroix C, Ropert A, Guglielmi JM, Said G. Symptomatic diabetic and nondiabetic neuropathies in a series of 100 diabetic patients. *J Neurol.* 2002;249(5):569–575.

295. Thakkar RS, Del Grande F, Thawait GK, Andreisek G, Carrino JA, Chhabra A. Spectrum of high-resolution MRI findings in diabetic neuropathy. *AJR Am J Roentgenol.* 2012;199(2):407–412.

296. Breiner A, Qrimli M, Ebadi H, et al. Peripheral nerve high-resolution ultrasound in diabetes. *Muscle Nerve.* 2017;55(2):171–178.

297. Malik RA. Pathology of human diabetic neuropathy. *Handb Clin Neurol.* 2014;126:249–259.

298. Kyle RA, Therneau TM, Rajkumar SV, et al. Prevalence of monoclonal gammopathy of undetermined significance. *N Engl J Med.* 2006;354(13):1362–1369.

299. Pascual-Goni E, Martin-Aguilar L, Lleixa C, et al. Clinical and laboratory features of anti-MAG neuropathy without monoclonal gammopathy. *Sci Rep.* 2019;9(1):6155.

300. Latov N. Biomarkers of CIDP in patients with diabetes or CMT1. *J Peripher Nerv Syst.* 2011;16(Suppl 1):14–17.

301. Rodriguez Y, Vatti N, Ramirez-Santana C, et al. Chronic inflammatory demyelinating poly-neuropathy as an autoimmune disease. *J Autoimmun.* 2019;102:8–37.

302. Bortoluzzi A, Silvagni E, Furini F, Piga M, Govoni M. Peripheral nervous system involvement in systemic lupus erythematosus: a review of the evidence. *Clin Exp Rheumatol.* 2019;37(1):146–155.

303. Thawani SP, Brannagan 3rd TH, Lebwohl B, Green PH, Ludvigsson JF. Risk of neuropathy among 28,232 patients with biopsy-verified celiac disease. *JAMA Neurol.* 2015;72(7):806–811.

304. Singhal NS, Irodenko VS, Margeta M, Layzer RB. Sarcoid polyneuropathy masquerading as chronic inflammatory demyelinating polyneuropathy. *Muscle Nerve.* 2015;52(4):664–668.

305. Said G. Sarcoidosis of the peripheral nervous system. *Handb Clin Neurol.* 2013;115:485–495.

306. Kimura K, Nezu A, Kimura S, et al. A case of myasthenia gravis in childhood associated with chronic inflammatory demyelinating polyradiculoneuropathy. *Neuropediatrics.* 1998;29(2):108–112.

307. Mori M, Kuwabara S, Nemoto Y, Tamura N, Hattori T. Concomitant chronic inflammatory demyelinating polyneuropathy and myasthenia gravis following cytomegalovirus infection. *J Neurol Sci.* 2006;240(1–2):103–106.

308. Bolz S, Totzeck A, Amann K, Stettner M, Kleinschnitz C, Hagenacker T. CIDP, myasthenia gravis, and membranous glomerulonephritis—three autoimmune disorders in one patient: a case report. *BMC Neurol.* 2018;18(1):113.

309. Quan W, Xia J, Tong Q, et al. Myasthenia gravis and chronic inflammatory demyelinating polyneuropathy in the same patient—a case report. *Int J Neurosci.* 2018;128(6):570–572.

310. Rajabally YA, Attarian S. Chronic inflammatory demyelinating polyneuropathy and malignancy: a systematic review. *Muscle Nerve.* 2018;57(6):875–883.

311. Callaghan BC, Xia R, Banerjee M, et al. Metabolic syndrome components are associated with symptomatic polyneuropathy independent of glycemic status. *Diabetes Care.* 2016;39(5):801–807.

312. Gabbai AA, Castelo A, Oliveira AS. HIV peripheral neuropathy. *Handb Clin Neurol.* 2013;115:515–529.

313. Taylor BV, Wijdicks EF, Poterucha JJ, Weisner RH. Chronic inflammatory demyelinating polyneuropathy complicating liver transplantation. *Ann Neurol.* 1995;38(5):828–831.

314. Shiota G, Harada K, Oyama K, et al. Severe exacerbation of hepatitis after short-term corticosteroid therapy in a patients with "latent" chronic hepatitis B. *Liver.* 2000;20(5):415–420.

315. Corcia P, Barbereau D, Guennoc AM, de Toffol B, Bacq Y. Improvement of a CIDP associated with hepatitis C virus infection using antiviral therapy. *Neurology.* 2004;63(1):179–180.

316. Aktas B, Basyigit S, Yilmaz B, Akturk T, Nazligul Y. Dramatic improvement of chronic inflammatory demyelinating polyneuropathy through Tenofovir treatment in a patient infected with hepatitis B virus. *J Neuroimmune Pharmacol.* 2015;10(2):191–192.

317. Lim JY, Lim YH, Choi EH. Acute-onset chronic inflammatory demyelinating polyneuropathy in hantavirus and hepatitis B virus coinfection: a case report. *Medicine (Baltimore).* 2016;95(49):e5580.

318. Tsuzaki K, Someda H, Inoue M, Tachibana N, Hamano T. Remission of chronic inflammatory demyelinating polyneuropathy after hepatitis C virus eradication with sofosbuvir and ledipasvir therapy. *Muscle Nerve.* 2018;58(5):E34–E36.

319. Lunemann JD, Tackenberg B, Stein A, et al. Dysregulated Epstein-Barr virus infection in patients with CIDP. *J Neuroimmunol.* 2010;218(1–2):107–111.

320. Rajabally YA, Fraser M, Critchley P. Chronic inflammatory demyelinating polyneuropathy after mycoplasma pneumoniae infection. *Eur J Neurol.* 2007;14(7):e20–e21.

321. Meyer Sauteur PM, Roodbol J, Hackenberg A, et al. Severe childhood Guillain-Barre syndrome associated with mycoplasma pneumoniae infection: a case series. *J Peripher Nerv Syst.* 2015;20(2):72–78.

322. Alshekhlee A, Basiri K, Miles JD, Ahmad SA, Katirji B. Chronic inflammatory demyelinating polyneuropathy associated with tumor necrosis factor-alpha antagonists. *Muscle Nerve.* 2010;41(5):723–727.

323. Foulkes AC, Wheeler L, Gosal D, Griffiths CE, Warren RB. Development of chronic inflammatory demyelinating polyneuropathy in a patient receiving infliximab for psoriasis. *Br J Dermatol.* 2014;170(1):206–209.

324. Nakao M, Asano Y, Nakamura K, et al. The development of chronic inflammatory demyelinating polyneuropathy during adalimumab treatment in a patient with psoriasis vulgaris. *Eur J Dermatol.* 2016;26(4):404–405.

325. Argyriou AA, Iconomou G, Kalofonos HP. Bortezomib-induced peripheral neuropathy in multiple myeloma: a comprehensive review of the literature. *Blood.* 2008;112(5):1593–1599.

326. Pitarokoili K, Yoon MS, Kroger I, Reinacher-Schick A, Gold R, Schneider-Gold C. Severe refractory CIDP: a case series of 10 patients treated with bortezomib. *J Neurol.* 2017;264(9): 2010–2020.

327. Bhagavati S, Maccabee P, Muntean E, Sumrani NB. Chronic sensorimotor polyneuropathy associated with tacrolimus immunosuppression in renal transplant patients: case reports. *Transplant Proc.* 2007;39(10):3465–3467.

328. Labate A, Morelli M, Palamara G, Pirritano D, Quattrone A. Tacrolimus-induced polyneuropathy after heart transplantation. *Clin Neuropharmacol.* 2010;33(3):161–162.

329. Renard D, Gauthier T, Venetz JP, Buclin T, Kuntzer T. Late onset tacrolimus-induced life-threatening polyneuropathy in a kidney transplant recipient patient. *Clin Kidney J.* 2012;5(4):323–326.

330. McCombe PA, van der Kreek SA, Pender MP. Neuropathological findings in chronic relapsing experimental allergic neuritis induced in the Lewis rat by inoculation with intradural root myelin and treatment with low dose cyclosporin A. *Neuropathol Appl Neurobiol.* 1992;18(2):171–187.

331. Taniguchi J, Sawai S, Mori M, et al. Chronic inflammatory demyelinating polyneuropathy sera inhibit axonal growth of mouse dorsal root ganglion neurons by activation of Rho-kinase. *Ann Neurol.* 2009;66(5):694–697.

332. Querol L, Nogales-Gadea G, Rojas-Garcia R, et al. Antibodies to contactin-1 in chronic inflammatory demyelinating polyneuropathy. *Ann Neurol.* 2013;73(3):370–380.

333. Doppler K, Appeltshauser L, Wilhelmi K, et al. Destruction of paranodal architecture in inflammatory neuropathy with anti-contactin-1 autoantibodies. *J Neurol Neurosurg Psychiatry.* 2015;86(7):720–728.

334. Hashimoto Y, Ogata H, Yamasaki R, et al. Chronic inflammatory demyelinating polyneuropathy with concurrent membranous nephropathy: an anti-paranode and podocyte protein antibody study and literature survey. *Front Neurol.* 2018;9:997.

335. Taieb G, Le Quintrec M, Pialot A, et al. "Neuro-renal syndrome" related to anti-contactin-1 antibodies. *Muscle Nerve.* 2019;59(3):E19–E21.

336. Garg N, Park SB, Yiannikas C, et al. Neurofascin-155 IGG4 neuropathy: pathophysiological insights, spectrum of clinical severity and response to treatment. *Muscle Nerve.* 2018;57(5):848–851.

337. Eftimov F, Vermeulen M, van Doorn PA, Brusse E, van Schaik IN. Predict. Long-term remission of CIDP after pulsed dexamethasone or short-term prednisolone treatment. *Neurology.* 2012;78(14):1079–1084.

338. Hughes RA, Mehndiratta MM. Corticosteroids for chronic inflammatory demyelinating polyradiculoneuropathy. *Cochrane Database Syst Rev.* 2012;8:CD002062.

339. van Lieverloo GGA, Peric S, Doneddu PE, et al. Corticosteroids in chronic inflammatory demyelinating polyneuropathy: a retrospective, multicenter study, comparing efficacy and safety of daily prednisolone, pulsed dexamethasone, and pulsed intravenous methylprednisolone. *J Neurol.* 2018;265(9):2052–2059.

340. Nobile-Orazio E, Cocito D, Jann S, et al. Intravenous immunoglobulin versus intravenous methylprednisolone for chronic inflammatory demyelinating polyradiculoneuropathy: a randomised controlled trial. *Lancet Neurol.* 2012;11(6):493–502.

341. Rajabally YA, Seow H, Wilson P. Dose of intravenous immunoglobulins in chronic inflammatory demyelinating polyneuropathy. *J Peripher Nerv Syst.* 2006;11(4):325–329.

342. Lunn MP, Ellis L, Hadden RD, Rajabally YA, Winer JB, Reilly MM. A proposed dosing algorithm for the individualized dosing of human immunoglobulin in chronic inflammatory neuropathies. *J Peripher Nerv Syst.* 2016;21(1):33–37.

343. Markvardsen LH, Debost JC, Harbo T, et al. Subcutaneous immunoglobulin in responders to intravenous therapy with chronic inflammatory demyelinating polyradiculoneuropathy. *Eur J Neurol.* 2013;20(5):836–842.

344. Markvardsen LH, Harbo T, Sindrup SH, et al. Subcutaneous immunoglobulin preserves muscle strength in chronic inflammatory demyelinating polyneuropathy. *Eur J Neurol.* 2014;21(12):1465–1470.

345. Markvardsen LH, Sindrup SH, Christiansen I, et al. Subcutaneous immunoglobulin as first-line therapy in treatment-naive patients with chronic inflammatory demyelinating polyneuropathy: randomized controlled trial study. *Eur J Neurol.* 2017;24(2):412–418.

346. van Schaik IN, Bril V, van Geloven N, et al. Subcutaneous immunoglobulin for maintenance treatment in chronic inflammatory demyelinating polyneuropathy (PATH): a randomised, double-blind, placebo-controlled, phase 3 trial. *Lancet Neurol.* 2018;17(1):35–46.

347. Mehndiratta MM, Hughes RA, Pritchard J. Plasma exchange for chronic inflammatory demyelinating polyradiculoneuropathy. *Cochrane Database Syst Rev.* 2015;8:CD003906.

348. Hughes R, Dalakas MC, Merkies I, et al. Oral fingolimod for chronic inflammatory demyelinating polyradiculoneuropathy (FORCIDP trial): a double-blind, multicenter, randomised controlled trial. *Lancet Neurol.* 2018;17(8):689–698.

349. Rajabally YA. Unconventional treatments for chronic inflammatory demyelinating polyneuropathy. *Neurodegener Dis Manag.* 2017;7(5):331–342.

350. Bus S, Zambreanu L, Abbas A, et al. *OPTIC Trial: intravenous immunoglobulin and intravenous methylprednisolone as induction treatment in CIDP – study update.* In: *Annual Peripheral Nerve Society Meeting, Genoa*; 2019.

351. Rajabally YA. Tailoring of therapy for chronic inflammatory demyelinating polyneuropathy. *Neural Regen Res.* 2015;10(9):1399–1400.

352. Rajabally YA. Long-term immunoglobulin therapy for chronic inflammatory demyelinating polyradiculoneuropathy. *Muscle Nerve.* 2015;51(5):657–661.

353. Graham RC, Hughes RA. A modified peripheral neuropathy scale: the overall neuropathy limitations scale. *J Neurol Neurosurg Psychiatry.* 2006;77(8):973–976.

354. Merkies IS, Schmitz PI, van der Meche FG, van Doorn PA. Psychometric evaluation of a new sensory scale in immune-mediated polyneuropathies. Inflammatory neuropathy cause and treatment (INCAT) group. *Neurology.* 2000;54(4):943–949.

355. Chan YC, Allen DC, Fialho D, Mills KR, Hughes RA. Predicting response to treatment in chronic inflammatory demyelinating polyradiculoneuropathy. *J Neurol Neurosurg Psychiatry.* 2006;77(1):114–116.

356. Merkies IS, Schmitz PI, Samijn JP, Meche FG, Toyka KV, van Doorn PA. Assessing grip strength in healthy individuals and patients with immune-mediated polyneuropathies. *Muscle Nerve*. 2000;23(9):1393–1401.

357. Allen JA, Pasnoor M, Burns T, et al. *IVIg treatment-related fluctuations in CIDP patients using daily grip strength measurements (GRIPPER): study update*. In: *Annual Peripheral Nerve Society Meeting, Genoa*; 2019.

358. Hadden R, Doneddu PE. *Assessing the best MCID threshold for grip strength in chronic inflammatory neuropathies*. In: *Annual Peripheral Nerve Society Meeting, Genoa*; 2019.

359. Christiansen I, Markvardsen LH, Jakobsen J. Comparisons in fluctuation of muscle strength and function in patients with immune-mediated neuropathy treated with intravenous versus subcutaneous immunoglobulin. *Muscle Nerve*. 2018;57(4):610–614.

360. Kreutzfeldt M, Jensen HB, Ravnborg M, Markvardsen LH, Andersen H, Sindrup SH. The six-spot-step test—a new method for monitoring walking ability in patients with chronic inflammatory polyneuropathy. *J Peripher Nerv Syst*. 2017;22(2):131–138.

361. Vanhoutte EK, Draak TH, Gorson KC, et al. Impairment measures versus inflammatory RODS in GBS and CIDP: a responsiveness comparison. *J Peripher Nerv Syst*. 2015;20(3):289–295.

362. Provan D, Chapel HM, Sewell WA, O'Shaughnessy D, Group UKIEW. Prescribing intravenous immunoglobulin: summary of Department of Health guidelines. *BMJ*. 2008;337:a1831.

Chapter 4

Multifocal motor neuropathy

Katie Beadon, Jean-Marc Léger

National Referral Center for Neuromuscular Diseases, Institut Hospitalo-Universitaire (IHU) de Neurosciences, University Hospital Pitié Salpêtrière, Paris, France

Introduction

Multifocal motor neuropathy (MMN) is a pure motor neuropathy characterized by progressive multifocal weakness that typically begins and predominates in the distal upper extremities. MMN is rare with a prevalence of about 0.6 per 100,000 people. The description of a multifocal motor syndrome with conduction block was first published by two separate groups in 1986.[1,2] MMN was formally named by Pestronk's group, who additionally reported its association with serum antibody IgM antiganglioside GM-1 and response to immunomodulatory therapy.[3,4] These descriptions distinguished MMN from both motor neuron diseases (MND) and other chronic immune-mediated neuropathies (CIN) such as chronic inflammatory demyelinating polyradiculoneuropathy (CIDP) and demyelinating neuropathy associated with monoclonal gammopathy. MMN remains a distinct entity given its lack of response to immunomodulatory medications efficacious in these other disorders.

Despite significant advances in the understanding of MMN as a disease affecting the nodal and paranodal regions of motor nerves, the pathophysiology of MMN and the role of antiganglioside antibodies in the development of the disease remain incompletely understood. High-dose intravenous immunoglobulin (IVIg) and subcutaneous immunoglobulin (SCIg) have been shown to improve weakness in MMN by randomized controlled trials (RCT) and are therefore the gold standard treatment.

However, the response to immunoglobulin may decline after years of treatment and the disability may progress despite immunoglobulin treatment, highlighting the need for further studies into the development of disease-modifying treatments.

In this chapter, we outline the epidemiology, diagnosis, pathophysiology, monitoring, and long-term treatment of MMN.

Dysimmune Neuropathies. https://doi.org/10.1016/B978-0-12-814572-2.00004-2

Epidemiology

MMN is a rare disorder with prevalence studies ranging from 0.29 to 0.70 per 100,000[5-7] compared to >6 per 100,000 in CIDP.[6] Median age of onset is 40–42[8,9] with 80% of patients between the ages of 20–50 at diagnosis.[10] MMN affects men more than women with a ratio of 2.7:1.[8] MMN is frequently difficult to diagnose and symptoms may be present for years prior to diagnosis.[8,9]

MMN typically affects adults but has been described in children in several case reports.[11-13] These children became symptomatic between the ages of 6–8 (two males, one female). They showed clinical features consistent with adult forms and responded to IVIg therapy. One had positive anti-GM1 antibodies.[13]

MMN has been associated with immunotherapy with tumor necrosis factor alpha (TNFα) inhibitor infliximab for Crohn's disease,[14,15] rheumatoid arthritis,[16] and psoriatic arthritis.[17] Some cases developed within months of initiating therapy[17] while others were after treatment for several years.[14] Many cases presented with fulminant disease with upper and lower extremity involvement developing within weeks. The medication was discontinued in all reported cases and most received IVIg. Patients had partial or full recovery over months to years.

Clinical features

The main clinical diagnostic criteria of MMN are weakness that is slowly or stepwise progressive, multifocal involvement of one or more nerves, and the absence of upper motor neuron findings or significant sensory symptoms (Table 1).

Case series have helped clarify the frequency of the classical and atypical signs and symptoms.[8,9] In a national cross-sectional descriptive study of 88 patients with MMN, onset of weakness was in the distal arm (61%) or distal leg (34%), and occasionally in the upper arm, but never in the upper leg.[8] Symptom onset was more frequent in the dominant hand. On neurological examination, reflexes were usually diminished or abolished in the affected territories, but brisk reflexes were found in 8%. A review of 47 patients with MMN found differential motor deficit across muscles supplied by a common terminal motor nerve in about 54% of patients and differential finger extension weakness as a frequent early manifestation, likely reflecting vulnerabilities of terminal branches of the posterior interosseous nerve[9] (Fig. 1).

Cramps and fasciculations are frequent in affected motor nerves. Marked motor deficits with little or no muscle atrophy are a hallmark of MMN and are the clinical reflection of CB.[9] Muscle weakness is often exacerbated by cold, which may be due to alteration in sodium channels.[19] Patients report increased weakness or fatigue after muscular effort, which may correlate with increased temporal dispersion and CB post exercise in motor nerve conduction studies.[20]

TABLE 1 Clinical criteria for multifocal motor neuropathy (EFNS/PNS Task Force 2010).[18]

Core criteria (both must be present):

1. slowly progressive or stepwise progressive, focal, asymmetric limb weakness[a] with motor involvement in the motor nerve distribution of at least two nerves for > 1 month (usually, > 6 months). If symptoms and signs are present in the distribution of only one nerve, a possible diagnosis can be made

2. no objective sensory abnormalities except for minor vibration sense abnormalities in the lower limbs[b]

Supportive clinical criteria:

1. predominant upper limb involvement

2. decreased or absent tendon reflexes in the affected limb[c]

3. absence of cranial nerve involvement

4. cramps and fasciculations in the affected limb

5. response in terms of disability or muscle strength to immunomodulatory treatment

Exclusion criteria:

1. upper motor neuron signs

2. marked bulbar involvement

3. sensory impairment more marked than minor vibration loss in the lower limbs

4. diffuse symmetric weakness during the initial weeks

[a] A difference of 1 Medical Research Council Score (MRC) grade if strength is MRC > 3 and 2 MRC grades if strength is MRC ≤ 3.
[b] Sensory signs and symptoms may develop over the course of MMN.
[c] Slightly increased reflexes have been reported and do not exclude the diagnosis of MMN provided there are no upper motor neuron signs.

Cranial nerve involvement is rare but hypoglossal and abducens nerve involvement have been reported.[21–23] Vestibular dysfunction has also been seldomly reported.[24] Autonomic dysfunction has not been associated with MMN.

Transient sensory symptoms may exist in some patients, but are not usually accompanied by any significant objective findings outside of decreased vibratory threshold in the distal lower extremities. Abnormal vibration in the legs was present in 22% of MMN patients in one series.[8] The paucity of sensory involvement in MMN may be explained on the basis of sensory nerves being less vulnerable to damage following anti-GM1 antibody binding.[25]

Patients are frequently disabled by their weakness. Cats et al.'s cross-sectional review of 88 patients with MMN found scores on the Overall Disability Sum Scores (ODSS) consistent with severe disability in the arms in 21%

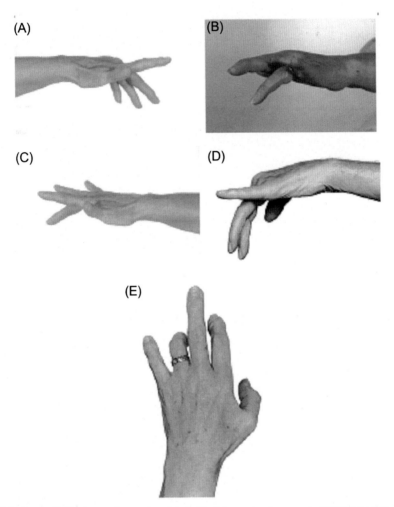

FIG. 1 (A–E) Weakness of extension of individual fingers is often seen in MMN reflecting differential conduction block in posterior interosseous nerve terminal motor branches.[9]

(ODSS >= 3), moderate disability in 61% (ODSS 2), and minimal or no disability in the arms in 18% (ODSS 0 or 1).[8] In the same series, fatigue severity scale (FSS) responses averaged 4.7 with >50% of patients describing severe fatigue (FSS > 5). More severe disability was associated with greater axonal loss, years untreated, symptom onset in the legs, and the presence of anti-GM1 IgM antibodies in univariate analysis, but only axonal loss was an independent determinant of disability in multivariate analysis.

MMN is typically slowly progressive but some have a step-wise course. Rarely, MMN can present with acute-onset mimicking acute inflammatory demyelinating polyneuropathy (AIDP), but the course and response to treatment follow that of classical MMN.[26] Fulminant progression leading to respiratory failure and death has been reported.[27] Rare patients have been reported with spontaneous remission.[8,28]

Electrophysiologic features

The hallmark of MMN is the presence of CB in motor nerves outside of typical compression sites without sensory changes. CB may be absent in patients with otherwise typical MMN. This may reflect conduction block in nerve segments that are not evaluated with routine electrodiagnostic studies or activity-dependent conduction block.[18]

Conduction block is defined as a significant reduction in the amplitude or area of the compound muscle action potential (CMAP) when stimulating proximally compared to distally (Fig. 2).

CB was initially defined as a 20%–30% reduction in amplitude or area if there was no significant increase in CMAP duration (< 15% greater than normal). However, an animal model of temporal dispersion and computer modeling of CB have shown that proximal to distal CMAP area reduction of up to 50% can be due to interphase cancellation alone.[29] The distal CMAP duration and prolongation of proximal CMAP duration are important factors in the definition of conduction block: the shorter the distal durations and proximal duration prolongation, the less amplitude reduction is required to diagnose CB. The EFNS/PNS guidelines define conduction block as definite or probable depending on the degree of area reduction (50% versus 30%) and the CMAP amplitude and duration (Table 2).

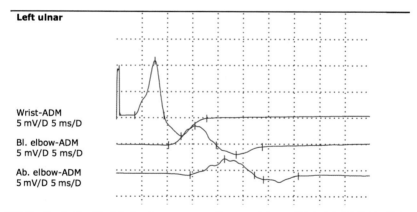

FIG. 2 Conduction block in the ulnar nerve recording over abductor digiti minimi (ADM). CMAP amplitude (10.4 mV) and area (27.2 ms*mV) are normal with distal stimulation (Wrist-ADM). Stimulation below the elbow shows definite conduction block with 64% drop in CMAP amplitude and 66% drop in CMAP area with stimulation below the elbow (Bl. Elbow-ADM). There is no significant conduction block across the elbow (Ab. Elbow-ADM).

TABLE 2 Electrodiagnostic criteria for conduction block[a] (EFNS/PNS guideline).[18]

1. Definite motor conduction block:

- negative peak CMAP area reduction on proximal versus distal stimulation of at least 50% whatever the nerve segment length (median, ulnar, and peroneal)
- distal negative peak CMAP amplitude in the segment with CB must be:
  - o 20% of the lower limit of normal and
  - o 1 mV
- the negative peak CMAP duration must increase by 30% or less between proximal and distal stimulation

2. Probable motor conduction blocks:

- negative peak CMAP area reduction of at least 30% over a long segment (e.g., wrist to elbow or elbow to axilla) of an upper limb nerve with increase of proximal to distal negative peak CMAP duration of 30% or less

OR

- negative peak CMAP area reduction of at least 50% (same as definite) with an increase of proximal to distal negative peak CMAP duration > 30%

3. Normal sensory nerve conduction in the upper limb segments with conduction block

[a] Conduction block must be outside of typical entrapment/compression sites.

In a retrospective study of 88 patients, the authors found that 81% had at least one definite CB, and 18% had no definite but at least one probable CB. CB was most often detected in the ulnar (80%) and median (77%) nerves.[8] Other electrophysiological alterations may be found such as prolonged distal motor latencies, prolonged or absent F-waves, mild slowing of motor nerve conduction velocities, and temporal dispersion.[30] Electromyography may show fasciculations and fibrillation potentials, usually detected in muscles with marked atrophy, consistent with secondary axonal degeneration.[30]

Sensory potentials are usually normal, but have rarely been studied in long-term follow-up. In a retrospective study of 21 patients with MMN with a mean follow-up of 7 ± 2.5 years, 13 patients (62%) had a reduction of the amplitude of at least one sensory potential, of whom four patients had abnormalities of two or more sensory potentials while eight patients had no abnormality.[31] No significant differences were found for gender, age at onset, number of involved motor nerves, presence of IgM anti-GM1 antibodies, or response to IVIg between the groups.

Advanced techniques to increase the detection of conduction block have been developed. Transcutaneous cervical root stimulation can be used with comparison to stimulation at more distal sites (e.g., Erb's point, axilla, elbow, and wrist) with recording over distal muscles to look for proximal conduction block. Triple stimulation aims to detect CB between the nerve root and Erb's point by comparing the results of transcranial magnetic stimulation (TMS) to standard electrical stimulation of the brachial plexus at Erb's point and distal nerve stimulation.[32–34] While these techniques may be helpful to document CB with increased sensitivity, they are not widely available.

Supportive criteria and diagnostic categories

Supportive criteria, including the detection of IgM anti-GM1 antibodies and MRI abnormalities in the brachial plexus, are listed in Table 3.

MRI imaging in patients with MMN shows T2 hyperintensities in the brachial plexus in 40%–50% of patients.[35] These abnormalities are usually asymmetric in MMN in contrast to CIDP where similar changes are seen but are often symmetric.[35] Contrast enhancement of the brachial plexus or nerve root enlargement can also be seen.[35] Diffuse nerve enlargement can be seen in the median and ulnar nerves of MMN patients by MRI or high-resolution ultrasound (HRUS).[36] MRI hyperintensities and nerve enlargement are not specific to MMN and also occur in other inflammatory and hereditary demyelinating neuropathies. However, MRI and HRUS can be used to support the diagnosis of MMN and distinguish MMN from amyotrophic lateral sclerosis (ALS), which can present with a similar clinical picture but typically has reduced nerve diameters when compared to controls.[36]

Summarizing the diagnostic criteria above, and factoring in the response to IVIg, the EFNS/PNS guideline agreed on defining diagnostic categories as definite, probable, and possible (Table 4).

Other features

MMN has been associated with other autoimmune conditions such as celiac disease and Hashimoto's thyroiditis.[37] First-degree family members of patients with MMN have a higher incidence of type 1 diabetes, celiac disease, and Hashimoto's thyroiditis. These associations may suggest a common

---

TABLE 3 Supportive criteria for multifocal motor neuropathy (EFNS/PNS guideline).[18]

1. Elevated IgM antiganglioside GM1 antibodies

2. Increased cerebrospinal fluid (CSF) protein (< 1 g/L)

3. MRI showing increased signal intensity on T2-weighted imaging

4. Objective clinical improvement following IVIg treatment

TABLE 4 Definitions of definite, probable, and possible multifocal motor neuropathy (EFNS/PNS guideline).

Definite	Probable	Possible	Possible
Both core clinical criteria	Both core clinical criteria	Both core clinical criteria	Core clinical criteria in a single nerve
No exclusion criteria	No exclusion criteria	No exclusion criteria	No exclusion criteria
Normal sensory studies in upper limb segments with CB	Normal sensory studies in upper limb segments with CB	Normal sensory studies in upper limb segments with CB	Normal sensory studies in upper limb segments with CB
Definite motor CB	Probable motor CB	Objective improvement following IVIG	Definite or probable CB
	2 supportive criteria		

pathogenic mechanism and underline the importance of searching for co-morbid conditions that may contribute to impairment of quality of life. A higher frequency of HLA-DRB1*15 was found in patients with MMN, which may suggest a similar pathogenic pathway to other diseases such as multiple sclerosis and CIDP that also share a higher incidence of this specific HLA haplotype than in control groups.[38] No correlations have been found between HLA type and disease specifics such as age of onset, clinical course, or disease severity.

Differential diagnosis

The differential diagnosis for MMN includes MND such as ALS variants progressive muscular atrophy (PMA) and brachial amyotrophic diplegia, monomelic amyotrophy (Hirayama's syndrome), CIDP and its Lewis-Sumner variant, and hereditary neuropathies such as hereditary neuropathy with liability to pressure palsy (HNPP) and motor forms of Charcot-Marie-Tooth disease (Table 5). Other considerations are pure motor neuropathies due to lead and dapsone toxicity, postpolio syndrome, and hexoaminidase-A deficiency (Sandhoff disease). In a case series of 88 patients with MMN, 65% of patients were initially misdiagnosed.[8] The alternate diagnoses included MND (32%), polyneuropathy (15%), mononeuropathy (13%), radiculopathy (2%), CIDP (1%), hereditary neuropathy (1%), and minor stroke (1%).

TABLE 5 Differential diagnosis of MMN.

Chronic inflammatory demyelinating polyradiculoneuropathy (CIDP)

• Lewis Sumner variant of CIDP

Hereditary neuropathy with liability to pressure palsy (HNPP)

Motor forms of Charcot-Marie-Tooth neuropathy

Amyotrophic lateral sclerosis

• Progressive muscular atrophy

Monomelic amyotrophy (Hirayama's Syndrome)

Lead neuropathy

Dapsone toxicity

Postpolio syndrome

Hexoaminidase-A deficiency (Sandhoff disease)

Pathophysiology

The pathophysiology of MMN has become better understood in the last decade. The two main areas of research have focused on determining the mechanisms underlying conduction block and the role of antiganglioside antibodies.

Conduction block leads to motor weakness in MMN

Motor CB is the electrophysiologic hallmark of MMN. In recent years, the understanding of MMN has been revolutionized by the idea that nerve dysfunction is probably due to antibody-mediated attack of the node of Ranvier and/or the paranodal region.[39–41] Saltatory conduction is dependent on multiple proteins in the nodal, paranodal, and juxtaparanodal regions. Uncini et al. proposed the term nodopathy-paranodopathy to describe neuropathies in which disruption of these regions leads to CB.[42] CB may occur due to myelin detachment at the paranode, nodal lengthening, disruption of voltage gated sodium channels, altered ion homeostasis, or inexcitability of the axolemma due to disorganized polarization.[40,41] These physiologic and structural changes may explain the presence of CB without true demyelination and help to explain patients' rapid response to IVIg.

The role of antiganglioside antibodies

A number of research articles have been published in recent years on the role of gangliosides at the nodes of Ranvier, as potential target antigens in motor neuropathies such as axonal variants of Guillain-Barré syndrome (GBS), acute motor axonal neuropathy (AMAN), acute motor-sensory neuropathy (AMSAN), and MMN.[43]

Ganglioside GM1 is ubiquitous but is more abundant on peripheral motor nerves than sensory nerves. GM1 localizes to both the axolemma and myelin of the peripheral nerves with the greatest abundance at the nodes of Ranvier and adjacent paranodes.[44,45]

GM1 concentrates in cholesterol-enriched domains of the plasma membrane thought to be related to paranodal stabilization and clustering of ion channels.[46] GM1 provides an anchor for potassium channels, concentrates sodium channels, and facilitates tight junctions through paranodal stabilization. These factors are important for the propagation of action potentials and the maintenance of conduction velocity. Disruption of these functions may lead to paranodal failure of conduction.

There has been debate as to whether antiganglioside antibodies are causative autoantibodies or represent a biomarker resulting from the inflammatory cascade leading to nerve injury. A number of studies have implicated antiganglioside antibodies as pathogenic in MMN. Several studies have shown that anti-GM1 IgM antibodies activate complement in vitro.[25,47,48] One study found that anti-GM1 antibodies from the serum of MMN patients bind to GM1 and activate complement.[45] The depositions of complement were highly correlated with anti-GM1 antibody titer and were reduced by treatment of the serum with IVIg. Another study found that serum from patients with MMN may disrupt the blood-nerve barrier by altering protein expression and transendothelial electrical resistance, which would allow for circulating inflammatory cells to interact with peripheral nerves.[49]

A recent study showed that stem cell-derived motor neurites exposed to the serum of anti-GM1 positive MMN patients showed complement dependent structural changes in motor neurites and alterations in calcium homeostasis[25] (Fig. 3). The serum of MMN patients without anti-GM1 antibodies also showed complement activation and IgM binding to motor neurites, indicating that they may have antibodies to the same or similar epitopes. These changes were significantly decreased when the serum was pretreated with IVIg. Sensory neurites showed less marked structural changes and no alteration in calcium homeostasis after exposure to MMN serum.

No animal model of MMN currently exists, but the aforementioned studies suggest that damage from IgM GM1 could be similar to that observed in a rabbit model of AMAN.[50] In this model, IgM GM1 activates the complement cascade and leads to the production of membrane attack complexes (MAC). This leads to compromised membrane integrity, spreads to internodal regions of the nerve, disrupts sodium channels, and allows for binding of antibodies to the axolemma. Complement inhibitors decrease the antiganglioside mediated damage in animal models, further supporting the role of a complement dependent pathology.

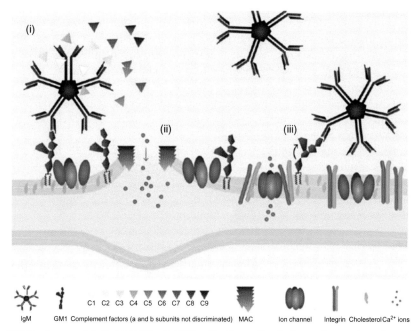

FIG. 3 Immunoglobulin M (IgM) anti-GM1 antibodies mediate both complement-dependent and complement-independent pathogenicity to motor neurons. Model shows putative modes of anti-GM1 antibody pathogenicity, with direct IgM anti-GM1 antibody and complement-dependent pathogenic effect, to neurons. (i) Binding of IgM anti-GM1 antibodies to GM1 gangliosides results in activation of complement and deposition of the membrane attack complex (MAC). (ii) Formation and deposition of the MAC may lead to nonspecific pore formation and focal swelling as a consequence of uncontrolled ion fluxes (e.g., Ca^{2+}). Disturbance of the membrane integrity at the paranodal regions may lead to further disruption of ion channel clustering. (iii) Acute direct effects of IgM anti-GM1 antibody binding may be caused by cross-linking of GM1 gangliosides, leading to Ca^{2+} influx and subsequent activation of voltage-independent ion channels.

Significant titers of serum IgM antibodies to GM1 are present in 40%–60% of cases of MMN. In the largest series reported, the prevalence of anti-GM1 antibodies was 43%.[8] The prevalence of anti-GM1 antibodies varies greatly between reported series, likely due to methodological differences. Testing should be done in a reference laboratory for standardization and should be interpreted with caution in patients who do not have significantly high titers. Testing for GM1/galactocerebroside (GM1/GalC) complexes may increase the positivity to 70%.[51,52] Cats et al. looked at the light chain profile of anti-GM1 positive patients with MMN and GBS and found that 90% of 42 MMN patients had a single type of light chain detected, whereas only 39% of GBS patients were monoclonal.[53] This suggests that antibodies are produced by a single or few B cell clones in MMN.

The relationship between antiganglioside antibody positivity and clinical phenotype or response to treatment is not clear. A recent study tested for anti-GM1 and anti-GD1b antibodies in chronic inflammatory neuropathies and found that of 60 MMN patients, 79% of seropositive patients responded to immunotherapy versus 46% of seronegative patients.[54] The seropositive patients also had a more sustained treatment response. However, prior studies have shown no correlation between treatment response and antibody status.[28]

Other antibodies are less frequently positive, including asialo-GM1, GD1A, and GM2. Autoantibodies to novel nodal and paranodal antigens that have been found in CIDP such as neurofascin-155, contactin-1, neurofascin-186, and gliomedin have not been found in MMN.[55]

The evaluation of complement profiles of patients with MMN has led to differing results. One study found elevated levels of cytokines related to B cell function (IL-1Ra, IL-2, G-CSF, TNFα, TNFR1)[56] while another study did not find any increase in IL-2, TNF-a, G-CSF, or the other cytokines studied.[57]

In summary, it is probable that multiple processes at the nodes of Ranvier, rather than simply demyelination, are important in the development of conduction block. The detection and role of antiganglioside antibodies remains an area of research and the activation of complement contributes to the pathogenesis of MMN.

Monitoring of patients with multifocal motor neuropathy

It is important to use outcome measures to follow the clinical course of patients, their response to treatment, and for clinical trials. Patients will often report an improvement in subjective symptoms with IVIg, but more objective measures are necessary to determine if there is a meaningful response to treatment and direct alterations in therapy. Past studies have used various subjective or objective scales such as the Modified Rankin scale, the Neuropathy Impairment Score-Motor subset, Medical Research Council (MRC) grading, the MRC sum score, grip strength, Guy's Neurological Disability Score (GNDS), and self-evaluation scores. The responsiveness of these measures was only seen in less than one-third of patients.[58] There has not been consensus in what primary outcome measures should be used in clinical trials or clinical practice.

Several outcome measures aimed at the impairment as well as activity and participation levels have been proposed for use in future trials of MMN. The Peripheral Neuropathy Outcome Measures Standardization (PeriNomS) study group developed an MMN-specific scale that consists of an interval questionnaire with 25 questions measuring disability at the activity level, the Rasch-built overall disability scale for patients with MMN (MMN-RODS)[59] (Table 6). This scale has been shown to have acceptable reliability and validity and focuses on the minimum clinically important difference (MCID) to define responders.

The PeriNomS group suggests that future trials in MMN should include multiple scores including the MMN-RODS to measure activity and participation, measures to define impairment such as grip strength with a Martin vigorimeter and/or MRC sum scores, and a quality of life measure such as the Rasch-built Quality of Life in Inflammatory Neuropathies (IN-QoL) scale.

TABLE 6 MMN-RODS questionnaire.

Are you able to:

1. Read a book?

2. Make a telephone call?

3. Eat?

4. Open and close a door?

5. Dress your upper body?

6. Brush your teeth?

7. Drink out of a mug/glass?

8. Turn a key in a lock?

9. Use a knife/fork (spoon)?

10. Clean after toilet?

11. Fill in a form/write?

12. Zip your trousers?

13. Get money from a cash point?

14. Do your own cooking?

15. Pick up a small object

16. Work on a computer?

17. Do the bed?

18. Fold laundry?

19. Throw an object (e.g., ball)?

20. Slice vegetables?

21. Peel an apple/orange?

22. Handle small objects (e.g., coin)?

23. Tie your laces?

24. Clip your fingernails?

25. Button your shirt/blouse?

Patients are instructed to answer if they are able to complete without difficulty (2 points), able to complete with difficulty (1 point), or unable to complete (0 points) each item for their affected limb(s).

Conduction block should not be used as an outcome measure in MMN. Some patients have clear resolution or improvement of conduction block as their clinical status ameliorates while others have stable or even progressive conduction block despite clinical improvement.[28] Electrophysiologic methods such as the motor unit number derived from CMAP amplitude have been reported but are not widely used.[60]

Treatment

MMN has no curative treatment and the goal of treatment of this slowly progressive disorder is to reduce motor deficit along with conduction block, slow down axonal degeneration, and promote reinnervation and remyelination. A minority of patients will have prolonged remission after initial treatment, but the majority of patients will require long-term therapy. In a retrospective study of 40 patients with MMN with a mean follow-up of 2.2 ± 2.0 years, only eight patients (22%) maintained clinical improvement over 6 months without further treatment after 6 months of IVIg while 25 patients (68%) were dependent on maintenance IVIg.[28] Another retrospective study of 88 MMN patients with a mean follow-up of 6 years (range 0–17) found similar results with 76% of patients receiving IVIg maintenance therapy at the time of the study and only 9% with a stable disease course without ongoing treatment.[8]

IVIG is the first-line treatment for MMN. Patients may be interested in increased treatment autonomy and home infusion of IVIg or subcutaneous IVIg, which may be good alternatives for well-selected patients. Steroid treatment and plasmapheresis are not recommended due to lack of efficacy and sometimes worsening of motor signs in MMN. In patients who are unresponsive or progress despite immunoglobulin treatment, other immunosupressive agents may be tried, although none have been shown to be clearly effective in MMN.

Intravenous immunoglobulin

Multiple randomized, double-blind, placebo-controlled trials have shown the benefit of IVIg in the treatment in MMN.[61–65] In a metaanalysis of four trials involving a total of 34 patients, 78% of patients receiving IVIg had improvement in motor strength in the weeks following treatment compared to 4% in the placebo group.[66] IVIg at a total dose of 2 g/kg was effective in 70% of 22 treatment-naive patients in one retrospective study[28] and 94% of 88 MMN patients in another retrospective study,[8] as defined by an increase in MRC grade in at least two muscles with no decrease in other muscles. A trend toward increased effectiveness in patients with lower MRC scores at inclusion and female gender was seen in the first study, but the results were not significant ($P = .07$ and .08, respectively). There was no correlation between clinical improvement and CB or the presence of anti-GM1 antibodies. In a randomized controlled study in 44 patients, IVIg was shown to be effective in improving both muscle strength and reducing disability in MMN patients versus the placebo.[62] Earlier treatment with IVIg after symptom onset may reduce permanent deficits from axonal loss.[8]

The mechanisms of immune modulation by IVIg are not clearly understood. It may alter the immune processes through various mechanisms, including neutralizing pathogenic antibodies and superantigens, inhibiting the B cell production of antibodies and accelerating antibody catabolism, suppressing pro-inflammatory mediators produced by T cells, inhibiting complement-mediated inflammation and damage, inducing a blockade of Fc receptors on macrophages, and regulating the proliferation and adhesion of T cells.[67–70]

Good practice points for treatment recommend an initial dose of 2 g/kg given over 2–5 consecutive days, and if effective, maintenance therapy, ideally 1 g/kg every 2–4 weeks or 2 g/kg every 1–2 months[18] (Table 7).

Although IVIg therapy is effective in most patients with MMN, treatment does not prevent a gradual decline in muscle strength over time. Several studies with long-term follow-up have shown this challenge. In a study of 11 patients with MMN followed for 4–8 years, patients were treated initially with one full course of IVIg (2 g/kg), then 0.4 g/kg every week, followed by maintenance therapy ranging from one infusion every 1–7 weeks.[71] Patients were assessed by an MRC sum score of 20 muscle groups, hand-held dynamometry on a selection of weak muscle groups, electrophysiological studies, and GNDS. Muscle strength improved significantly within 3 weeks of starting IVIg treatment and was significantly better at the last follow-up examination than before treatment. However, scores decreased slightly and significantly during the follow-up period. During follow-up, CB disappeared in six nerve segments but new CB appeared in eight nerve segments. Improvement in electrophysiology with

---

TABLE 7 EFNS/PNS good practice points for the treatment of MMN.[18]

1. IVIg (2 g/kg given over 2–5 days) should be the first-line treatment (level A) when disability is sufficiently severe to warrant treatment.

2. Corticosteroids are not recommended.

3. If an initial treatment with IVIg is effective, repeated IVIg treatment should be considered in selected patients (level C).

4. The frequency of IVIg maintenance therapy should be guided by the response. Typical treatment regimens are 1 g/kg every 2–4 weeks or 2 g/kg every 1–2 months.

5. If IVIg is not sufficiently effective, then immunosuppressive treatment may be considered. However, no agent has been shown to be beneficial in a clinical trial and data from case series are conflicting.

6. Toxicity makes cyclophosphamide a less-desirable option.

remyelination or reinnervation occurred in 13 nerves during follow-up while progression with demyelination or axonal loss occurred in 14 nerves. The authors concluded that IVIg maintenance therapy had a beneficial long-term effect on muscle strength and upper limb disability, but may not prevent a slight decrease in muscle strength over time. The electrophysiological findings implied that IVIg treatment favorably influenced the mechanisms of remyelination or reinnervation, but that axon loss cannot be prevented. Similar results were found by other authors who reported follow-up in 10 MMN patients responding to an initial course of IVIg with periodic infusions for 5–12 years (mean 8.2 years).[72] At the last follow-up, only two patients had maintained the maximal improvement achieved during therapy while eight worsened despite IVIg therapy. This decline started after 3–7 years (mean 4.8 years) of therapy and correlated with a reduction of distal CMAP amplitudes. Conversely, a third study reported significant and sustained improvement in muscle strength (assessed by MRC in eight muscle groups), disability (assessed by a Modified Rankin score), CB, and signs of axonal degeneration on electrophysiological studies in 10 MMN patients, with a follow-up of 3.5–12 years (mean 7.25 years).[73] The authors concluded that long-term IVIg therapy improved muscle strength and functional disability, decreased the number of CBs and the extent of axonal degeneration, and promoted reinnervation. The difference from previous findings may be explained by the different IVIg regimens, as the patients in this last study were treated with significantly higher IVIg maintenance doses.

Many different brands of IVIg exist. A retrospective review that included seven patients with MMN found no difference in efficacy or tolerability between four types of IVIg used in their center (Flebogamma, IgVena, Gammagard, and Kiovig).[74] However, individual patients may have differing side effects with different agents and modifications to therapy may be necessary.

IVIg is generally well tolerated but can lead to headache, aseptic meningitis, and rash and infusion reactions with fever and chills. Side effects can be mitigated by pretreatment with analgesics and antihistamines.

Long-term IVIg therapy may be limited by adverse effects, including thromboembolic events, anaphylactic reactions, difficult venous access, and renal tubular necrosis. Renal effects may be avoided by the detection of preexisting renal disease and adequate hydration.

Subcutaneous immunoglobulin

Subcutaneous immunoglobulin (SCIg) has been used for primary immune deficiency (PID) for > 20 years. In this population, SCIg has been shown to be efficacious as well as increase patient satisfaction over IV treatment and be cost effective. The use of SCIg in inflammatory neuropathies such as CIDP and MMN has been explored in the last decade, given the improved patient autonomy and the theoretical improvement in steady-state immunoglobulin levels with weekly injections over periodic infusions. The recently published PATH study randomized 172 IVIg-responsive CIDP patients to low-dose (0.2 g/kg per week) and high-dose (0.4 g/kg per week) SCIg or placebo and found SCIg to be efficacious and well tolerated, making it a good alternative to IVIg for maintenance therapy.[75] These findings probably apply to MMN. Several small studies have shown the safety and efficacy of SCIg in MMN.[76–78] A recent metaanalysis of SCIg for chronic autoimmune neuropathies included 50 patients with MMN and found no difference in muscle strength between IVIg and SCIg treatment over follow-up periods of 1–2 years.[79] However, in an Italian cohort of CIDP and MMN patients who received SCIg with a follow-up of 2 years, 40% of 21 MMN patients required increases in SCIg, combining SCIg and IVIg, or transition back to IVIg to stabilize the clinical condition versus only 13% of 45 CIDP patients who required changes in SCIg treatment.[80] Consequently, there is a need for further studies into the long-term efficacy of SCIg in MMN.

SCIg is associated with lower incidences of headache and nausea than IVIg.[76,81] The most common side effects of SCIg treatment are malaise, injection site swelling, erythema, or soreness, which usually resolve within 24 h of treatment.[76] These adverse effects can be mitigated by rotating injection sites, changing needle size, or reducing the infusion rate.[76] Patients are typically able to learn infusion techniques and complete them independently or with a caregiver within a few training sessions.[82] Most patients report increased satisfaction of managing therapy autonomously, but proper patient selection is important.

The optimal dosing of SCIg is not clear. The bioavailability of SCIg measured in serum was shown to be 65%–70% of IVIg in PID and the dosing of SCIg in that population is therefore 1.2–1.53 that of IVIg. Some studies of SCIg in MMN have used a 1:1 ratio of SCIg:IVIg and others 1.53:1 when possible, but this is limited given the restriction of maximum dosing of <2 g/kg per month.[76] There is no clear evidence for which dose is most efficacious or tolerable at present.

Other immunomodulatory treatments

Corticosteroids and plasma exchange, which are effective in CIDP, are not recommended in MMN and may lead to worsening of motor functions.[18] Consequently, they should not be considered a therapeutic option in patients with MMN.

However, a minority of patients with MMN do not respond to IVIg, require increasingly frequent IVIg infusions to maintain remission, or have an involvement of new motor nerves despite IVIg therapy. The use of various immunomodulatory agents has therefore been trialed in MMN either as an adjunct to IVIg or as an alternative when IVIg is ineffective or poorly tolerated. To date, cyclophosphamide and mycophenolate mofetil are the most frequently reported. Eculizumab has also been proposed as a targeted therapy.

Cyclophosphamide

Several uncontrolled studies, including a historical one,[3] have suggested the efficacy of cyclophosphamide as an alternative therapy. However, the

EFNS/PNS guidelines concluded that cyclophosphamide is a less desirable option, primarily due to its toxicity and the lack of evidence of efficacy.[18] As an adjunctive treatment, only one uncontrolled study showed a reduction of the frequency of IVIg infusions in six patients, but three patients presented severe side effects.[83]

Mycophenolate mofetil

Previous small case series have reported reduced IVIg dosing when mycophenolate mofetil is used as an adjunctive therapy.[84,85] However, a single randomized, placebo-controlled study of mycophenolate mofetil 1 g twice a day for 1 year in addition to IVIg treatment in 28 MMN patients failed to show benefits in terms of a reduction in the IVIg dose or a difference in muscle strength, functional scores, and IgM anti-GM1 antibody titers between patients having received mycophenolate mofetil or a placebo.[86] This study was evaluated in a Cochrane review of immunomodulatory treatment for MMN, which concluded that it was significantly underpowered to definitively rule out a clinically important effect of mycophenolate mofetil.[87]

Other agents such as cyclosporine, azathioprine, interferon beta-1a, and rituximab have been reported, but none have shown clear benefit.

Eculizumab

Experimental studies have shown that the pathogenic effect of anti-GM1 antibodies is complement-mediated (see above). Inhibition of the complement may therefore prevent damage to motor nerves in MMN. Eculizumab is a monoclonal antibody that binds complement component C5 and inhibits terminal complement activation and membrane lysis via MAC.[88] Its safety and efficacy were first shown in complement-mediated diseases including paroxysmal nocturnal hemoglobinuria, and it has recently been approved for the treatment of refractory antibody positive myasthenia gravis.[89,90] A 2011 open-label study investigated eculizumab in 13 patients with MMN for 14 weeks.[88] A trend was seen toward improvement in patient-rated subjective scores and increased muscle strength measured by myometry. A small decrease in CB was also seen. Eculizumab was well tolerated in this study.

Eculizumab was investigated for the treatment of GBS in two recent randomized trials.[91,92] Both randomized trials included acute GBS patients unable to walk independently to receive IVIg and eculizumab or IVIg and placebo infusions. The first study included seven patients and found that eculizumab adjunctive therapy was safe and well tolerated, but no clear trends in efficacy were seen.[91] The second study included 34 patients.[92] The primary efficacy outcome was the ability to walk independently at 4 weeks. This occurred in 61% of patients treated with eculizumab and 40% of the placebo group, but did not achieve the predefined threshold response rate. No significant differences were seen in the secondary outcomes of performance on assessment scales or electrophysiologic parameters. There was an improvement in the ability to run at 24 weeks. The most common side effects were infections and decreased liver function.[92] Complement inhibition may hold promise as a new approach in the treatment of MMN, but further research is required.

Conclusion

MMN is a rare chronic immune-mediated neuropathy that can have a significant impact on a patient's quality of life. Progressive multifocal weakness without significant sensory alterations and the presence of CB are the hallmarks of the disease. The pathogenesis of MMN involves activation of the complement cascade. Anti-GM1 IgM antibodies likely play a primary role in the activation of complement. A continued focus on experimental models to study the pathophysiology of MMN could lead to a better understanding of the disease and may direct new approaches to the treatment of MMN. The standardization of monitoring tools with more disease-specific scales such as the MMN-RODS is important for the evaluation of disease course and treatment.

IVIg remains the mainstay of treatment of MMN, but does not prevent the progression of motor deficits or axonal loss. SCIg is an efficacious alternative to IVIg for maintenance therapy in patients interested in increased treatment autonomy. Complement inhibition with monoclonal antibody eculizumab has been investigated for the treatment of GBS and needs further study in MMN. Other immunomodulatory agents such as mycophenolate mofetil have been trialed in patients who do not respond to IVIg or progress despite treatment, but none have shown clear efficacy in prospective trials. Further studies are required to identify disease-modifying therapies in MMN.

Acknowledgments

None.

Financial support and sponsorship

No financial support or sponsorship was received for this review.

Conflict of interest

J.M. Léger was the primary investigator for a monocentric randomized controlled trial conducted in MMN patients with Endobulin (Immuno AG, then Baxter SA), a monocentric retrospective study conducted in MMN patients treated with Tégéline (Laboratoire Français du Biofractionnement: LFB), and the LIME study comparing two different brands of IVIg in the treatment of MMN, supported by LFB.

K. Beadon has no conflicts of interest.

References

1. Roth G, Rohr J, Magistris MR, Ochsner F. Motor neuropathy with proximal multifocal persistent conduction block, fasciculations and myokymia. Evolution to tetraplegia. *Eur Neurol.* 1986;25(6):416–423.

2. Chad DA, Hammer K, Sargent J. Slow resolution of multifocal weakness and fasciculation: a reversible motor neuron syndrome. *Neurology.* 1986;36(9):1260–1263.

3. Pestronk A, Cornblath DR, Ilyas AA, et al. A treatable multifocal motor neuropathy with antibodies to GM1 ganglioside. *Ann Neurol.* 1988;24(1):73–78.

4. Feldman EL, Bromberg MB, Albers JW, Pestronk A. Immunosuppressive treatment in multifocal motor neuropathy. *Ann Neurol.* 1991;30(3):397–401.

5. Mahdi-Rogers M, Hughes RA. Epidemiology of chronic inflammatory neuropathies in Southeast England. *Eur J Neurol.* 2014;21(1):28–33.

6. Lefter S, Hardiman O, Ryan AM. A population-based epidemiologic study of adult neuromuscular disease in the republic of Ireland. *Neurology.* 2017;88(3):304–313.

7. Matsui N. Multifocal motor neuropathy: current review of epidemiology and treatment. *Rinsho Shinkeigaku.* 2012;52(11):920–922.

8. Cats EA, van der Pol WL, Piepers S, et al. Correlates of outcome and response to IVIg in 88 patients with multifocal motor neuropathy. *Neurology.* 2010;75(9):818–825.

9. Slee M, Selvan A, Donaghy M. Multifocal motor neuropathy: the diagnostic spectrum and response to treatment. *Neurology.* 2007;69(17):1680–1687.

10. Nobile-Orazio E, Cappellari A, Priori A. Multifocal motor neuropathy: current concepts and controversies. *Muscle Nerve.* 2005;31(6):663–680.

11. Moroni I, Bugiani M, Ciano C, Bono R, Pareyson D. Childhood-onset multifocal motor neuropathy with conduction blocks. *Neurology.* 2006;66(6):922–924.

12. Kamata A, Muramatsu K, Sawaura N, et al. Demyelinating neuropathy in a 6-year-old girl with autism spectrum disorder. *Pediatr Int.* 2017;59(8):951–954.

13. Ishigaki H, Hiraide T, Miyagi Y, et al. Childhood-onset multifocal motor neuropathy with immunoglobulin M antibodies to gangliosides GM1 and GM2: a case report and review of the literature. *Pediatr Neurol.* 2016;62:51–57.

14. Rowan CR, Tubridy N, Cullen G. Multifocal motor neuropathy associated with infliximab. *J Crohns Colitis.* 2015;9(12):1174–1175.

15. Fernandez-Menendez S, Gonzalez Nafria N, Redondo-Robles L, Sierra-Ausin M, Garcia-Santiago R, Saponaro-Gonzalez A. Multifocal-motor-neuropathy-like disease associated with infliximab treatment in a patient with Crohn's disease. *J Neurol Sci.* 2015;349(1–2):246–248.

16. Theibich A, Dreyer L, Magyari M, Locht H. Demyelinizing neurological disease after treatment with tumor necrosis factor alpha-inhibiting agents in a rheumatological outpatient clinic: description of six cases. *Clin Rheumatol.* 2014;33(5):719–723.

17. Landais A, Fanhan R. A case of multifocal-motor-neuropathy-like disease with conduction blocks under infliximab with spontaneous progressive recovery. *Presse Med.* 2018;47(3): 298–301.

18. van Schaik IN, Leger JM, Nobile-Orazio E, et al. European Federation of Neurological Societies/Peripheral Nerve Society guideline on management of multifocal motor neuropathy. Report of a joint task force of the European Federation of Neurological Societies and the Peripheral Nerve Society – first revision. *J Periph Nerv Syst.* 2010;15(4):295–301.

19. Straver D, van Asseldonk J, Notermans N, Wokke J, van den Berg L, Franssen H. Cold paresis in multifocal motor neuropathy. *J Neurol.* 2011;258(2):212–217.

20. Straver DCG, van den Berg, Leonard H, van den Berg-Vos, Renske M, Franssen H. Activity-dependent conduction block in multifocal motor neuropathy. *Muscle Nerve.* 2011;43(1): 31–36.

21. Galassi G, Albertini G, Valzania F, Barbieri A. Cranial nerve involvement as presenting sign of multifocal motor neuropathy. *J Clin Neurosci.* 2012;19(12):1733–1735.

22. Kaji R, Shibasaki H, Kimura J. Multifocal demyelinating motor neuropathy: cranial nerve involvement and immunoglobulin therapy. *Neurology.* 1992;42(3 Pt 1):506–509.

23. Axelsson G, Liedholm LJ. Multifocal motor neuropathy-unusual cause of hypoglossal palsy. *Lakartidningen.* 2002;99(13):1448–1450.

24. Blanquet M, Petersen JA, Palla A, et al. Vestibulo-cochlear function in inflammatory neuropathies. *Clin Neurophysiol.* 2018;129(4):863–873.

25. Harschnitz O, van den Berg LH, Johansen LE, et al. Autoantibody pathogenicity in a multifocal motor neuropathy induced pluripotent stem cell-derived model. *Ann Neurol.* 2016;80(1): 71–88.

26. Galassi G, Girolami F. Acute-onset multifocal motor neuropathy (AMMN): how we meet the diagnosis. *Int J Neurosci.* 2012;122(8):413–422.

27. Galassi G, Girolami F, Ariatti A, Monelli M, Sola P. Fulminant multifocal motor neuropathy: a report of two cases. *Int J Neurosci.* 2012;122(7):395–400.

28. Léger JM, Viala K, Cancalon F, et al. Intravenous immunoglobulin as short- and long-term therapy of multifocal motor neuropathy: a retrospective study of response to IVIg and of its predictive criteria in 40 patients. *J Neurol Neurosurg Psychiatry.* 2008;79(1):93–96.

29. Rhee EK, England JD, Sumner AJ. A computer simulation of conduction block: effects produced by actual block versus interphase cancellation. *Ann Neurol.* 1990;28(2):146–156.

30. Beadon K, Guimaraes-Costa R, Léger JM. Multifocal motor neuropathy. *Curr Opin Neurol.* 2018;31(5):559–564.

31. Lievens I, Fournier E, Viala K, Maisonobe T, Bouche P, Léger JM. Multifocal motor neuropathy: a retrospective study of sensory nerve conduction velocities in long-term follow-up of 21 patients. *Rev Neurol (Paris).* 2009;165(3):243–248.

32. Attarian S, Azulay JP, Verschueren A, Pouget J. Magnetic stimulation using a triple-stimulation technique in patients with multifocal neuropathy without conduction block. *Muscle Nerve.* 2005;32(6):710–714.

33. Deroide N, Uzenot D, Verschueren A, Azulay JP, Pouget J, Attarian S. Triple-stimulation technique in multifocal neuropathy with conduction block. *Muscle Nerve.* 2007;35(5):632–636.

34. Xu YS, Zheng JY, Zhang S, Fan DS. Diagnostic role of triple stimulation technique in patients with multifocal motor neuropathy. *Zhonghua Yi Xue Za Zhi.* 2012;92(7):456–459.

35. Jongbloed BA, Bos JW, Rutgers D, van der Pol WL, van den Berg LH. Brachial plexus magnetic resonance imaging differentiates between inflammatory neuropathies and does not predict disease course. *Brain Behav.* 2017;7(5):e00632.

36. Jongbloed BA, Haakma W, Goedee HS, et al. Comparative study of peripheral nerve mri and ultrasound in multifocal motor neuropathy and amyotrophic lateral sclerosis. *Muscle Nerve.* 2016;54(6):1133–1135.

37. Cats EA, Bertens AS, Veldink JH, van den Berg LH, van der Pol WL. Associated autoimmune diseases in patients with multifocal motor neuropathy and their family members. *J Neurol.* 2012;259(6):1137–1141.

38. Sutedja NA, Otten HG, Cats EA, et al. Increased frequency of HLA-DRB1*15 in patients with multifocal motor neuropathy. *Neurology.* 2010;74(10):828–832.

39. Fehmi J, Scherer SS, Willison HJ, Rinaldi S. Nodes, paranodes and neuropathies. *J Neurol Neurosurg Psychiatry.* 2018;89(1):61–71.

40. Uncini A, Kuwabara S. Nodopathies of the peripheral nerve: an emerging concept. *J Neurol Neurosurg Psychiatry.* 2015;86(11):1186–1195.
41. Franssen H. The node of Ranvier in multifocal motor neuropathy. *J Clin Immunol.* 2014;34(Suppl 1):105.
42. Uncini A, Susuki K, Yuki N. Nodo-paranodopathy: beyond the demyelinating and axonal classification in anti-ganglioside antibody-mediated neuropathies. *Clin Neurophysiol.* 2013;124(10):1928–1934.
43. Yuki N. Acute motor axonal neuropathy and multifocal motor neuropathy: more in common than not. *Muscle Nerve.* 2013;48(5):693–695.
44. Willison HJ, Plomp JJ. Anti-ganglioside antibodies and the presynaptic motor nerve terminal. *Ann N Y Acad Sci.* 2008;1132:114–123.
45. Yuki N, Watanabe H, Nakajima T, Spath PJ. IVIg blocks complement deposition mediated by anti-GM1 antibodies in multifocal motor neuropathy. *J Neurol Neurosurg Psychiatry.* 2011;82(1):87–91.
46. Susuki K, Rasband MN, Tohyama K, et al. Anti-GM1 antibodies cause complement-mediated disruption of sodium channel clusters in peripheral motor nerve fibers. *J Neurosci.* 2007;27(15):3956–3967.
47. Sudo M, Miyaji K, Späth PJ, Morita-Matsumoto K, Yamaguchi Y, Yuki N. Polyclonal IgM and IgA block in vitro complement deposition mediated by anti-ganglioside antibodies in autoimmune neuropathies. *Int Immunopharmacol.* 2016;40:11–15.
48. Vlam L, Cats E, Harschnitz O, et al. Complement activity is associated with disease severity in multifocal motor neuropathy. *Neurol Neuroimmunol Neuroinflamm.* 2015;2(4):e119.
49. Shimizu F, Omoto M, Sano Y, et al. Sera from patients with multifocal motor neuropathy disrupt the blood-nerve barrier. *J Neurol Neurosurg Psychiatry.* 2014;85(5):526–537.
50. O'Hanlon GM, Humphreys PD, Goldman RS, et al. Calpain inhibitors protect against axonal degeneration in a model of anti-ganglioside antibody-mediated motor nerve terminal injury. *Brain.* 2003;126(Pt 11):2497–2509.
51. Nobile-Orazio E, Giannotta C, Musset L, Messina P, Léger JM. Sensitivity and predictive value of anti-GM1/galactocerebroside IgM antibodies in multifocal motor neuropathy. *J Neurol Neurosurg Psychiatry.* 2014;85(7):754–758.
52. Delmont E, Halstead S, Galban-Horcajo F, Yao D, Desnuelle C, Willison H. Improving the detection of IgM antibodies against glycolipids complexes of GM1 and galactocerebroside in multifocal motor neuropathy using glycoarray and ELISA assays. *J Neuroimmunol.* 2015;278:159–161.
53. Cats EA, van der Pol WL, Tio-Gillen AP, Diekstra FP, van den Berg LH, Jacobs BC. Clonality of anti-GM1 IgM antibodies in multifocal motor neuropathy and the Guillain-Barre syndrome. *J Neurol Neurosurg Psychiatry.* 2015;86(5):502–504.
54. Martinez-Thompson JM, Snyder MR, Ettore M, et al. Composite ganglioside autoantibodies and immune treatment response in MMN and MADSAM. *Muscle Nerve.* 2018;57(6):1000–1005.
55. Doppler K, Appeltshauser L, Kramer HH, et al. Contactin-1 and neurofascin-155/-186 are not targets of auto-antibodies in multifocal motor neuropathy. *PLoS One.* 2015;10(7):e0134274.
56. Furukawa T, Matsui N, Fujita K, et al. Increased proinflammatory cytokines in sera of patients with multifocal motor neuropathy. *J Neurol Sci.* 2014;346(1–2):75–79.
57. Vlam L, Stam M, de Jager W, Cats EA, van den Berg LH, van der Pol WL. Cytokine profiles in multifocal motor neuropathy and progressive muscular atrophy. *J Neuroimmunol.* 2015;286:1–4.
58. Pruppers MH, Draak TH, Vanhoutte EK, et al. Outcome measures in MMN revisited: further improvement needed. *J Peripher Nerv Syst.* 2015;20(3):306–318.

59. Vanhoutte EK, Faber CG, van Nes SI, et al. Rasch-built overall disability scale for multifocal motor neuropathy (MMN-RODS((c))). *J Peripher Nerv Syst.* 2015;20(3):296–305.

60. Philibert M, Grapperon AM, Delmont E, Attarian S. Monitoring the short-term effect of intravenous immunoglobulins in multifocal motor neuropathy using motor unit number index. *Clin Neurophysiol.* 2017;128(1):235–240.

61. Federico P, Zochodne DW, Hahn AF, Brown WF, Feasby TE. Multifocal motor neuropathy improved by IVIg: randomized, double-blind, placebo-controlled study. *Neurology.* 2000;55(9):1256–1262.

62. Hahn AF, Beydoun SR, Lawson V, et al. A controlled trial of intravenous immunoglobulin in multifocal motor neuropathy. *J Peripher Nerv Syst.* 2013;18(4):321–330.

63. Léger JM, Chassande B, Musset L, Meininger V, Bouche P, Baumann N. Intravenous immunoglobulin therapy in multifocal motor neuropathy: a double-blind, placebo-controlled study. *Brain.* 2001;124(Pt 1):145–153.

64. Van den Berg LH, Kerkhoff H, Oey PL, et al. Treatment of multifocal motor neuropathy with high dose intravenous immunoglobulins: a double blind, placebo controlled study. *J Neurol Neurosurg Psychiatry.* 1995;59(3):248–252.

65. Azulay JP, Blin O, Pouget J, et al. Intravenous immunoglobulin treatment in patients with motor neuron syndromes associated with anti-GM1 antibodies: a double-blind, placebo-controlled study. *Neurology.* 1994;44(3 Pt 1):429–432.

66. van Schaik IN, van den Berg LH, de Haan R, Vermeulen M. Intravenous immunoglobulin for multifocal motor neuropathy. *Cochrane Database Syst Rev.* 2005;2:CD004429.

67. Kazatchkine MD, Kaveri SV. Immunomodulation of autoimmune and inflammatory diseases with intravenous immune globulin. *N Engl J Med.* 2001;345(10):747–755.

68. Dalakas MC. Mechanisms of action of IVIg and therapeutic considerations in the treatment of acute and chronic demyelinating neuropathies. *Neurology.* 2002;59(12 Suppl 6):13.

69. Dalakas MC. Pathogenesis of immune-mediated neuropathies. *Biochim Biophys Acta.* 2015;1852(4):658–666.

70. Kumar A, Patwa HS, Nowak RJ. Immunoglobulin therapy in the treatment of multifocal motor neuropathy. *J Neurol Sci.* 2017;375:190–197.

71. Van den Berg-Vos RM, Franssen H, Wokke JH, Van den Berg LH. Multifocal motor neuropathy: long-term clinical and electrophysiological assessment of intravenous immunoglobulin maintenance treatment. *Brain.* 2002;125(Pt 8):1875–1886.

72. Terenghi F, Cappellari A, Bersano A, Carpo M, Barbieri S, Nobile-Orazio E. How long is IVIg effective in multifocal motor neuropathy? *Neurology.* 2004;62(4):666–668.

73. Vucic S, Black KR, Chong PS, Cros D. Multifocal motor neuropathy: decrease in conduction blocks and reinnervation with long-term IVIg. *Neurology.* 2004;63(7):1264–1269.

74. Gallia F, Balducci C, Nobile-Orazio E. Efficacy and tolerability of different brands of intravenous immunoglobulin in the maintenance treatment of chronic immune-mediated neuropathies. *J Peripher Nerv Syst.* 2016;21(2):82–84.

75. van Schaik IN, Bril V, van Geloven N, et al. Subcutaneous immunoglobulin for maintenance treatment in chronic inflammatory demyelinating polyneuropathy (PATH): a randomised, double-blind, placebo-controlled phase 3 trial. *Lancet Neurol.* 2018;17(1):35–46.

76. Katzberg HD, Rasutis V, Bril V. Subcutaneous immunoglobulin for treatment of multifocal motor neuropathy. *Muscle Nerve.* 2016;54(5):856–863.

77. Harbo T, Andersen H, Hess A, Hansen K, Sindrup SH, Jakobsen J. Subcutaneous versus intravenous immunoglobulin in multifocal motor neuropathy: a randomized, single-blinded crossover trial. *Eur J Neurol.* 2009;16(5):631–638.

78. Christiansen I, Markvardsen LH, Jakobsen J. Comparisons in fluctuation of muscle strength and function in patients with immune-mediated neuropathy treated with intravenous versus subcutaneous immunoglobulin. *Muscle Nerve*. 2018;57(4):610–614.

79. Racosta JM, Sposato LA, Kimpinski K. Subcutaneous versus intravenous immunoglobulin for chronic autoimmune neuropathies: a meta-analysis. *Muscle Nerve*. 2017;55(6):802–809.

80. Cocito D, Merola A, Romagnolo A, et al. Subcutaneous immunoglobulin in CIDP and MMN: a different long-term clinical response? *J Neurol Neurosurg Psychiatry*. 2016;87(7):791–793.

81. Markvardsen LH, Christiansen I, Andersen H, Jakobsen J. Headache and nausea after treatment with high-dose subcutaneous versus intravenous immunoglobulin. *Basic Clin Pharmacol Toxicol*. 2015;117(6):409–412.

82. Rasutis VM, Katzberg HD, Bril V. High-dose subcutaneous immunoglobulin in patients with multifocal motor neuropathy: a nursing perspective. *J Infus Nurs*. 2017;40(5):305–312.

83. Meucci N, Cappellari A, Barbieri S, Scarlato G, Nobile-Orazio E. Long term effect of intravenous immunoglobulins and oral cyclophosphamide in multifocal motor neuropathy. *J Neurol Neurosurg Psychiatry*. 1997;63(6):765–769.

84. Benedetti L, Grandis M, Nobbio L, et al. Mycophenolate mofetil in dysimmune neuropathies: a preliminary study. *Muscle Nerve*. 2004;29(5):748–749.

85. Umapathi T, Hughes R. Mycophenolate in treatment-resistant inflammatory neuropathies. *Eur J Neurol*. 2002;9(6):683–685.

86. Piepers S, Van den Berg-Vos R, Van der Pol WL, Franssen H, Wokke J, Van den Berg L. Mycophenolate mofetil as adjunctive therapy for MMN patients: a randomized, controlled trial. *Brain*. 2007;130(Pt 8):2004–2010.

87. Umapathi T, Hughes RA, Nobile-Orazio E, Léger JM. Immunosuppressant and immunomodulatory treatments for multifocal motor neuropathy. *Cochrane Database Syst Rev*. 2015;3:CD003217.

88. Fitzpatrick AM, Mann CA, Barry S, Brennan K, Overell JR, Willison HJ. An open label clinical trial of complement inhibition in multifocal motor neuropathy. *J Periph Nerv Syst*. 2011;16(2):84–91.

89. Howard JF, Utsugisawa K, Benatar M, et al. Safety and efficacy of eculizumab in anti-acetylcholine receptor antibody-positive refractory generalised myasthenia gravis (REGAIN): a phase 3, randomised, double-blind, placebo-controlled, multicentre study. *Lancet Neurol*. 2017;16(12):976–986.

90. Dhillon S. Eculizumab: a review in generalized myasthenia gravis. *Drugs*. 2018;78(3):367–376.

91. Davidson AI, Halstead SK, Goodfellow JA, et al. Inhibition of complement in Guillain-Barré syndrome: the ICA-GBS study. *J Periph Nerv Syst*. 2017;22(1):4–12.

92. Misawa S, Kuwabara S, Sato Y, et al. Safety and efficacy of eculizumab in Guillain-Barre syndrome: a multicentre, double-blind, randomised phase 2 trial. *Lancet Neurol*. 2018;17(6):519–529.

Chapter 5

Monoclonal gammopathy associated neuropathy: Focusing on IgM M-protein associated neuropathy

Mariëlle H.J. Pruppers[a,b], Ingemar S.J. Merkies[b,c], Nicolette C. Notermans[a]

[a]Department of Neurology, University Medical Center Utrecht, Utrecht, The Netherlands,
[b]Department of Neurology, Maastricht University Medical Center, Maastricht, The Netherlands,
[c]Department of Neurology, Sint-Elisabeth Hospital, Willemstad, Curaçao

Introduction

A man, first seen in the outpatient clinic at the age of 60 years, experiences a numb feeling in both feet, which started > 2 years ago in his toes and has slowly progressed since. He also feels insecure when walking in the dark or when walking down the stairs. Apart from that, he has no other symptoms and has always been healthy with no family history of neuromuscular disorders. Because you suspect a polyneuropathy, you perform an extensive laboratory investigation and electrophysiological studies. The laboratory workup is normal except for an M-protein of the IgM type, and electrophysiological studies show a polyneuropathy with distal demyelination. This case describes an example of a patient with IgM monoclonal protein (M-protein) associated neuropathy.

Neuropathies associated with M-proteins are a complex and difficult to classify group of disorders. This is mainly due to their heterogeneous characteristics and their different neurological and hematological aspects. This chapter aims to give background information on neuropathies associated with M-proteins, with special focus on IgM M-protein associated neuropathy, and gives a guideline on how to diagnose and treat patients with IgM M-protein associated neuropathy.

Dysimmune Neuropathies. https://doi.org/10.1016/B978-0-12-814572-2.00005-4
109

Background

M-proteins

M-proteins are immunoglobulins produced in excess by an abnormal clonal proliferation of B-lymphocytes or plasma cells.[1] This M-protein is characteristic for a group of disorders variously called monoclonal gammopathies, paraproteinaemias, or plasma cell dyscrasias. These disorders comprise a spectrum of premalignant and malignant hematological conditions, such as monoclonal gammopathy of undetermined significance (MGUS), lymphoplasmacytic lymphoma (LPL)/Waldenström macroglobulinemia (WM), multiple myeloma (MM), cryoglobulinemia, lymphoma, amyloidosis, and POEMS (polyneuropathy, organomegaly, endocrinopathy, M-protein, and skin manifestations) syndrome.[1]

The most common monoclonal gammopathy is the premalignant condition MGUS, accounting for two-thirds of M-proteins.[2] The term MGUS was coined by Robert Kyle in 1978 after the observation that asymptomatic patients with an M-protein had a higher risk of developing LPL/WM, MM, and amyloidosis, which are progressive conditions with a potentially fatal outcome.[3] Although the term MGUS might indicate that the patient is asymptomatic, MGUS can be accompanied by neuropathy or nephropathy.[4] The diagnosis MGUS requires the absence of hypercalcaemia, renal failure, anemia, and bone lesions (referred to as CRAB features) that could be caused by an underlying malignant monoclonal gammopathy.[5] One does not know at the time of diagnosis whether the M-protein will remain stable and benign or will develop into a symptomatic malignant variant.[2]

MGUS can be classified into two major biological subtypes, IgM and non-IgM, because of the difference in the clonal cell that is involved and the nature of progression between these two types.[6] IgM-MGUS typically arises from a CD20 + lymphoplasmacytic cell that has not undergone switch recombination, and this disease type is associated with a risk of progression to LPL or WM. In contrast, non-IgM MGUS typically arises from mature plasma cells that have undergone switch recombination and is associated with a risk of progression to multiple myeloma. Both disease types can progress to amyloidosis.[6]

M-proteins and neuropathy

Neuropathies can occur in patients across the spectrum of monoclonal gammopathies.[7,8] The mere presence of an M-protein in a patient with neuropathy does not immediately imply a causal relationship. In fact, the association is most often coincidental, simply reflecting the relatively high prevalence of both the M-protein and neuropathy in the general population.[8] However, a causal relation is considered between the IgM subclass of the M-protein and neuropathy, with approximately 30%–60% of neuropathies associated with M-proteins being IgM related.[2,9] This disease is named IgM M-protein associated neuropathy.

Not only does the causality between the M-protein and neuropathy separate IgM M-protein associated neuropathy from IgG or IgA neuropathies, but there are also clinical, pathological, and immunological differences.[10]

IgM M-protein associated neuropathy presents in general as a slowly progressive, symmetric, predominantly sensory ataxic neuropathy with relatively mild or no weakness.[11] This so-called "classical phenotype" is also the phenotype most strongly associated with IgM antibodies to myelin-associated glycoprotein (anti-MAG, see Section "Pathophysiology"). In contrast, non-IgM monoclonal proteins can be seen in the full spectrum of neuropathy phenotypes, including both demyelinating and axonal neuropathies. Approximately 50%–60% of patients with IgM M-protein associated neuropathy have high titers of IgM anti-MAG antibodies or other antibodies such as anti-GM1, anti-GM2, anti-GQ1b, anti-GD1a, or anti-GD1b.[12]

Epidemiology

Monoclonal gammopathies are relatively common in the general population, occurring in 3%–4% in people over 50 years of age.[13] The prevalence increases with age, as indicated by a prevalence of 5.3% in people over 70 years, 10% in people over 80 years, and 14% in people over 90 years. The disease is more common in men than in women.[13–15]

The prevalence of neuropathy rises with age as well, reaching up to 8% of people over 60 years of age.[15] Given the high prevalence of both MGUS and neuropathy at a higher age, neuropathies associated with an M-protein are frequently encountered in clinical practice, affecting predominantly elderly patients.[8] In patients with neuropathy, an M-protein can be detected in approximately 3%–5% of patients, especially when they are referred to a tertiary care center.[8,16] Among patients with peripheral neuropathy, in whom no cause is apparent, the prevalence of an M-protein may be as high as 10%.[15,16]

Etiology

Life style/environmental exposure

No lifestyle or environmental exposure factors have been identified that are consistently linked to either an increased risk of MGUS or MM or the transition between the two.[17] There is emerging evidence to support a role for autoimmunity, infections, and inflammation in the etiology of MGUS and MM. Potentially, immune-mediated conditions might act as triggers for MGUS and MM development.[18]

Genetics

The genetics of IgM M-protein associated neuropathy are largely unknown. Familial occurrence of monoclonal gammopathy and neuropathy has only been described in case reports.[19–21] Busis et al.[20] described the occurrence of monoclonal gammopathy and neuropathy in a mother and son. However, these investigators could not definitely rule out hereditary motor and sensory neuropathy (HMSN). Manschot et al.[19] described three pairs of first-degree relatives with monoclonal gammopathy and neuropathy. They concluded that if there is a familial history of neuropathy and HMSN type 1 can be ruled out as a cause, it is important to search for the presence of a monoclonal gammopathy.

Familial clustering of MGUS, WM/LPL, and MM has also been described in case reports.[10,18,22–25] Lynch et al.[23] studied a family that comprised a sibship of seven persons of whom three siblings had MM and two siblings had MGUS. Fine et al.[24] described three out of five siblings that were diagnosed with WM, with two of them developing WM after having first been diagnosed with MGUS. Population-based studies have found excess risk for MGUS among first-degree relatives of MM or LPL/WM patients,[26] and a three-fold increased risk of MGUS and a four-fold increased risk of LPL/WM among first-degree relatives of MGUS patients.[18] These observations suggest the potential significance of inherited genetic factors in MGUS and malignant forms of monoclonal gammopathies.

Mutations in the MYD88 (L265P) gene are often present in patients with WM, and also occur in approximately 50% of patients with IgM MGUS.[27,28] Patients with this mutation have significantly higher levels of IgM compared to patients with wild-type MYD88 (L265P).[27] Furthermore, patients with MGUS and neuropathy with the MYD88 (L265P) mutation have a shorter time to progression to WM than those with the wild-type genotype.[28]

Malignant transformation

In general, MGUS is associated with a 0.5%–1.5% per year risk of progression to related malignancies and the risk of malignant transformation persists even after 30 years of follow-up.[29–33] The mechanisms that underlie the transition are not yet well understood and there are no reliable biologic markers that are able to predict which individual with MGUS will progress to a malignancy. In the absence of such markers, MGUS is currently risk stratified based on clinical variables identified through epidemiological studies.[29]

The most important independent prognostic factor for malignant transformation in patients with MGUS without neuropathy is the M-protein level.[34,35] Other prognostic factors are an M-protein of the IgA or IgM isotype, the abnormal serum free light chain (FLC) ratio, an increase of M-protein level during follow up, light-chain proteinuria, age over 70 years, and kappa light chain.[36–40]

Malignant transformation in patients with MGUS and neuropathy might be even higher, as Eurelings et al.[41] described a 2.7% risk per year in a prospective study of 193 patients with neuropathy and associated monoclonal gammopathy. They also described unexplained weight loss, rapid progression of neuropathy, unexplained fever or night sweats, and the M-protein level as independent predictors of malignant transformation.

Pathophysiology

The exact pathophysiology of IgM M-protein associated neuropathy is not well understood. As discussed earlier, there is a known coexistence between neuropathy and monoclonal gammopathy. Furthermore, there is strong evidence for a pathogenic role of IgM antibodies in neuropathy development.[42] However, when no antibodies are found, a relationship between M-protein and the neuropathy is debatable.

IgM anti-MAG antibodies

Monoclonal IgM antibodies can target specific antigens expressed in nerves, such as antimyelin associated glycoprotein (MAG).[43–45] MAG is a transmembrane glycoprotein selectively localized in the periaxonal membranes of Schwann cells, where it is important for normal formation and maintenance of myelinated axons.[46–48] About 50%–60% of patients with IgM M-protein associated neuropathy have antibodies against MAG, the so-called anti-MAG antibodies.[12] That anti-MAG antibodies have the capacity to cause demyelination was first shown by intraneural injection of serum from three patients with IgM M-protein associated neuropathy with anti-MAG antibodies in cats.[49,50] However, the pathology bears little resemblance to that seen in human neuropathy.[50] Sural nerve biopsies from patients with IgM M-protein associated neuropathy demonstrate deposits of IgM and complement on myelin sheaths as well as widening of myelin lamellae, indicating their role in demyelination.[51–53] There is also a correlation between the IgM anti-MAG penetration into myelinated fibers and the extent of widening.[52,54] The suggested pathogenic mechanism is that monoclonal antibodies react with nerve sheath components, leading to complement activation and resulting in myelin damage.

Although the presence of IgM anti-MAG antibodies is significantly associated with neuropathy, the correlation between IgM anti-MAG titers and neuropathy severity is debated. The severity of the neuropathy does not always correlate with serum antibody levels and only some uncontrolled studies treating small numbers of patients with rituximab or cytostatics suggest that the decrease of IgM anti-MAG titers is associated with a decrease of neuropathy severity.[55,56]

IgM antiganglioside antibodies

IgM antibodies against gangliosides, specifically glycolipids on the nerve cell surface such as GM1, GM2, GD1a, GD1b, and GQ1b, have been found in patients without anti-MAG antibodies.[57] Stork et al.[58] detected IgM antibodies against gangliosides in sera from 28% of patients with IgM M-protein associated neuropathy without anti-MAG antibodies. Eurelings et al.[57] showed that the antiganglioside reactivity was significantly associated with a demyelinating neuropathy and an IgM monoclonal gammopathy. Furthermore, IgM anti-GQ1b antibodies were specifically reported in patients with chronic, predominantly sensory neuropathy and a monoclonal gammopathy.[59] Willison et al.[45] described a syndrome associated with antidisialosyl IgM antibodies. The clinical picture comprises a chronic neuropathy with marked sensory ataxia and areflexia, and with relatively preserved motor function in the limbs. In addition, motor weakness affecting the oculomotor and bulbar muscles is often present. When present altogether, these clinical features have been described previously under the acronym CANOMAD: chronic ataxic neuropathy, ophthalmoplegia, IgM paraprotein, cold agglutinins, and disialosyl antibodies.

Antiganglioside antibodies may play a role in the pathogenesis of IgM M-protein associated neuropathy; however, the specific mechanism is yet unknown. There is convincing evidence that antiganglioside antibodies play a role in the pathogenesis of inflammatory neuropathies because antiganglioside IgM, IgA, and IgG antibodies are associated with acute axonal forms of Guillain-Barre syndrome, Miller Fisher syndrome, and multifocal motor neuropathy (MMN).[45,60–62]

Clinical spectrum

The most frequently described phenotype of IgM M-protein associated neuropathy includes a slowly progressive, symmetric, predominantly sensory ataxic neuropathy with relatively mild or no weakness. This is also the phenotype most strongly associated with the presence of IgM anti-MAG antibodies.[11]

The first symptoms patients experience are mostly slowly progressive distal paraesthesiae prominent in the feet and/or impaired balance. The disease can further lead to impaired proprioception, pseudoathetosis, sensory ataxia, tremors, unsteady gait, and a varying degree of distal muscle weakness.[63–66] Also, pain in hands and/or feet was reported by 80% of subjects, with the most common subtype being paraesthesiae and dysaesthesiae (70%). Cramps were reported in > 60% of patients.[67] Deep tendon reflexes are absent in the majority of patients and the cranial nerves and autonomic functions are usually spared.[68]

Prominent tremor and ataxia have been emphasized as particular features in IgM M-protein associated neuropathy, especially in patients with anti-MAG antibodies.[9,69–71] A tremor is reported to occur in about 30%–90% of patients.[65,66,71–74] This tremor is generally coarse, irregular, and unrelated to proprioception loss, muscle weakness, fatigue, or a coexisting cerebellar disease.[63,71] Both a more severe neuropathy as well as peripheral demyelination are associated with the higher occurrence of a tremor while increasing age is not associated with tremor occurrence.[74] There is no relationship between tremor and weakness or sensory loss.[73]

Not only is the clinical spectrum of IgM M-protein associated neuropathy highly variable, but so is the extent to which patients experience limitations. Whereas some patients may only have minor distal paraesthaesiae, not interfering with their daily activities, others may suffer from a variable combination of sensory ataxia, impaired gait, and/or distal weakness, experiencing major difficulties and restrictions in their activities of daily living.[63] Disability rates vary between 22% and 42% after around 10 years of neuropathy.[73,75,76] The risk of disability is highest when there is a demyelinating neuropathy because these patients showed more severe sensory disturbances and muscle weakness than those with axonal neuropathy.[65]

Whether patients with IgM anti-MAG antibodies represent a separate clinical subgroup is still highly debatable. Gorson and Ropper[64] noted that anti-MAG antibodies occurred more often in demyelinating than in axonal neuropathy. Pestronk et al.[77] also determined that patients with anti-MAG antibodies had predominantly demyelinating features on physiologic testing compared to patients without antibodies. Both studies supported the notion that anti-MAG antibodies may be relatively specific for demyelinating neuropathies.[64] In line with these results, Maisonobe et al.[78] noted that the length-dependent demyelinating neuropathy was significantly more prominent in patients with anti-MAG antibodies compared to patients without anti-MAG antibodies. On the other hand, Notermans et al.[75] found no physiologic differences between patients with and without anti-MAG antibodies. Simovic et al.[79] were similarly unable to determine significant clinical features separating the two. Additionally, Svahn et al.[80] recently found that the clinical spectrum showed no significant differences between low, medium, or high anti-MAG antibody titers. To date, the importance of anti-MAG antibodies as clinical markers distinguishing patients with IgM M-protein associated neuropathy remains unproven.

Diagnostics

When diagnosing IgM M-protein associated neuropathy, it is of importance to estimate the probability of causality between the IgM M-protein and the neuropathy. The joint taskforce of the European Federation of Neurological Societies (EFNS) and the Peripheral Nerve Society (PNS)[11] developed guidelines to help determine the causal relationship between M-proteins and neuropathy. Based on these guidelines, we have developed three categories of possible causality between the IgM M-protein and the neuropathy: highly probable, probable, and possible (see Table 1).

In order to investigate the possibility of a causal relationship, first determine whether there are no other causes for the neuropathy other than the detected M-protein. Causes such as diabetes mellitus, alcohol abuse, chronic renal insufficiency, medication, genetics, etc., should be excluded by extensive laboratory investigation.[81] Then determine whether there are features to

TABLE 1 Causal relationship between IgM M-proteins and neuropathy.[11]

Highly probable

- IgM M-protein (MGUS or Waldenström's), **and**
- Titers of IgM anti-MAG antibodies

Supportive features are:

   o Distal demyelinating polyneuropathy
   o Nerve biopsy showing IgM or complement deposits on myelin, or widely spaced myelin on electron microscopy

Probable

- IgM M-protein (MGUS or Waldenström's), **and**
- Titers of IgM antibodies to other neural antigens (GM1, GM2, GD1a, GD1b), **and**
- Slowly progressive predominantly distal symmetrical sensory neuropathy

Possible

- IgM M-protein (MGUS), **and**
- Polyneuropathy
- **Without** titers of IgM antibodies to neural antigens

MAG, myelin associated glycoprotein; *MGUS*, monoclonal gammopathy of undetermined significance.

support the diagnosis of IgM M-protein associated neuropathy. Fig. 1 shows a flowchart of the work-up of patients with suspected IgM M-protein associated neuropathy and specific clues for which to look. As the clinical picture was discussed above, we will discuss the different components of the diagnostic process separately below.

M-protein detection

Serum protein electrophoresis should be done for any patient with a peripheral neuropathy of unknown cause.[2] Immunofixation should be used to confirm the presence of an M-protein and to distinguish the immunoglobulin type and its light chain class. Immunofixation is a more sensitive method than immunoelectrophoresis when searching for a small monoclonal immunoglobulin or light chain in the serum.[2] Analysis of urine to search for an M-protein is also essential for patients with monoclonal gammopathies.[2]

Diagnostics of antibodies

Testing for antibodies to MAG should be considered in all patients with an IgM M-protein and a neuropathy.[82] If negative, then testing for IgM antibodies against antigangliosides, including GQ1b, GM1, GM2, GD1a, and GD1b,

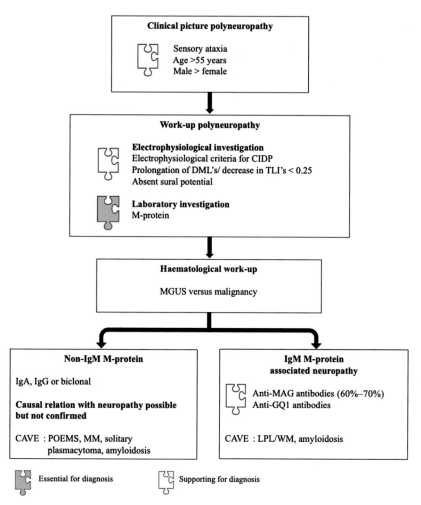

FIG. 1 Work-up of IgM M-protein associated neuropathy. *DML*, distal motor latency; *CIDP*, chronic inflammatory demyelinating polyneuropathy; *LPL*, lymphoplasmacytic lymphoma; *MAG*, myelin associated glycoprotein; *MGUS*, monoclonal gammopathy of undetermined significance; *MM*, multiple myeloma; *POEMS*, polyneuropathy, organomegaly, endocrinopathy, M-protein, and skin manifestations; *TLI*, terminal latency index; and *WM*, Waldenström's macroglobulinemia.

should be considered. The presence of these antibodies increases the probability, but does not prove, a pathogenic link between the IgM M-protein and the neuropathy.[11]

An enzyme-linked immunosorbent essay (ELISA) is the principal method for detecting autoantibodies.[83] Kuijf et al.[84] investigated the detection of serum antibodies to MAG in patients with demyelinating neuropathy and IgM monoclonal gammopathy using ELISA. Their findings suggested that ELISA is more sensitive than western blot (WB) for identifying patients with an anti-MAG-related neuropathy and should at least be used as a first screening method in the clinical workup of patients with chronic demyelinating neuropathy and an IgM M-protein.

Nerve conduction studies

There is considerable evidence indicating that IgM M-protein associated neuropathy is primarily demyelinating.[9,85] Patients with IgM M-protein associated neuropathy meeting the definite electrophysiological criteria for chronic inflammatory demyelinating polyneuropathy (CIDP) have a high probability of a relation between the IgM M-protein and the neuropathy.[11] IgM M-protein associated neuropathy distinguishes itself from CIDP as it is assumed to be a length-dependent process and there are some electrophysiological length dependency features for which to look.[86–88] Typical features comprise: (1) uniform symmetrical reduction of conduction velocities, with more severe sensory than motor involvement; (2) disproportionately prolonged distal motor latency (DML), which may be quantified as the terminal latency index (TLI) [ratio of distal distance/motor conduction velocity × distal motor latency] ≤ 0.25; (3) absent sural potential (i.e., less likely to have the "abnormal median, normal sural" sensory action potential pattern); and (4) partial motor conduction block and marked distal compound muscle action potential (CMAP) dispersion are very rare.[11,89,90]

However, not all patients with an IgM M-protein and a neuropathy will have demyelination. In a prospective study of 15 patients with an IgM M-protein associated neuropathy by Notermans et al.[75] three had findings consistent with demyelination, four with pure axonal degeneration, and eight with both. Ponsford et al.[66] described 24 patients with an IgM M-protein associated neuropathy after long-term follow-up where two had a pure axonal neuropathy and the other 22 had a predominantly demyelinating neuropathy. This suggests that there might be a subset of patients with electrophysiological distinguishing features from the primarily demyelinating variant. This heterogeneity of electrophysiological features may also reflect different pathogenic mechanisms of the axonal neuropathy in patients with the IgM M-protein.[64] To date, we are still questioning whether IgM M-protein associated neuropathy might be one distinct disease or whether there are several syndromes.

Hematological evaluation

When diagnosing IgM M-protein associated neuropathy, one of the main goals is to ensure that the gammopathy is MGUS and not a sign of an underlying malignant gammopathy. The hematologist will look for signs of malignancy by performing a physical examination looking for peripheral lymphadenopathy, hepatosplenomegaly, macroglossia, and signs of POEMS syndrome.

Furthermore, an extensive laboratory examination will be performed including full blood count, renal and liver function, calcium, phosphate, erythrocyte sedimentation rate, C-reactive protein, uric acid, beta 2-microglobulin, lactate dehydrogenase, rheumatoid factor, serum cryoglobulins, and vascular endothelial growth factor level (VEGF-level).[11,91] A radiographic x-ray skeletal survey or CT will usually not be performed to look for lytic or sclerotic bone lesions because this is more common in IgG/IgA M-proteins. A bone marrow examination should be considered for every patient with an IgM MGUS because even low M-protein levels could indicate a malignancy.[11,92]

Therapy

Treatment

Treatment choices are influenced by the burden of the disease and evidence for benefit and cost.[93] Treatment in IgM M-protein associated neuropathy is preferably started when there is measurable progressive disease causing disability in combination with relatively short disease duration (preferably <2 years from onset) or rapid progression of the neuropathy; the decision to treat is often made on a case-by-case judgment.

Through the years, many different therapeutic options have been investigated, such as intravenous immunoglobulin (IVIg),[94–96] interferon alfa-2a,[96,97] plasma exchange,[98,99] rituximab,[100–105] corticosteroids,[106] chemotherapeutic (or cytotoxic) therapies,[98] and cyclophosphamide and prednisolone combination.[107] Lunn and Nobile-Orazio have analyzed the evidence for therapeutic options in IgM anti-MAG associated neuropathy.[108,109] They concluded that the eight published randomized controlled trials of immunotherapy in IgM M-protein associated neuropathy were all either too small, too short, or too flawed to draw confident conclusions about the efficacy of individual treatments or comparisons between them. There is low-quality evidence that rituximab is of benefit in stabilizing or improving IgM anti-MAG associated neuropathy.[109] The statistically significant short-term benefit from IVIg may not be clinically relevant. In patients having significant or progressive disability associated with an IgM M-protein associated neuropathy, immunosuppressive or immunomodulatory treatment may be considered as an alternative to rituximab, depending on availability, comorbidity, and patient preference.[108]

Even though strong evidence for therapeutic options is lacking, some of these treatments clearly have positive results in individual patients, emphasizing the shortcomings in study designs of previous studies.

Outcome measures

Through platforms such as the Inflammatory Neuropathy Cause and Treatment (INCAT) group and the Peripheral Neuropathy Outcome Measures

Standardization (PeriNomS) group for inflammatory neuropathies, major shortcomings in study designs and outcome measures in clinical studies of inflammatory neuropathies have been exposed.[110–112] The longstanding commitment of these group members has resulted in an international consensus for most inflammatory neuropathies at the various levels of assessing outcome.[112] IgM M-protein associated neuropathy is an exception. Because this is a rarer and more indolent disease, previous attempts did not succeed in collecting a large cohort of patients that could be observed over a longer period of time.

In brief, outcome measures should be at the interval or ratio level because their level of assessment precision is higher than those of the nominal and ordinal level. Nominal and ordinal outcome measures provide a description of the observed quality of interest and have no numerical values.[113,114] Therefore, calculated sum scores will not be linear and cannot be analyzed using parametric methods. Interval and ratio outcome measures, on the other hand, do have a "fixed" numerical value and therefore sum scores can be calculated and analyzed using parametric testing.[113] Inappropriate analyses of generated summed scores of multiitem ordinal outcome measures may lead to false-negative or false-positive results in randomized controlled trials. This might, in both cases, expose patients to unnecessary and potentially serious risks.[115] Rasch analyses can be used to transform an ordinal outcome measure into a linear interval outcome measure, as long as the data fit Rasch model expectations.[116,117] Also, clinimetric aspects such as being simple, valid, reliable, and particularly responsive are important in creating outcome measures.[116,118,119] The latter is pivotal to capture relevant changes over time.

None of the clinical trials in IgM M-protein associated neuropathy has led to a significantly positive treatment effect.[108,120] This lack of significant effect can be assigned to multiple factors and ultimately results in the lack of international consensus on how to assess and treat patients. Most of the problems relate to flawed study designs, including short follow-up periods (despite the indolent disease course), examining a relatively low number of patients, adopting treatment dosages that might not be aggressive enough, differences in the definition of a "responder," and the use of inappropriate, often ordinal, and nonresponsive outcome measures.[120] Also, problems can arise from the choice for outcome measures that are of little relevance to the patient, for example improved electrophysiological nerve conduction may not reflect reduced disability for the patient.[93]

The IMAGiNe study is currently being carried out. It is a collaborative effort in creating an IgM M-protein associated neuropathy registry.[93] The main aim is to create a unique cohort of prospectively collected and highly standardized clinical data of a large group of well-defined patients with IgM M-protein associated neuropathy. Also, an IgM-specific outcome measure at the activity and participation level is under construction.

References

1. Rison RA, Beydoun SR. Paraproteinemic neuropathy: a practical review. *BMC Neurol.* 2016;16:13.
2. Kyle RA, Dyck PJ. Neuropathy associated with the monoclonal gammopathies. In: *Peripheral Neuropathy.* 4th ed.Philadelphia: Elsevier Saunders; 2005:2255–2276.
3. Thomsen H, Campo C, Weinhold N, et al. Genomewide association study on monoclonal gammopathy of unknown significance (MGUS). *Eur J Haematol.* 2017;99(1):70–79.
4. Leung N, Bridoux F, Hutchison CA, et al. Monoclonal gammopathy of renal significance: when MGUS is no longer undetermined or insignificant. *Blood.* 2012;120(22):4292–4295.
5. Rajkumar SV, Dimopoulos MA, Palumbo A, et al. International myeloma working group updated criteria for the diagnosis of multiple myeloma. *Lancet Oncol.* 2014;15(12):e538–e548.
6. Kyle RA, Larson DR, Therneau TM, et al. Long-term follow-up of monoclonal gammopathy of undetermined significance. *N Engl J Med.* 2018;378(3):241–249.
7. Levine T, Pestronk A, Florence J, et al. Peripheral neuropathies in Waldenstrom's macroglobulinaemia. *J Neurol Neurosurg Psychiatry.* 2006;77(2):224–228.
8. Chaudhry HM, Mauermann ML, Rajkumar SV. Monoclonal gammopathy-associated peripheral neuropathy: diagnosis and management. *Mayo Clin Proc.* 2017;92(5):838–850.
9. Yeung KB, Thomas PK, King RH, et al. The clinical spectrum of peripheral neuropathies associated with benign monoclonal IgM, IgG and IgA paraproteinaemia. Comparative clinical, immunological and nerve biopsy findings. *J Neurol.* 1991;238(7):383–391.
10. Lynch HT, Watson P, Tarantolo S, et al. Phenotypic heterogeneity in multiple myeloma families. *J Clin Oncol.* 2005;23(4):685–693.
11. Joint Task Force of the EFNS and the PNS. European Federation of Neurological Societies/Peripheral Nerve Society Guideline on management of paraproteinemic demyelinating neuropathies. Report of a Joint Task Force of the European Federation of Neurological Societies and the Peripheral Nerve Society – first revision. *J Peripher Nerv Syst.* 2010;15(3): 185–195.
12. Nobile-Orazio E, Manfredini E, Carpo M, et al. Frequency and clinical correlates of antineural IgM antibodies in neuropathy associated with IgM monoclonal gammopathy. *Ann Neurol.* 1994;36(3):416–424.
13. Kyle RA, Therneau TM, Rajkumar SV, et al. Prevalence of monoclonal gammopathy of undetermined significance. *N Engl J Med.* 2006;354(13):1362–1369.
14. Crawford J, Eye MK, Cohen HJ. Evaluation of monoclonal gammopathies in the "well" elderly. *Am J Med.* 1987;82(1):39–45.
15. Martyn CN, Hughes RA. Epidemiology of peripheral neuropathy. *J Neurol Neurosurg Psychiatry.* 1997;62(4):310–318.
16. Kelly Jr JJ, Kyle RA, O'Brien PC, Dyck PJ. Prevalence of monoclonal protein in peripheral neuropathy. *Neurology.* 1981;31(11):1480–1483.
17. Weinhold N, Johnson DC, Rawstron AC, et al. Inherited genetic susceptibility to monoclonal gammopathy of unknown significance. *Blood.* 2014;123(16):2513–2517 [quiz 2593].
18. Landgren O, Kristinsson SY, Goldin LR, et al. Risk of plasma cell and lymphoproliferative disorders among 14621 first-degree relatives of 4458 patients with monoclonal gammopathy of undetermined significance in Sweden. *Blood.* 2009;114(4):791–795.
19. Manschot SM, Notermans NC, van den Berg LH, Verschuuren JJ, Lokhorst HM. Three families with polyneuropathy associated with monoclonal gammopathy. *Arch Neurol.* 2000;57(5):740–742.

20. Busis NA, Halperin JJ, Stefansson K, et al. Peripheral neuropathy, high serum IgM, and paraproteinemia in mother and son. *Neurology.* 1985;35(5):679–683.

21. Grant JA, Blumenschein GR, Buckley 3rd CE. Familial paraproteinemia. *Arch Intern Med.* 1971;128(3):427–431.

22. Bizzaro N, Pasini P. Familial occurrence of multiple myeloma and monoclonal gammopathy of undetermined significance in 5 siblings. *Haematologica.* 1990;75(1):58–63.

23. Lynch HT, Sanger WG, Pirruccello S, Quinn-Laquer B, Weisenburger DD. Familial multiple myeloma: a family study and review of the literature. *J Natl Cancer Inst.* 2001;93(19): 1479–1483.

24. Fine JM, Lambin P, Massari M, Leroux P. Malignant evolution of asymptomatic monoclonal IgM after seven and fifteen years in two siblings of a patient with Waldenstrom's macroglobulinemia. *Acta Med Scand.* 1982;211(3):237–239.

25. Treon SP, Hunter ZR, Aggarwal A, et al. Characterization of familial Waldenstrom's macroglobulinemia. *Ann Oncol.* 2006;17(3):488–494.

26. Kristinsson SY, Bjorkholm M, Goldin LR, McMaster ML, Turesson I, Landgren O. Risk of lymphoproliferative disorders among first-degree relatives of lymphoplasmacytic lymphoma/Waldenstrom macroglobulinemia patients: a population-based study in Sweden. *Blood.* 2008;112(8):3052–3056.

27. Varettoni M, Arcaini L, Zibellini S, et al. Prevalence and clinical significance of the MYD88 (L265P) somatic mutation in Waldenstrom's macroglobulinemia and related lymphoid neoplasms. *Blood.* 2013;121(13):2522–2528.

28. Correa JG, Cibeira MT, Tovar N, et al. Prevalence and prognosis implication of MYD88 L265P mutation in IgM monoclonal gammopathy of undetermined significance and smouldering Waldenstrom macroglobulinaemia. *Br J Haematol.* 2017;179(5):849–851.

29. Merlini G, Palladini G. Differential diagnosis of monoclonal gammopathy of undetermined significance. *Hematology Am Soc Hematol Educ Program.* 2012;2012:595–603.

30. Cesana C, Klersy C, Barbarano L, et al. Prognostic factors for malignant transformation in monoclonal gammopathy of undetermined significance and smoldering multiple myeloma. *J Clin Oncol.* 2002;20(6):1625–1634.

31. Kyle RA, Rajkumar SV. Epidemiology of the plasma-cell disorders. *Best Pract Res Clin Haematol.* 2007;20(4):637–664.

32. Turesson I, Kovalchik SA, Pfeiffer RM, et al. Monoclonal gammopathy of undetermined significance and risk of lymphoid and myeloid malignancies: 728 cases followed up to 30 years in Sweden. *Blood.* 2014;123(3):338–345.

33. Kyle RA, Therneau TM, Rajkumar SV, Larson DR, Plevak MF, Melton 3rd LJ. Long-term follow-up of 241 patients with monoclonal gammopathy of undetermined significance: the original Mayo Clinic series 25 years later. *Mayo Clin Proc.* 2004;79(7):859–866.

34. Kyle RA, Therneau TM, Rajkumar SV, et al. A long-term study of prognosis in monoclonal gammopathy of undetermined significance. *N Engl J Med.* 2002;346(8):564–569.

35. Kyle RA, Therneau TM, Rajkumar SV, et al. Long-term follow-up of IgM monoclonal gammopathy of undetermined significance. *Blood.* 2003;102(10):3759–3764.

36. Rajkumar SV, Kyle RA, Therneau TM, et al. Serum free light chain ratio is an independent risk factor for progression in monoclonal gammopathy of undetermined significance. *Blood.* 2005;106(3):812–817.

37. Blade J, Lopez-Guillermo A, Rozman C, et al. Malignant transformation and life expectancy in monoclonal gammopathy of undetermined significance. *Br J Haematol.* 1992;81(3): 391–394.

38. Baldini L, Guffanti A, Cesana BM, et al. Role of different hematologic variables in defining the risk of malignant transformation in monoclonal gammopathy. *Blood.* 1996;87(3):912–918.

39. Vuckovic J, Ilic A, Knezevic N, Marinkovic M, Zemunik T, Dubravcic M. Prognosis in monoclonal gammopathy of undetermined significance. *Br J Haematol.* 1997;97(3):649–651.

40. van de Poel MH, Coebergh JW, Hillen HF. Malignant transformation of monoclonal gammopathy of undetermined significance among out-patients of a community hospital in southeastern Netherlands. *Br J Haematol.* 1995;91(1):121–125.

41. Eurelings M, Lokhorst HM, Kalmijn S, Wokke JH, Notermans NC. Malignant transformation in polyneuropathy associated with monoclonal gammopathy. *Neurology.* 2005;64(12):2079–2084.

42. Notermans NC. Monoclonal gammopathy and neuropathy. *Curr Opin Neurol.* 1996;9(5):334–337.

43. Latov N, Braun PE, Gross RB, Sherman WH, Penn AS, Chess L. Plasma cell dyscrasia and peripheral neuropathy: identification of the myelin antigens that react with human paraproteins. *Proc Natl Acad Sci U S A.* 1981;78(11):7139–7142.

44. Braun PE, Frail DE, Latov N. Myelin-associated glycoprotein is the antigen for a monoclonal IgM in polyneuropathy. *J Neurochem.* 1982;39(5):1261–1265.

45. Willison HJ, O'Leary CP, Veitch J, et al. The clinical and laboratory features of chronic sensory ataxic neuropathy with anti-disialosyl IgM antibodies. *Brain.* 2001;124(Pt 10):1968–1977.

46. Quarles RH. Myelin-associated glycoprotein (MAG): past, present and beyond. *J Neurochem.* 2007;100(6):1431–1448.

47. Willison HJ, Yuki N. Peripheral neuropathies and anti-glycolipid antibodies. *Brain.* 2002;125(Pt 12):2591–2625.

48. Quarles RH, Weiss MD. Autoantibodies associated with peripheral neuropathy. *Muscle Nerve.* 1999;22(7):800–822.

49. Hays AP, Latov N, Takatsu M, Sherman WH. Experimental demyelination of nerve induced by serum of patients with neuropathy and an anti-MAG IgM M-protein. *Neurology.* 1987;37(2):242–256.

50. Willison HJ, Trapp BD, Bacher JD, Dalakas MC, Griffin JW, Quarles RH. Demyelination induced by intraneural injection of human antimyelin-associated glycoprotein antibodies. *Muscle Nerve.* 1988;11(11):1169–1176.

51. Hays AP, Lee SS, Latov N. Immune reactive C3d on the surface of myelin sheaths in neuropathy. *J Neuroimmunol.* 1988;18(3):231–244.

52. Ritz MF, Erne B, Ferracin F, Vital A, Vital C, Steck AJ. Anti-MAG IgM penetration into myelinated fibers correlates with the extent of myelin widening. *Muscle Nerve.* 1999;22(8):1030–1037.

53. Takatsu M, Hays AP, Latov N, et al. Immunofluorescence study of patients with neuropathy and IgM M proteins. *Ann Neurol.* 1985;18(2):173–181.

54. Vital C, Vital A, Deminiere C, Julien J, Lagueny A, Steck AJ. Myelin modifications in 8 cases of peripheral neuropathy with Waldenstrom's macroglobulinemia and anti-MAG activity. *Ultrastruct Pathol.* 1997;21(6):509–516.

55. Renaud S, Fuhr P, Gregor M, et al. High-dose rituximab and anti-MAG-associated polyneuropathy. *Neurology.* 2006;66(5):742–744.

56. Nobile-Orazio E, Baldini L, Barbieri S, et al. Treatment of patients with neuropathy and anti-MAG IgM M-proteins. *Ann Neurol.* 1988;24(1):93–97.

57. Eurelings M, Ang CW, Notermans NC, Van Doorn PA, Jacobs BC, Van den Berg LH. Antiganglioside antibodies in polyneuropathy associated with monoclonal gammopathy. *Neurology.* 2001;57(10):1909–1912.

58. Stork AC, Jacobs BC, Tio-Gillen AP, et al. Prevalence, specificity and functionality of anti-ganglioside antibodies in neuropathy associated with IgM monoclonal gammopathy. *J Neuroimmunol*. 2014;268(1–2):89–94.

59. Carpo M, Pedotti R, Lolli F, et al. Clinical correlate and fine specificity of anti-GQ1b antibodies in peripheral neuropathy. *J Neurol Sci*. 1998;155(2):186–191.

60. Nobile-Orazio E, Giannotta C, Briani C. Anti-ganglioside complex IgM antibodies in multifocal motor neuropathy and chronic immune-mediated neuropathies. *J Neuroimmunol*. 2010;219(1–2):119–122.

61. Kaida K, Kanzaki M, Morita D, et al. Anti-ganglioside complex antibodies in Miller Fisher syndrome. *J Neurol Neurosurg Psychiatry*. 2006;77(9):1043–1046.

62. Kaida K, Morita D, Kanzaki M, et al. Anti-ganglioside complex antibodies associated with severe disability in GBS. *J Neuroimmunol*. 2007;182(1–2):212–218.

63. Dalakas MC. Advances in the diagnosis, immunopathogenesis and therapies of IgM-anti-MAG antibody-mediated neuropathies. *Ther Adv Neurol Disord*. 2018;11. 1756285617746640.

64. Gorson KC, Ropper AH. Axonal neuropathy associated with monoclonal gammopathy of undetermined significance. *J Neurol Neurosurg Psychiatry*. 1997;63(2):163–168.

65. Niermeijer JM, Fischer K, Eurelings M, Franssen H, Wokke JH, Notermans NC. Prognosis of polyneuropathy due to IgM monoclonal gammopathy: a prospective cohort study. *Neurology*. 2010;74(5):406–412.

66. Ponsford S, Willison H, Veitch J, Morris R, Thomas PK. Long-term clinical and neurophysiological follow-up of patients with peripheral, neuropathy associated with benign monoclonal gammopathy. *Muscle Nerve*. 2000;23(2):164–174.

67. Rajabally YA, Delmont E, Hiew FL, et al. Prevalence, correlates and impact of pain and cramps in anti-MAG neuropathy: a multicentre European study. *Eur J Neurol*. 2018;25(1):135–141.

68. Gorson KC. Clinical features, evaluation, and treatment of patients with polyneuropathy associated with monoclonal gammopathy of undetermined significance (MGUS). *J Clin Apher*. 1999;14(3):149–153.

69. Smith IS, Kahn SN, Lacey BW, et al. Chronic demyelinating neuropathy associated with benign IgM paraproteinaemia. *Brain*. 1983;106(Pt 1):169–195.

70. Kelly Jr JJ. Polyneuropathies associated with plasma cell dyscrasias. *Semin Neurol*. 1987;7(1):30–39.

71. Dalakas MC, Teravainen H, Engel WK. Tremor as a feature of chronic relapsing and dysgammaglobulinemic polyneuropathies. Incidence and management. *Arch Neurol*. 1984;41(7): 711–714.

72. Bain PG, Britton TC, Jenkins IH, et al. Tremor associated with benign IgM paraproteinaemic neuropathy. *Brain*. 1996;119(Pt 3):789–799.

73. Smith IS. The natural history of chronic demyelinating neuropathy associated with benign IgM paraproteinaemia. A clinical and neurophysiological study. *Brain*. 1994;117(Pt 5):949–957.

74. Ahlskog MC, Kumar N, Mauermann ML, Klein CJ. IgM-monoclonal gammopathy neuropathy and tremor: a first epidemiologic case control study. *Parkinsonism Relat Disord*. 2012;18(6):748–752.

75. Notermans NC, Wokke JH, Lokhorst HM, Franssen H, van der Graaf Y, Jennekens FG. Polyneuropathy associated with monoclonal gammopathy of undetermined significance. A prospective study of the prognostic value of clinical and laboratory abnormalities. *Brain*. 1994;117(Pt 6):1385–1393.

76. Nobile-Orazio E, Meucci N, Baldini L, Di Troia A, Scarlato G. Long-term prognosis of neuropathy associated with anti-MAG IgM M-proteins and its relationship to immune therapies. *Brain*. 2000;123(Pt 4):710–717.

77. Pestronk A, Li F, Griffin J, et al. Polyneuropathy syndromes associated with serum antibodies to sulfatide and myelin-associated glycoprotein. *Neurology.* 1991;41(3):357–362.

78. Maisonobe T, Chassande B, Verin M, Jouni M, Leger JM, Bouche P. Chronic dysimmune demyelinating polyneuropathy: a clinical and electrophysiological study of 93 patients. *J Neurol Neurosurg Psychiatry.* 1996;61(1):36–42.

79. Simovic D, Gorson KC, Ropper AH. Comparison of IgM-MGUS and IgG-MGUS polyneuropathy. *Acta Neurol Scand.* 1998;97(3):194–200.

80. Svahn J, Petiot P, Antoine JC, et al. Anti-MAG antibodies in 202 patients: clinicopathological and therapeutic features. *J Neurol Neurosurg Psychiatry.* 2018;89(5):499–505.

81. Vrancken AF, Kalmijn S, Buskens E, et al. Feasibility and cost efficiency of a diagnostic guideline for chronic polyneuropathy: a prospective implementation study. *J Neurol Neurosurg Psychiatry.* 2006;77(3):397–401.

82. Nobile-Orazio E, Gallia F, Terenghi F, Allaria S, Giannotta C, Carpo M. How useful are anti-neural IgM antibodies in the diagnosis of chronic immune-mediated neuropathies? *J Neurol Sci.* 2008;266(1–2):156–163.

83. Willison HJ, Veitch J, Swan AV, et al. Inter-laboratory validation of an ELISA for the determination of serum anti-ganglioside antibodies. *Eur J Neurol.* 1999;6(1):71–77.

84. Kuijf ML, Eurelings M, Tio-Gillen AP, et al. Detection of anti-MAG antibodies in polyneuropathy associated with IgM monoclonal gammopathy. *Neurology.* 2009;73(9):688–695.

85. Mendell JR, Sahenk Z, Whitaker JN, et al. Polyneuropathy and IgM monoclonal gammopathy: studies on the pathogenetic role of anti-myelin-associated glycoprotein antibody. *Ann Neurol.* 1985;17(3):243–254.

86. Franssen H, Notermans NC. Length dependence in polyneuropathy associated with IgM gammopathy. *Ann Neurol.* 2006;59(2):365–371.

87. Capasso M, Torrieri F, Di Muzio A, De Angelis MV, Lugaresi A, Uncini A. Can electrophysiology differentiate polyneuropathy with anti-MAG/SGPG antibodies from chronic inflammatory demyelinating polyneuropathy? *Clin Neurophysiol.* 2002;113(3):346–353.

88. Kaku DA, England JD, Sumner AJ. Distal accentuation of conduction slowing in polyneuropathy associated with antibodies to myelin-associated glycoprotein and sulphated glucuronyl paragloboside. *Brain.* 1994;117(Pt 5):941–947.

89. Notermans NC, Franssen H, Eurelings M, Van der Graaf Y, Wokke JH. Diagnostic criteria for demyelinating polyneuropathy associated with monoclonal gammopathy. *Muscle Nerve.* 2000;23(1):73–79.

90. Rajabally YA. Neuropathy and paraproteins: review of a complex association. *Eur J Neurol.* 2011;18(11):1291–1298.

91. Pihan M, Keddie S, D'Sa S, et al. Raised VEGF: High sensitivity and specificity in the diagnosis of POEMS syndrome. *Neurol Neuroimmunol Neuroinflamm.* 2018;5(5):e486.

92. Eurelings M, Notermans NC, Van de Donk NW, Lokhorst HM. Risk factors for hematological malignancy in polyneuropathy associated with monoclonal gammopathy. *Muscle Nerve.* 2001;24(10):1295–1302.

93. Pruppers MHJ, Merkies ISJ, Lunn MPT, Notermans NC, Group IMS. 230th ENMC international workshop: improving future assessment and research in IgM anti-MAG peripheral neuropathy: a consensus collaborative effort, Naarden, The Netherlands, 24–26 February 2017. *Neuromuscul Disord.* 2017;27(11):1065–1072.

94. Comi G, Roveri L, Swan A, et al. A randomised controlled trial of intravenous immunoglobulin in IgM paraprotein associated demyelinating neuropathy. *J Neurol.* 2002;249(10):1370–1377.

95. Dalakas MC, Quarles RH, Farrer RG, et al. A controlled study of intravenous immunoglobulin in demyelinating neuropathy with IgM gammopathy. *Ann Neurol.* 1996;40(5):792–795.

96. Mariette X, Chastang C, Clavelou P, Louboutin JP, Leger JM, Brouet JC. A randomised clinical trial comparing interferon-alpha and intravenous immunoglobulin in polyneuropathy associated with monoclonal IgM. The IgM-associated Polyneuropathy Study Group. *J Neurol Neurosurg Psychiatry.* 1997;63(1):28–34.

97. Mariette X, Brouet JC, Chevret S, et al. A randomised double blind trial versus placebo does not confirm the benefit of alpha-interferon in polyneuropathy associated with monoclonal IgM. *J Neurol Neurosurg Psychiatry.* 2000;69(2):279–280.

98. Oksenhendler E, Chevret S, Leger JM, Louboutin JP, Bussel A, Brouet JC. Plasma exchange and chlorambucil in polyneuropathy associated with monoclonal IgM gammopathy. IgM-associated Polyneuropathy Study Group. *J Neurol Neurosurg Psychiatry.* 1995;59(3):243–247.

99. Dyck PJ, Low PA, Windebank AJ, et al. Plasma exchange in polyneuropathy associated with monoclonal gammopathy of undetermined significance. *N Engl J Med.* 1991;325(21):1482–1486.

100. Benedetti L, Briani C, Grandis M, et al. Predictors of response to rituximab in patients with neuropathy and anti-myelin associated glycoprotein immunoglobulin M. *J Peripher Nerv Syst.* 2007;12(2):102–107.

101. Benedetti L, Briani C, Franciotta D, et al. Long-term effect of rituximab in anti-mag polyneuropathy. *Neurology.* 2008;71(21):1742–1744.

102. Goldfarb AR, Weimer LH, Brannagan 3rd TH. Rituximab treatment of an IgM monoclonal autonomic and sensory neuropathy. *Muscle Nerve.* 2005;31(4):510–515.

103. Dalakas MC, Rakocevic G, Salajegheh M, et al. Placebo-controlled trial of rituximab in IgM anti-myelin-associated glycoprotein antibody demyelinating neuropathy. *Ann Neurol.* 2009;65(3):286–293.

104. Leger JM, Viala K, Nicolas G, et al. Placebo-controlled trial of rituximab in IgM anti-myelin-associated glycoprotein neuropathy. *Neurology.* 2013;80(24):2217–2225.

105. Gorson KC, Natarajan N, Ropper AH, Weinstein R. Rituximab treatment in patients with IVIg-dependent immune polyneuropathy: a prospective pilot trial. *Muscle Nerve.* 2007;35(1):66–69.

106. Notermans NC, Vermeulen M, Lokhorst HM, et al. Pulsed high-dose dexamethasone treatment of polyneuropathy associated with monoclonal gammopathy. *J Neurol.* 1997;244(7):462–463.

107. Niermeijer JM, Eurelings M, van der Linden MW, et al. Intermittent cyclophosphamide with prednisone versus placebo for polyneuropathy with IgM monoclonal gammopathy. *Neurology.* 2007;69(1):50–59.

108. Lunn MP, Nobile-Orazio E. Immunotherapy for IgM anti-myelin-associated glycoprotein paraprotein-associated peripheral neuropathies. *Cochrane Database Syst Rev.* 2012;5:CD002827.

109. Lunn MP, Nobile-Orazio E. Immunotherapy for IgM anti-myelin-associated glycoprotein paraprotein-associated peripheral neuropathies. *Cochrane Database Syst Rev.* 2016;10:CD002827.

110. Merkies IS, Lauria G. 131st ENMC international workshop: selection of outcome measures for peripheral neuropathy clinical trials 10–12 December 2004, Naarden, The Netherlands. *Neuromuscul Disord.* 2006;16(2):149–156.

111. Lunn MP, Leger JM, Merkies IS, et al. 151st ENMC international workshop: Inflammatory neuropathy consortium 13th–15th April 2007, Schiphol, The Netherlands. *Neuromuscul Disord.* 2008;18(1):85–89.

112. Vanhoutte EK, Faber CG, Merkies IS, PeriNomS study group. 196th ENMC international workshop: outcome measures in inflammatory peripheral neuropathies 8–10 February 2013, Naarden, The Netherlands. *Neuromuscul Disord.* 2013;23(11):924–933.

113. Stevens SS. On the theory of scales of measurement. *Science*. 1946;103(2684):677–680.
114. DeVellis RF. Classical test theory. *Med Care*. 2006;44(11 Suppl 3):S50–S59.
115. Grimby G, Tennant A, Tesio L. The use of raw scores from ordinal scales: time to end malpractice? *J Rehabil Med*. 2012;44(2):97–98.
116. Tennant A, Conaghan PG. The Rasch measurement model in rheumatology: what is it and why use it? When should it be applied, and what should one look for in a Rasch paper? *Arthritis Rheum*. 2007;57(8):1358–1362.
117. Rasch G. *Probabilistic Models for some Intelligence and Attainment Tests*. Vol. 1. Copenhagen: Danmarks Paedagogiske Institut; 1960.
118. Liang MH. Evaluating measurement responsiveness. *J Rheumatol*. 1995;22(6):1191–1192.
119. Streiner D, Norman G. *Health Measurement Scales: A Practical Guide to their Development and Use*. 2nd ed. New York: Oxford University Press; 1998.
120. Pruppers MH, Merkies IS, Notermans NC. Recent advances in outcome measures in IgM-anti-MAG + neuropathies. *Curr Opin Neurol*. 2015;28(5):486–493.

Chapter 6

POEMS syndrome

Chiara Briani[a], Marta Campagnolo[a], Marco Luigetti[b,c], Federica Lessi[d], Fausto Adami[d]

[a]Department of Neuroscience, University of Padova, Padova, Italy, [b]Catholic University of the Sacred Heart, Rome, Italy, [c]Neurology Unit, University Hospital A. Gemelli—IRCCS, Rome, Italy, [d]Hematology and Clinical Immunology Unit, Department of Medicine, University of Padova, Padova, Italy

Introduction

POEMS (polyneuropathy, organomegaly, endocrinopathy, monoclonal gammopathy, skin changes) is a rare, likely paraneoplastic syndrome due to an underlying plasma cell disorder.

Other than polyneuropathy, which is the hallmark of the disease, a wide range of organ involvement and pleiotropic clinical features exists that contributes to the enigma of POEMS syndrome.

The syndrome is hematologic in nature, but its pathogenesis is still unclear. It is deemed that clinical features are largely attributable to the high concentrations of serum vascular endothelial growth factor (sVEGF)[1–3] although normal or nearly normal sVEGF levels have been described in a few POEMS patients[4,5] and sVEGF levels do not always reflect the disease course.[6,7] Other cytokines such as IL-12,[8] Il-6, TNF-α,[9] bFGF, and HGF[10] appear to be upregulated in POEMS syndrome and may contribute to the clinical picture. In patients with the Castleman variant of POEMS (see below), IL-6 is the predominantly elevated cytokine.[3] Plasma cells, both monoclonal and polyclonal, are thought to be the main source of the excessive concentrations of sVEGF and other cytokines, both in the bone marrow[11,12] and lymph nodes of Castleman's disease.[13] It is presently unclear how this deregulated cytokine network may drive the modifications of the involved organs and determine the clinical picture. VEGF is thought to be the main actor on the scene: it targets endothelial cells as well as induces angiogenesis and a reversible increase of the microvascular permeability, thus leading to interstitial edema, but how these actions may contribute to the neuropathy, endocrinopathy, and skin changes is under debate or largely unexplained.

Dysimmune Neuropathies. https://doi.org/10.1016/B978-0-12-814572-2.00006-6

Pathological background

In POEMS syndrome, bone marrow infiltration by clonal plasma cells is scanty (median ≈5%, 90% lambda). Moreover, in a minority of patients, the plasma cells do not appear clonal. In about half of cases, there is a thin rim of plasma cells around lymphoid aggregates, a finding virtually never seen in the bone marrow of other plasma cell diseases. Megakaryocyte hyperplasia and clustering may also be present, reminiscent of myeloproliferative diseases, but the JAK2V617 mutation is consistently lacking.[14] In about one-third of patients, there are no clonal plasma cells on the standard bone marrow biopsy; such patients usually present with one or more "solitary plasmacytoma." Up to 30% of POEMS patients have slightly enlarged lymph nodes that display the histopathologic features of Castleman's disease, both in its hyaline-vascular and multicentric variants.[15–17] Patients diagnosed with Castleman's disease with signs and symptoms of POEMS syndrome but lacking both the neuropathy and a formal demonstration of a clonal plasma cell disease are referred to as having a Castleman disease variant of the POEMS syndrome.[18, 19]

Clinical picture

Hematologic involvement

POEMS syndrome implies pleiotropic and nonstereotypical organ involvement. As expected from a disease originating from plasma cells, there is bone involvement—mostly multiple—in up to 95% of the patients but, different from multiple myeloma, the pattern is osteosclerotic or mixed lytic-sclerotic rather than osteolytic.[20] A whole body CT scan is deemed the appropriate tool to explore the bone disease,[21] even more accurate that the FDG-uptake at ^{18}F-FDG PET/CT, which may be not sensitive in patients with purely sclerotic bone lesions.[22] About 85% of the patients display a serum monoclonal component (MC)[23] (see specific paragraph).

Polyneuropathy

Polyneuropathy, a mandatory major criterion and often the presenting feature of POEMS syndrome, is usually a sensory-motor symmetrical polyneuropathy with subacute or acute onset, sensory disturbances, and rapidly progressing distal weakness, with patients becoming wheelchair-bound quite early in the course of the disease.[24, 25] A distinctive and common feature in POEMS syndrome is the presence of neuropathic pain (55%–76%),[26] which is usually severe, associated with hyperalgesia and allodynia, and sometimes unresponsive to common pain medications.[27] Neurophysiological studies disclose a mixed axonal and demyelinating pattern involving preferentially the lower limbs, with slowing of motor and sensory conduction velocities (predominant in intermediate nerve segments) and prolonged distal latencies (Fig. 1). Temporal dispersion has been reported in around 13% of patients and conduction blocks in 7%. Nerve amplitudes are reduced early in the

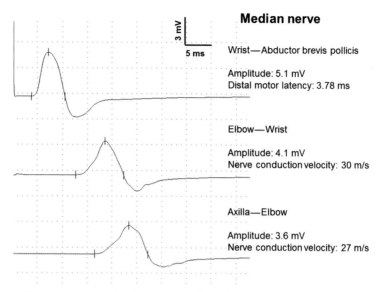

FIG. 1 Nerve conduction study of median nerve. Neurophysiological study reveals low-borderline amplitude of median nerve with normal values of distal motor latency and reduced nerve conduction velocity in intermediate segments. No conduction blocks or excessive temporal dispersion are detectable.

course of the disease, indicating axonal loss, with predominant involvement of lower limbs.[28] Nerve biopsies disclose prominent axonal degeneration, diffuse myelinated fiber loss, uncompacted myelin lamellae, and increased epineurial blood vessels[27, 29] (Fig. 2A–D). High serum VEGF and high peripheral nerve VEGF were all associated with more severe endoneurial vessel involvement and nerve damage. Furthermore, sural nerve biopsies from POEMS patients have disclosed increased thickness of the basal lamina, narrowing of the lumina of endoneurial vessels at light microscopy, and proliferation of endothelial cells with opening of tight junctions at electron microscopy, supporting the role of angiogenic factors in the pathogenesis of neuropathy in POEMS syndrome.[3] Despite the availability of specific diagnostic criteria[23], including a highly sensitive biomarker such as VEGF, misdiagnosis or delayed diagnosis in POEMS syndrome remains a common problem. A number of reasons have been suggested, including the clinical and neurophysiological characteristics of the peripheral neuropathy that frequently mimics chronic inflammatory demyelinating polyradiculoneuropathy (CIDP), with more than 60% of patients being misdiagnosed at onset.[26] However, some distinctive features have been suggested to help achieve a correct diagnosis. Neuropathic pain can be reported in CIDP but represents a less-frequent feature, usually pointing toward a diagnosis of POEMS syndrome. In CIDP, a more diffuse pattern with both proximal and distal weakness is described while POEMS syndrome is characterized by a predominant distal involvement. From a neurophysiological point of view, CIDP, differently from POEMS syndrome, presents with slowing of conduction velocities involving

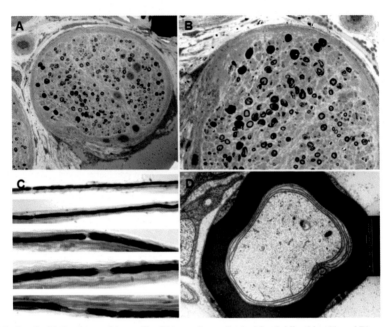

FIG. 2 (A–D) Sural nerve biopsy. Semithin section stained with toluidine blue (A and B) reveals moderate reduction of fiber density (A: magnification 10×) with abundant axonal degenerations (B: magnification 20×). Teased fiber analysis (C) shows normal myelinated fibers with occasional paranodal demyelination (fibers at bottom). Ultrastructural analysis at electron microscope shows typical uncompact myelin lamellae (D).

mostly the distal nerve segments, frequent detection of conduction blocks, and a more diffuse distribution involving both upper and lower limbs. Despite some differences in the two conditions, neurophysiological findings need to be appropriately interpreted in the general clinical context in order to reach a correct diagnosis. Immunomodulatory therapies including intravenous immunoglobulins (IV Ig), steroids, and plasma exchange are routinely used in CIDP and are effective in more than 80% of patients. On the contrary, neuropathy in POEMS syndrome shows no response to IV Ig or plasma exchange, with only mild or transient benefit after steroid administration. The absence of benefit in a patient with a CIDP-like pattern should raise concerns about the diagnosis and lead to further investigations to rule out possible POEMS syndrome.[30] Moreover, accompanying systemic features may be helpful to point toward a correct diagnosis. Subtle bone marrow abnormalities can be easily overlooked, contributing to an incorrect diagnosis and highlighting the importance of a thorough and extensive diagnostic work-up. An additional confounding factor may be the detection of a serum monoclonal component, which has been reported in up to 20% of CIDP patients. Thrombocytosis can be detected in more than 50% of patients with POEMS while it is often absent in CIDP.[31] Other symptoms or signs indicating a possible underlying multisystemic disease such as weight loss and skin changes are frequently reported in POEMS syndrome and are crucial for a correct diagnosis. Cerebrospinal fluid examination is usually performed, but it can provide misleading information because albumin-cytological is a common finding in both CIDP and POEMS syndrome.

Organomegaly

A variable proportion (25%–75%) of the patients is reported to have enlarged liver, spleen, and lymph nodes.[15, 17, 23, 32] A biopsy of the involved lymph nodes shows a Castleman's disease pattern mostly of the hyaline vascular type. Little is known about the histopathologic changes in the liver and spleen.

Endocrinopathy

Endocrinopathy occurs in up to 85% of the patients.[33] Most patients experience multiple endocrine abnormalities, with gonadal dysfunction being the most frequent. Gynecomastia in men may also be present. The involvement of thyroid function, glucose metabolism alterations, and adrenal insufficiency may also be associated. Given the high incidence of isolated glucose metabolism alterations and thyroid dysfunctions in the general population, only multiple endocrinopathies associated with neuropathy are reliably attributable to POEMS syndrome. Most of the time, endocrine dysfunctions persist even after long-lasting hematologic and sVEGF remission (personal observation).

Monoclonal plasmaproliferative disorder

The demonstration of a plasma cell clone is one of the two mandatory criteria required to establish the diagnosis. In about 85% of the patients, the clone is witnessed by a serum MC, which is IgG or IgA—rarely IgM—but lambda-restricted in almost 90% of the cases. The serum MC is usually small (median 1 g/L). Serum-free light chains are reported to be elevated in the majority of patients with POEMS syndrome, but the κ/λ ratio is usually within normal values.[34] Very small amounts (median $\leq$ 100 mg/24 h) of urine MC (i.e., Bence Jones protein) is reported in less than 50% of the patients.[23] The size of the serum MC does not parallel sVEGF levels[1] and it reflects very roughly the course of the disease. The clinical, laboratory, and histological features of the plasma cell clone may be so elusive that a sensitive immunohistochemistry on a biopsy specimen from an osteosclerotic bone or bone marrow and serum and urine immunofixation are needed to uncover them.

Skin changes

Also, the skin changes are heterogeneous and include hyperpigmentation, hypertricosis, acrocianosis, thickening, clubbing and white discoloration of the nails, and recent onset of multiple hemangiomas[35–37] (Fig. 3). The most common histopathologic alterations of the dermis consist of microvascular abnormalities such as dilated and frequently anastomotic vessels.[38, 39]

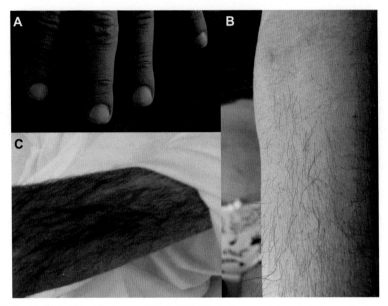

FIG. 3 Characteristic skin abnormalities in POEMS syndrome: white nails (A); massive hypertrichosis at lower limbs in a female patient (B and C).

Papilledema

More than 60% of a cohort of 33 patients referred for ophthalmologic examination complained of ocular signs and symptoms such as blurred vision and diplopia, and about 50% of them had papilledema.[40] Papilledema has been found to have an adverse prognostic significance.[41]

Extravascular volume overload

The main manifestations of extravascular volume overload consist of peripheral edema, ascites, and pleural (most often) and pericardial effusions. In most instances, ascitic and pleural fluid have been found to have exudative features.[2, 34]

Respiratory manifestations

Respiratory involvement has multiform manifestations, including pleural effusions, impaired diffusion capacity of carbon monoxide (DLCO), restrictive lung disease (about 10% of the patients),[18] and pulmonary hypertension (about 25% of the patients),[42, 43] the latter being more likely to occur in patients with extravascular volume overload, although a cytokine-mediated mechanism has been postulated.[43] Both papilledema and reduced DLCO have been associated with shorter overall survival.[41]

Thrombosis

About 20% of the patients experience thrombotic events, both arterial and venous in nature. Stroke, myocardial, and intestinal infarction have been described[41,44,45] as well as the Budd-Chiari syndrome.[23] About 10% of the patients present with a cerebrovascular event that is embolic or related to vessel dissection,[46,47] and may also be the symptom at onset.[48] Thrombocytosis, polyglobulia, hyperfibrinogenemia,[45] bone marrow plasmacytosis, high levels of inflammatory cytokines, and alterations in the coagulation cascade[48] are considered risk factors for thrombotic events.

Renal findings

In most patients, the renal function is somewhat impaired, as witnessed by high serum levels of cystatin C.[49] Significant proteinuria and raised serum creatinine are uncommon ($<10\%$ of the patients). Renal disease is more frequent in patients with coexisting Castleman's disease.[20] The renal histologic findings are heterogeneous, and most of the time they are reminiscent of those seen in membranoproliferative glomerulonephritis.[50]

Pachymeningeal involvement

Patients with POEMS syndrome or osteosclerotic myeloma with cerebral or spinal pachymeningitis have occasionally been described.[51,52] Recently, we extensively investigated brain and spinal MRI in patients with POEMS syndrome and also performed meningeal histopathological studies, showing the frequent pachymeningeal, not inflammatory, involvement in POEMS syndrome (Fig. 4).[53] Meningeal histopathology revealed hyperplasia of meningothelial cells, neovascularization, and obstructive vessel remodeling without inflammatory signs, pointing to a role of VEGF in the meningeal manifestations. The dramatic pachymeningeal improvement in POEMS patients undergoing lenalidomide therapy further supports a possible role of angiogenic factors in the pachymeningeal involvement.[54]

Diagnosis

Owing to its intricate pathogenesis, no single test can establish the diagnosis of POEMS syndrome. It is now accepted that the diagnosis could be established if a number of differently relevant criteria are fulfilled, that is, both the two mandatory major criteria, one major criterion, and one of the six minor criteria are needed (see Table 1).

The relationship between Castleman's disease and POEMS syndrome is uncertain because some patients may share symptoms and signs of both diseases (including peripheral neuropathy) and 10%–30% of patients with POEMS syndrome have histologically proven Castleman's disease.[15,16,23] It is currently proposed

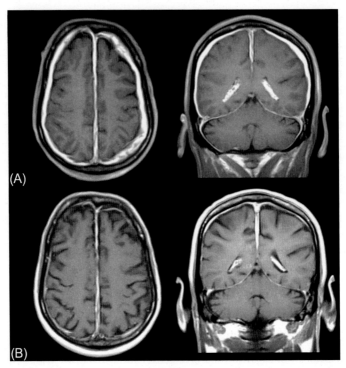

FIG. 4   Pachymeningeal involvement in POEMS. Brain MRI: (A) axial and coronal contrast-enhanced images in a 67-year-old male showing diffuse thickening of the supratentorial dura mater with moderate mass effect (note the relative sulcal effacement and the small lateral ventricles). (B) axial and coronal contrast-enhanced images at the same level of A, 4 years later after lenalinomide treatment: pachymeningeal thickening is strikingly less evident.

that patients with Castleman's disease and symptoms and signs of POEMS syndrome without both neuropathy and evidence of clonal plasma cell disease may be diagnosed with the "Castleman disease variant of the POEMS syndrome."[18, 19]

Therapy

Currently, there is not a standardized therapeutic algorithm because the rarity of the disease prevents large prospective randomized trials. Therapy is generally borrowed from the treatment of other plasma cell disorders, and includes both local radiotherapy and systemic chemotherapy including autologous stem cell transplantation (ASCT). Due to the rarity of the disease, there are no established upfront or second-line therapies, and comparison among different chemotherapeutic regimens is very difficult.

In about 25% of the patients, that is, those with a negative bone marrow biopsy and limited (usually less than two) sclerotic bone lesions, local radiation therapy is suitable and potentially curative or, at least, capable of inducing long-lasting

TABLE 1 Diagnostic criteria for POEMS syndrome.

Mandatory major criteria	1. Polyneuropathy
	2. Monoclonal plasma cell proliferative disorder
Other major criteria	3. Castleman's disease
	4. Sclerotic bone lesions
	5. Vascular endothelial growth factor elevation
Minor criteria	6. Organomegaly (hepatomegaly, splenomegaly or lymphadenopathy)
	7. Endocrinopathy (gonadal, thyroid, adrenal, pancreatic, pituitary)
	8. Skin changes (hyperpigmentation, hypertrichosis, acrocyanosis)
	9. Extravascular volume overload (edema, ascites, pleural effusions)
	10. Papilledema
	11. Erythrocytosis, thrombocytosis
Other	Weight loss, pulmonary hypertension, clubbing, diarrhea
	Low vitamin B_{12} values

clinical improvement in about 50% of patients.[39] Local radiation therapy may be used also in association with systemic chemotherapy should large lytic bone lesions be present. Once a disseminated disease is identified, systemic therapy is warranted. Corticosteroids, namely medium-to-high dose dexamethasone, are part of all regimens, despite their short-lived efficacy when used alone. The combination of melphalan and dexamethasone was first reported by Zhang et al.,[55] obtaining hematological, clinical, and sVEGF response in more than 80% of the 31 treated patients. Lenalidomide in combination with dexamethasone has shown good efficacy both in the "neoadiuvant" setting before radiotherapy and high dose chemotherapy and ASCT,[56] both in retrospective[57] and prospective studies.[58, 59] The reported response (VEGF and FDG-PET, clinical/neurological) rates range from 50% to 90%, with 46% of the responding patients obtaining a hematologic complete response.[59] Considerable concern, due to the well-known neurotoxicity of both drugs, prevented the large therapeutic use of both thalidomide and bortezomib. However, a number of studies showed that this concern is overestimated because thalidomide showed good efficacy and negligible neurotoxicity.[60–65] Similarly, also bortezomib and a bortezomib-based regimen appear to be manageable and effective. Most reports show that bortezomib improves symptoms and signs of peripheral neuropathy in responders,[66–72] even after long-lasting exposure and high cumulative doses (> 100 mg/m^2) (personal observation).

Role of autologous stem cell transplantation

Since 2001, a number of reports have dealt with high-dose chemotherapy (melphalan) and ASCT in patients with POEMS syndrome, showing a good efficacy.[73–76] The most recent papers on a higher number of patients confirm previous data and show that ASCT can induce high and long-lasting overall response rates, which translate into better progression-free survival (PFS) (65%–75% at 5 years) and overall survival (OS) (88% at 5 years).[77, 78] As a matter of fact, hematologic responses rates exceed 70% (CR ~ 50%) and the overall survival for patients treated with ASCT is at least 80% at 5 years. Moreover, ASCT improves the quality of life, ameliorating both the neurologic and the overall clinical conditions in nearly 100% of the responding patients.[77–80] In the last decade, the transplant-related mortality dropped to about 2%, owing to a more careful selection of patients. Although no standard selection criteria for ASCT has been established, age > 65, pulmonary hypertension, and arterial hypotension are deemed exclusion criteria. The mobilization-related morbidity—more often an acute renal failure—can be as high as 23%.[81] The engraftment syndrome (fever, pulmonary infiltrates, weight gain) is a serious complication of the ASCT procedure; whether the mobilization, which includes cyclophosphamide, can reduce the engraftment syndrome is a matter of debate.[78, 82] In conclusion, ASCT is a suitable option in patients with POEMS syndrome, and should be considered as the first-line therapy in young patients, provided that organ dysfunction is lacking.

In our institution, we favor the novel drugs such as those used in patients with multiple myeloma (bortezomib and lenalidomide) as the first-line therapy if ASCT criteria are not fulfilled or ASCT is refused by the patient.

Therapy response

The large majority of responding patients display clinically significant improvement months after the completion of therapy. This is especially true for the neuropathy whose maximal response may take 2–3 years while skin changes, papilledema, anasarca, sVEGF values, and FDG-PET may change sooner and anticipate the neurological response.[18]

Risk factors and prognosis

The course of the disease is chronic and there are no genetic or molecular markers predicting survival. A number of different adverse prognostic factors have been reported such as age > 50 years, pleural effusions and ascites, pulmonary hypertension and reduced DLCO, high sVEGF levels, and Castleman's disease. Patients with limited disease, candidates for local radiotherapy, and those with lower sVEGF levels are reported to have better survival.[17, 23, 42, 83]

Patients diagnosed and treated after 2003 show survival past 10 years (79%) versus those treated before 2003 (55%).[79] It is likely that the longer survival benefit comes from the new drugs available to patients with multiple myeloma (and used also in POEMS syndrome) and that this will also benefit patients not eligible for high-dose chemotherapy and ASCT.

References

1. Watanabe O, Maruyama I, Arimura K, et al. Overproduction of vascular endothelial growth factor/vascular permeability factor is causative in Crow-Fukase (POEMS) syndrome. *Muscle Nerve.* 1998;21(11):1390–1397 [Epub 1998/10/15].
2. Cui R-T, Yu S-Y, Huang X-S, et al. Incidence and risk factors of pleural effusions in patients with POEMS syndrome. *Hematol Oncol.* 2015;33(2):80–84.
3. Scarlato M, Previtali SC, Carpo M, et al. Polyneuropathy in POEMS syndrome: role of angiogenic factors in the pathogenesis. *Brain.* 2005;128(Pt 8):1911–1920 [Epub 2005/06/25].
4. Pulivarthi S, Gurram M. An atypical presentation of POEMS syndrome with IgG kappa type M protein and normal VEGF level: case report and review of literature. *J Cancer Res Ther.* 2018;14(3):679–681.
5. Misawa S, Sato Y, Katayama K, et al. Vascular endothelial growth factor as a predictive marker for POEMS syndrome treatment response: retrospective cohort study. *BMJ Open.* 2015;5(11):e009157 [Epub 2015/11/13].
6. Kuwabara S, Kanai K, Misawa S, Nakaseko C. Relapse of POEMS syndrome without increased level of VEGF. *Neuromuscul Disord.* 2009;19(10):740.
7. Imai N, Taguchi J, Yagi N, Konishi T, Serizawa M, Kobari M. Relapse of polyneuropathy, organomegaly, endocrinopathy, M-protein, and skin changes (POEMS) syndrome without increased level of vascular endothelial growth factor following successful autologous peripheral blood stem cell transplantation. *Neuromuscul Disord.* 2009;19(5):363–365.
8. Kanai K, Sawai S, Sogawa K, et al. Markedly upregulated serum interleukin-12 as a novel biomarker in POEMS syndrome. *Neurology.* 2012;79(6):575–582.
9. Nakayama-Ichiyama S, Yokote T, Hirata Y, et al. Multiple cytokine-producing plasmablastic solitary Plasmacytoma of bone with polyneuropathy, organomegaly, endocrinology, monoclonal protein, and skin changes syndrome. *J Clin Oncol.* 2012;30(7):e91–e94.
10. Yamada Y, Sawai S, Misawa S, et al. Multiple angiogenetic factors are upregulated in POEMS syndrome. *Ann Hematol.* 2013;92(2):245–248.
11. Wang C, Huang XF, Cai QQ, et al. Remarkable expression of vascular endothelial growth factor in bone marrow plasma cells of patients with POEMS syndrome. *Leuk Res.* 2016;50:78–84 [Epub 2016/10/27].
12. Nakajima H, Ishida S, Furutama D, et al. Expression of vascular endothelial growth factor by plasma cells in the sclerotic bone lesion of a patient with POEMS syndrome. *J Neurol.* 2007;254(4):531–533.
13. Nishi J, Arimura K, Utsunomiya A, et al. Expression of vascular endothelial growth factor in sera and lymph nodes of the plasma cell type of Castleman's disease. *Br J Haematol.* 1999;104(3):482–485 [Epub 1999/03/23].

14. Dao LN, Hanson CA, Dispenzieri A, Morice WG, Kurtin PJ, Hoyer JD. Bone marrow histopathology in POEMS syndrome: a distinctive combination of plasma cell, lymphoid, and myeloid findings in 87 patients. *Blood.* 2011;117(24):6438–6444 [Epub 2011/03/10].

15. Nakanishi T, Sobue I, Toyokura Y, et al. The Crow-Fukase syndrome: a study of 102 cases in Japan. *Neurology.* 1984;34(6):712–720 [Epub 1984/06/01].

16. Soubrier MJ, Dubost JJ, Sauvezie BJ. POEMS syndrome: a study of 25 cases and a review of the literature. French study group on POEMS syndrome. *Am J Med.* 1994;97(6):543–553 [Epub 1994/12/01].

17. Li J, Zhou DB, Huang Z, et al. Clinical characteristics and long-term outcome of patients with POEMS syndrome in China. *Ann Hematol.* 2011;90(7):819–826 [Epub 2011/01/12].

18. Dispenzieri A. POEMS syndrome: 2019 update on diagnosis, risk-stratification, and management. *Am J Hematol.* 2019;94(7):812–827.

19. Warsame R, Yanamandra U, Kapoor P. POEMS syndrome: an enigma. *Curr Hematol Malig Rep.* 2017;12(2):85–95.

20. Li J, Duan MH, Wang C, et al. Impact of pretransplant induction therapy on autologous stem cell transplantation for patients with newly diagnosed POEMS syndrome. *Leukemia.* 2017;31:1375.

21. Glazebrook K, Guerra Bonilla FL, Johnson A, Leng S, Dispenzieri A. Computed tomography assessment of bone lesions in patients with POEMS syndrome. *Eur Radiol.* 2015;25(2):497–504 [Epub 2014/09/26].

22. Pan Q, Li J, Li F, Zhou D, Zhu Z. Characterizing POEMS syndrome with 18F-FDG PET/CT. *J Nucl Med.* 2015;56(9):1334–1337 [Epub 2015/07/18].

23. Dispenzieri A, Kyle RA, Lacy MQ, et al. POEMS syndrome: definitions and long-term outcome. *Blood.* 2003;101(7):2496–2506 [Epub 2002/11/29].

24. Mauermann ML, Sorenson EJ, Dispenzieri A, Mandrekar J, Suarez GA, Dyck PJ. Uniform demyelination and more severe axonal loss distinguish POEMS syndrome from CIDP. *J Neurol Neurosurg Psychiatry.* 2012;83(5):480–486 [Epub 2012/03/08].

25. Karam C, Klein CJ, Dispenzieri A, et al. Polyneuropathy improvement following autologous stem cell transplantation for POEMS syndrome. *Neurology.* 2015;84(19):1981–1987 [Epub 2015/04/17].

26. Nasu S, Misawa S, Sekiguchi Y, et al. Different neurological and physiological profiles in POEMS syndrome and chronic inflammatory demyelinating polyneuropathy. *J Neurol Neurosurg Psychiatry.* 2012;83(5):476–479 [Epub 2012/02/18].

27. Koike H, Iijima M, Mori K, et al. Neuropathic pain correlates with myelinated fibre loss and cytokine profile in POEMS syndrome. *J Neurol Neurosurg Psychiatry.* 2008;79(10):1171–1179 [Epub 2008/03/22].

28. Mauermann ML. The peripheral neuropathies of POEMS syndrome and Castleman disease. *Hematol Oncol Clin North Am.* 2018;32(1):153–163 [Epub 2017/11/22].

29. Vital C, Vital A, Ferrer X, et al. Crow-Fukase (POEMS) syndrome: a study of peripheral nerve biopsy in five new cases. *J Peripher Nerv Syst.* 2003;8(3):136–144 [Epub 2003/08/09].

30. Keddie S, D'Sa S, Foldes D, Carr AS, Reilly MM, Lunn MPT. POEMS neuropathy: optimising diagnosis and management. *Pract Neurol.* 2018;18(4):278–290 [Epub 2018/03/08].

31. Naddaf E, Dispenzieri A, Mandrekar J, Mauermann ML. Thrombocytosis distinguishes POEMS syndrome from chronic inflammatory demyelinating polyneuropathy. *Muscle Nerve.* 2015;52(4):658–659 [Epub 2015/07/17].

32. Takatsuki K, Sanada I. Plasma cell dyscrasia with polyneuropathy and endocrine disorder: clinical and laboratory features of 109 reported cases. *Jpn J Clin Oncol.* 1983;13(3):543–555 [Epub 1983/09/01].

33. Gandhi GY, Basu R, Dispenzieri A, Basu A, Montori VM, Brennan MD. Endocrinopathy in POEMS syndrome: the Mayo Clinic experience. *Mayo Clin Proc.* 2007;82(7):836–842 [Epub 2007/07/04].

34. Cui RT, Yu SY, Huang XS, Zhang JT, Li F, Pu CQ. The characteristics of ascites in patients with POEMS syndrome. *Ann Hematol.* 2013;92(12):1661–1664.

35. Iwashita H, Ohnishi A, Asada M, Kanazawa Y, Kuroiwa Y. Polyneuropathy, skin hyper-pigmentation, edema, and hypertrichosis in localized osteosclerotic myeloma. *Neurology.* 1977;27(7):675–681 [Epub 1977/07/01].

36. Chan JK, Fletcher CD, Hicklin GA, Rosai J. Glomeruloid hemangioma. A distinctive cutane-ous lesion of multicentric Castleman's disease associated with POEMS syndrome. *Am J Surg Pathol.* 1990;14(11):1036–1046 [Epub 1990/11/01].

37. Barete S, Mouawad R, Choquet S, et al. Skin manifestations and vascular endothelial growth factor levels in POEMS syndrome: impact of autologous hematopoietic stem cell transplanta-tion. *Arch Dermatol.* 2010;146(6):615–623 [Epub 2010/06/23].

38. Ishikawa O, Nihei Y, Ishikawa H. The skin changes of POEMS syndrome. *Br J Dermatol.* 1987;117(4):523–526 [Epub 1987/10/01].

39. Humeniuk MS, Gertz MA, Lacy MQ, et al. Outcomes of patients with POEMS syndrome treated initially with radiation. *Blood.* 2013;122(1):68–73 [Epub 2013/05/24].

40. Kaushik M, Pulido JS, Abreu R, Amselem L, Dispenzieri A. Ocular findings in patients with polyneuropathy, organomegaly, endocrinopathy, monoclonal gammopathy, and skin changes syndrome. *Ophthalmology.* 2011;118(4):778–782 [Epub 2010/11/03].

41. Cui R, Yu S, Huang X, Zhang J, Tian C, Pu C. Papilloedema is an independent prognostic fac-tor for POEMS syndrome. *J Neurol.* 2014;261(1):60–65.

42. Li J, Tian Z, Zheng HY, et al. Pulmonary hypertension in POEMS syndrome. *Haematologica.* 2013;98(3):393–398 [Epub 2012/09/18].

43. Lesprit P, Godeau B, Authier FJ, et al. Pulmonary hypertension in POEMS syndrome: a new feature mediated by cytokines. *Am J Respir Crit Care Med.* 1998;157(3 Pt 1):907–911 [Epub 1998/03/28].

44. Zenone T, Bastion Y, Salles G, et al. POEMS syndrome, arterial thrombosis and thrombocy-thaemia. *J Intern Med.* 1996;240(2):107–109 [Epub 1996/08/01].

45. Kang K, Chu K, Kim DE, Jeong SW, Lee JW, Roh JK. POEMS syndrome associated with ischemic stroke. *Arch Neurol.* 2003;60(5):745–749 [Epub 2003/05/21].

46. Dupont SA, Dispenzieri A, Mauermann ML, Rabinstein AA, Brown Jr RD. Cerebral infarc-tion in POEMS syndrome: incidence, risk factors, and imaging characteristics. *Neurology.* 2009;73(16):1308–1312 [Epub 2009/10/21].

47. Dacci P, Lessi F, Dalla Bella E, Morbin M, Briani C, Lauria G. Ischemic stroke as clinical onset of POEMS syndrome. *J Neurol.* 2013;260(12):3178–3181 [Epub 2013/11/14].

48. Saida K, Kawakami H, Ohta M, Iwamura K. Coagulation and vascular abnormalities in Crow-Fukase syndrome. *Muscle Nerve.* 1997;20(4):486–492 [Epub 1997/04/01].

49. Stankowski-Drengler T, Gertz MA, Katzmann JA, et al. Serum immunoglobulin free light chain measurements and heavy chain isotype usage provide insight into disease biology in patients with POEMS syndrome. *Am J Hematol.* 2010;85(6):431–434 [Epub 2010/06/01].

50. Sanada S, Ookawara S, Karube H, et al. Marked recovery of severe renal lesions in POEMS syndrome with high-dose melphalan therapy supported by autologous blood stem cell trans-plantation. *Am J Kidney Dis.* 2006;47(4):672–679 [Epub 2006/03/28].

51. Watanabe M, Ushiyama O, Matsui M, Kakigi R, Kuroda Y. A case of crow-Fukase syndrome associated with chronic pachymeningitis. *Rinsho Shinkeigaku.* 1993;33(4):422–426 [Epub 1993/04/01].

52. Mazzeo A, Granata F, Vinci S, et al. Osteosclerotic myeloma with spinal leptomeningitis and severe polyneuropathy: a case report. *J Comput Assist Tomogr.* 2006;30(4):649–652 [Epub 2006/07/18].

53. Briani C, Fedrigo M, Manara R, et al. Pachymeningeal involvement in POEMS syndrome: MRI and histopathological study. *J Neurol Neurosurg Psychiatry.* 2012;83(1):33–37 [Epub 2011/06/10].

54. Briani C, Manara R, Lessi F, Citton V, Zambello R, Adami F. Pachymeningeal involvement in POEMS syndrome: dramatic cerebral MRI improvement after lenalidomide therapy. *Am J Hematol.* 2012;87(5):539–541 [Epub 2012/03/06].

55. Li J, Zhang W, Jiao L, et al. Combination of melphalan and dexamethasone for patients with newly diagnosed POEMS syndrome. *Blood.* 2011;117(24):6445–6449 [Epub 2011/03/12].

56. Jaccard A, Lazareth A, Karlin L, et al. A prospective phase II trial of Lenalidomide and dexamethasone (LEN-DEX) in POEMS syndrome. *Blood.* 2014;124(21):36.

57. Royer B, Merlusca L, Abraham J, et al. Efficacy of lenalidomide in POEMS syndrome: a retrospective study of 20 patients. *Am J Hematol.* 2013;88(3):207–212 [Epub 2013/01/22].

58. Nozza A, Terenghi F, Gallia F, et al. Lenalidomide and dexamethasone in patients with POEMS syndrome: results of a prospective, open-label trial. *Br J Haematol.* 2017;179(5):748–755 [Epub 2017/10/20].

59. Li J, Huang XF, Cai QQ, et al. A prospective phase II study of low dose lenalidomide plus dexamethasone in patients with newly diagnosed polyneuropathy, organomegaly, endocrinopathy, monoclonal gammopathy, and skin changes (POEMS) syndrome. *Am J Hematol.* 2018;93(6):803–809 [Epub 2018/04/01].

60. Kim SY, Lee SA, Ryoo HM, Lee KH, Hyun MS, Bae SH. Thalidomide for POEMS syndrome. *Ann Hematol.* 2006;85(8):545–546.

61. Kuwabara S, Misawa S, Kanai K, et al. Thalidomide reduces serum VEGF levels and improves peripheral neuropathy in POEMS syndrome. *J Neurol Neurosurg Psychiatry.* 2008;79(11):1255–1257.

62. Inoue D, Kato A, Tabata S, et al. Successful treatment of POEMS syndrome complicated by severe congestive heart failure with thalidomide. *Intern Med.* 2010;49(5):461–466 [Epub 2010/03/02].

63. Kawano Y, Nakama T, Hata H, et al. Successful treatment with rituximab and thalidomide of POEMS syndrome associated with Waldenstrom macroglobulinemia. *J Neurol Sci.* 2010;297(1–2):101–104 [Epub 2010/08/03].

64. Ohguchi H, Ohba R, Onishi Y, et al. Successful treatment with bortezomib and thalidomide for POEMS syndrome. *Ann Hematol.* 2011;90(9):1113–1114.

65. Misawa S, Sato Y, Katayama K, et al. Safety and efficacy of thalidomide in patients with POEMS syndrome: a multicentre, randomised, double-blind, placebo-controlled trial. *Lancet Neurol.* 2016;15(11):1129–1137 [Epub 2016/08/09].

66. Sobas MA, Alonso Vence N, Diaz Arias J, Bendaña Lopez A, Fraga Rodriguez M, Bello Lopez JL. Efficacy of bortezomib in refractory form of multicentric Castleman disease associated to poems syndrome (MCD-POEMS variant). *Ann Hematol.* 2009;89(2):217.

67. Tang X, Shi X, Sun A, et al. Successful bortezomib-based treatment in POEMS syndrome. *Eur J Haematol.* 2009;83(6):609–610.

68. Kaygusuz I, Tezcan H, Cetiner M, Kocakaya O, Uzay A, Bayik M. Bortezomib: a new therapeutic option for POEMS syndrome. *Eur J Haematol.* 2010;84(2):175–177.

69. Warsame R, Kohut IE, Dispenzieri A. Successful use of cyclophosphamide, bortezomib, and dexamethasone to treat a case of relapsed POEMS. *Eur J Haematol.* 2012;88(6):549–550.

70. Li J, Zhang W, Kang W-Y, Cao X-X, Duan M-H, Zhou D-B. Bortezomib and dexamethasone as first-line therapy for a patient with newly diagnosed polyneuropathy, organomegaly, endocrinopathy, M protein and skin changes syndrome complicated by renal failure. *Leuk Lymphoma*. 2012;53(12):2527–2529.

71. Zeng K, Yang J, Li J, et al. Effective induction therapy with subcutaneous administration of bortezomib for newly diagnosed POEMS syndrome: a case report and a review of the literature. *Acta Haematol*. 2013;129(2):101–105.

72. He H, Fu W, Du J, Jiang H, Hou J. Successful treatment of newly diagnosed POEMS syndrome with reduced-dose bortezomib based regimen. *Br J Haematol*. 2018;181(1):126–128 [Epub 2017/02/02].

73. Hogan WJ, Lacy MQ, Wiseman GA, Fealey RD, Dispenzieri A, Gertz MA. Successful treatment of POEMS syndrome with autologous hematopoietic progenitor cell transplantation. *Bone Marrow Transplant*. 2001;28:305.

74. Rovira M, Carreras E, Bladé J, et al. Dramatic improvement of POEMS syndrome following autologous haematopoietic cell transplantation. *Br J Haematol*. 2001;115(2):373–375.

75. Jaccard A, Royer B, Bordessoule D, Brouet J-C, Fermand J-P. High-dose therapy and autologous blood stem cell transplantation in POEMS syndrome. *Blood*. 2002;99(8):3057–3059.

76. Dispenzieri A, Moreno-Aspitia A, Suarez GA, et al. Peripheral blood stem cell transplantation in 16 patients with POEMS syndrome, and a review of the literature. *Blood*. 2004;104(10):3400–3407.

77. Kawajiri-Manako C, Sakaida E, Ohwada C, et al. Efficacy and long-term outcomes of autologous stem cell transplantation in POEMS syndrome: a nationwide survey in Japan. *Biol Blood Marrow Transplant*. 2018;24(6):1180–1186.

78. Cook G, Iacobelli S, van Biezen A, et al. High-dose therapy and autologous stem cell transplantation in patients with POEMS syndrome: a retrospective study of the Plasma Cell Disorder sub-committee of the Chronic Malignancy Working Party of the European Society for Blood & Marrow Transplantation. *Haematologica*. 2017;102(1):160–167.

79. Kourelis TV, Buadi FK, Kumar SK, et al. Long-term outcome of patients with POEMS syndrome: an update of the Mayo Clinic experience. *Am J Hematol*. 2016;91(6):585–589 [Epub 2016/03/15].

80. Gavriatopoulou M, Musto P, Caers J, et al. European myeloma network recommendations on diagnosis and management of patients with rare plasma cell dyscrasias. *Leukemia*. 2018;32(9):1883–1898.

81. Li J, D-b Z. New advances in the diagnosis and treatment of POEMS syndrome. *Br J Haematol*. 2013;161(3):303–315.

82. Jimenez-Zepeda VH, Trudel S, Reece DE, Chen C, Rabea AM, Kukreti V. Cyclophosphamide and prednisone induction followed by cyclophosphamide mobilization effectively decreases the incidence of engraftment syndrome in patients with POEMS syndrome who undergo stem cell transplantation. *Am J Hematol*. 2011;86(10):873–875.

83. Wang C, Huang XF, Cai QQ, et al. Prognostic study for overall survival in patients with newly diagnosed POEMS syndrome. *Leukemia*. 2017;31(1):100–106 [Epub 2016/06/25].

Chapter 7

Peripheral nervous system involvement in vasculitis

Stéphane Mathis[a,b], Mathilde Duchesne[c,d], Laurent Magy[d,e], Jean-Michel Vallat[d,e]

[a]*Department of Neurology, Nerve-Muscle Unit, CHU Bordeaux (Pellegrin University Hospital), University of Bordeaux, Bordeaux, France,* [b]*National Reference Center 'maladies neuromusculaires du grand sud-ouest', CHU Bordeaux (Pellegrin University Hospital), University of Bordeaux, Bordeaux, France,* [c]*Department of Pathology, University Hospital Dupuytren, Limoges, France,* [d]*Department of Neurology, University Hospital Dupuytren, Limoges, France,* [e]*National Reference Center 'neuropathies périphériques rares', University Hospital Dupuytren, Limoges, France*

Abbreviations

AAV	ANCA-associated vasculitis
ANCA	antineutrophil cytoplasmic antibody
C	complement (C3, C4, C5b9, etc.)
CB	conduction block
CD	cluster of differentiation (CD4, CD20, etc.)
CHCC	Chapel Hill consensus conference
CMV	cytomegalovirus
DLRPN	diabetic lomboradiculoplexus neuropathy
EGPA	eosinophilic granulomatosis with polyangiitis
EMG	electromyography
ESR	erythrocyte sedimentation rate
GCA	giant cell arteritis
GPA	granulomatosis with polyangiitis
HBV	hepatitis B virus
HCV	hepatitis C virus
HIV	human immunodeficiency virus
HSP	Henoch-Schönlein purpura
HTLV1	human T cell leukemia/lymphoma virus type 1
Ig	immunoglobulin (A, G, M)
IVIg	intravenous immunoglobulin
LCA	leukocyte common antigen
LRPN	lomboradiculoplexus neuropathy

Dysimmune Neuropathies. https://doi.org/10.1016/B978-0-12-814572-2.00007-8

145

μm	micrometer
MB	muscle biopsy
MM	multiple mononeuropathy (or 'mononeuritis multiplex')
MPA	microscopic polyangiitis
MPO	myeloperoxidase
MUP	motor unit potentials
NB	nerve biopsy
NCS	nerve conduction study
NMB	nerve-muscle biopsy (or 'neuromuscular biopsy')
NSVPN	nonsystemic vasculitic peripheral neuropathy
PAN	polyarteritis nodosa (or 'periarteritis nodosa')
PET	positron emission tomography
PLEX	plasma exchange
PNS	peripheral nervous system
PVS	primary vasculitis syndrome
RA	rheumatoid arthritis
RV	rheumatoid vasculitis
SLE	systemic lupus erythematosus
SMA	smooth muscle antigen
SNAP	sensory nerve action potentials
SVPN	systemic vasculitic peripheral neuropathy
SVS	secondary vasculitis syndrome
TAB	temporal artery biopsy
VPN	vasculitic peripheral neuropathy

Introduction

Vasculitis (or vasculitides), characterized by inflammation in and around vessels, is a series of disorders that may lead to fibrinoid necrosis, destroy blood vessel walls, and induce lumen thrombosis.[1] The clinical manifestations of systemic vasculitis (due to distal ischemia or rarely to bleeding) are highly variable, depending on tissue vulnerabilities, local immunologic environments, and, of course, the affected territory. Various organs may be involved such as the skin, kidneys, lungs, joints, nervous system, etc. There are two main categories of systemic vasculitis: primary vasculitis syndrome (PVS) and secondary vasculitis syndrome (SVS). PVS is directly caused by inflammation of blood vessels, whereas SVS is the consequence of an underlying condition such as connective tissue diseases, infections, drugs, or tumors.[1] However, both PVS and SVS are considered to be systemic autoimmune diseases. Most cases of vasculitis require treatment with corticosteroids, sometimes combined with other immunosuppressive treatments.

We agree with Collins and Dyck that *"peripheral nervous system (PNS) microvasculitis without vascular damage is a nonspecific alteration having only a weak association with clinico-pathologic surrogates of vasculitic neuropathy. It has been reported in such nonvasculitic disorders as chronic inflammatory demyelinating polyneuropathy, paraneoplastic and Sjogren's-related sensory neuronopathy, motor neuron disease, Buerger disease, diabetic polyneuropathy, infectious neuropathies, cholesterol emboli syndrome, celiac disease, and multiple entrapments".*[2]

History and classification of vasculitides

The inflammatory nature of some vascular disorders called "vasculitis" was clearly recognized by the end of the 18th and the beginning of the 19th century, first through the observations of purpura by Robert Wilan (1757–1812),[3] William Heberden (1710–1801),[4] Charles-Prosper Ollivier d'Angers (1796–1845),[5] and Johann Lukas Schönlein (1793–1864),[6] although arterial pathology had been recognized since antiquity.[7] After studies on veins and arteries by John Hunter (1728–1793),[8] Joseph Hodgson (1788–1869),[9] and others,[7] Karl von Rokitansky (1804–1878) thought that arteritis was an inflammatory process of the adventitia.[10] On the other hand, Rudolf Virchow (1821–1902)[11] observed inflammation in the intima, especially the intima-media interface.[12] In 1852, Rokitansky reported the case of a 23-year-old patient who presented, at autopsy, aneurysmal lesions with nodes in multiple arteries (excepted aorta and most of its more prominent root branches) that he considered dissecting aneurysms caused by spontaneous tears in the intima and media of smaller arteries.[13] With the development of microscopical and staining techniques in the second half of the 19th century, diseases such as vasculitis have been better characterized.[14] Thus, it was the German physicians Adolf Kussmaul (1822–1909) and Rudolf Robert Maier (1824–1888) who first fully described this new disease they named "periarteris nodosa,"[15] 14 years after Rokitansky.[13] It corresponds to the first complete description of this form of systemic necrotizing vasculitis, also known as "Kussmaul-Maier disease."[12] The 27-year-old patient described by Kussmaul and Maier presented acute febrile muscle weakness, nephritis, and subcutaneous nodules of the abdomen and chest. He died within one month, and upon autopsy, the microscopic examination of the nodularly thickened vessels showed dramatic inflammatory changes in the media and adventitia, with intact intima.[15,16] A few years later, Hans Eppinger (1848–1916), after analysis of anatomic specimens of Rokitansky's case (small bowel, mesenteric and coronary arteries), observed marked thickening of the intima and disruption of all wall layers.[17]

After these first descriptions of periarteritis nodosa, later called "*polyarteritis acuta nodosa*" (PAN),[18,19] many authors reported other forms of vasculitis under this term. For example, the term "*infantile periarteritis nodosa*" was used to describe early cases of Kawasaki disease;[20,21] some cases of microscopic polyangiitis (MPA) have also been classified as PAN in some studies.[22] Moreover, during the following decades, the debate about the nature of vasculitis centered on the question of the anatomic origin of arterial inflammation, especially with the description of many new forms of vasculitis.[23] After the observations of Eduard Heinrich Henoch (1820–1910) in 1874, the concept of Henoch-Schönlein purpura (HSP) emerged, without clear cause until 1973 and the identification of vascular immunoglobulin A (IgA) deposits.[24] In 1890, Jonathan Hutchinson (1828–1913) reported a *"peculiar form of thrombotic arteritis of the aged (that) is sometimes productive of gangrene,"*[25] corresponding to the disease described many years later by Bayard Taylor Horton (1895–1980),[26–28] nowadays known as "giant cell (temporal) arteritis." Takayasu's arteritis was described in 1908 by the Japanese physician Mikito Takayasu (1860–1938),[29] although other cases had previously been reported.[23] In 1936–39,[30, 31] after a first observation by Heinz Klinger (1907–?) a few years earlier,[32] Friedrich Wegener (1907–90) described the disease nowadays known as "Wegener's granulomatosis." In 1951, Jacob Churg (1910–2001) and Lotte Strauss (1913–85) reported on *"allergic granulomatosis, allergic angiitis, and periarteritis nodosa,"* [33] called "Churg-Strauss disease." In 1967, the Japanese pediatrician Tomisaku Kawasaki (1931) was the first to report another form of vasculitis with *"acute febrile mucocutaneous syndrome with lymphoid involvement with specific desquamation of the fingers and toes in children,"*[34] known as "Kawasaki's disease."

In 1930, PAN (a term at that time still used in a generic sense to encompass all types of vasculitis) was classified on pathological criteria into four stages by Aaron Arkin, according to the characteristic changes observed in the small arteries.[35] But, considering the great variety of necrotizing vasculitis, a first clinico-pathologic classification of vasculitis was proposed in the 1950s by Zeek et al., separating small-vessel vasculitis from PAN and other conditions affecting larger vessels. Zeek et al. divided them into periarteritis nodosa, allergic granulomatosis, Wegener's granulomatosis, eukocytoclastic angiitis (or hypersensitivity angiitis), and giant-cell arteritis.[36, 37] Another classification of vasculitides was proposed in 1976, with the five following categories: leukocytoclastic vasculitis, rheumatic vasculitis, granulomatous vasculitis, polyarteritis nodosa (PAN), and giant cell arteritis (GCA).[38] Over the years, the presence of circulating immune complexes and perivascular deposits of various immune globulins and complement suggested an immunologic cause, and older terms (such as microscopic polyarteritis) were resurrected, generating some confusion and a lack of standardized diagnostic terms and definitions.[14] In 1990, the American College of Rheumatology proposed seven categories of vasculitis for a standardized description of groups of patients in therapeutic, epidemiologic, or other studies: PAN, Churg-Strauss syndrome, Wegener's granulomatosis, hypersensitivity vasculitis, HSP, GCA, and Takayasu arteritis.[39] In 1994, a first consensus, the Chapel Hill consensus conference on the nomenclature of vasculitis (CHCC 1994), was obtained for a limited number (10) of primary vasculitis that were the most common ones, based on the size and histopathology of involved vessels.[40] But some limitations remained in this classification, such as the incomplete list of the various forms of vasculitis, no single-organ vasculitides, and the lack of the antineutrophil cytoplasmic antibodies (ANCA)-associated vasculitides (AAV). For these reasons, a new consensus methodology for the classification of AAV was developed and validated.[41] In 2012, the CHCC 1994 was finally revised (CHCC 2012), with the elimination of most of the eponyms and also the inclusion of secondary forms of vasculitis.[42] Vasculitis syndromes were still classified according to the size of the affected vessels, corresponding to the major criterion of classification.[42] They can be regrouped into large vessel (aorta and its branches; diameter > 100 μm), medium vessel (smaller than the major branches of the aorta, containing an internal elastic membrane and muscular media and adventitia; 40–100 μm of diameter), and small vessel (including capillaries and postcapillary venules and arterioles; diameter < 40 μm; small-vessel vasculitis is called microvasculitis) vasculitis (Table 1 and Fig. 1).[43]

Diagnostic criteria of vasculitis

The classification criteria for the various vasculitic syndromes (mainly proposed for research purposes) are finally not useful for the diagnosis of vasculitis, a still challenging and uncommon disease (annual incidence in adults: 140/1,000,000).[44] The most frequent forms of vasculitis are GCA, cutaneous vasculitides, rheumatoid vasculitis (RV), PAN, and the ANCA-associated vasculitides: granulomatosis with polyangiitis (GPA, Wegener's), eosinophilic granulomatosis with polyangiitis (EGPA, Churg-Strauss), and MPA.[45]

The first step for the diagnosis of vasculitis is the clinical examination, first based on the recognition of patterns or clusters of signs and symptoms: headache, scalp tenderness, jaw claudication, vision loss, and muscle stiffness (GCA); new-onset cough with hemoptysis and hematuria (pulmonary-renal syndrome in MPA); chronic sinus involvement or asthma and eosinophilia (GPA; EGPA); absence of a pulse or blood pressure, or its unilateral decrease in an arm (Takayasu's arteritis); Raynaud's phenomenon and palpable purpura in a patient with hepatitis C virus (cryoglobulinaemic vasculitis); skin rash and ulcers, myalgia, arthralgia, etc.[46] The age of syndrome onset may also be useful to orientate the diagnosis: for example, GCA usually occurs in patients over 50 years, whereas Kawasaki's disease develops almost exclusively in children.[46]

Function of the targeted organ(s) and the cause of vasculitis, patients may present anemia (usually normochromic and normocytic), thrombocytosis, eosinophilia, hematuria, proteinuria, elevated transaminases, crryoglobulinemia, elevated creatine kinase or aldolase, etc. The erythrocyte sedimentation rate (ESR) is often elevated, along with the C-reactive protein (CRP). However, some ancillary tests may be helpful to orientate the diagnosis in case of clinical symptoms suggestive of vasculitis. For example, cytoplasmic ANCA (cANCA) is seen most commonly in generalized GPA; perinuclear ANCA (pANCA) is observed most commonly in MPA. Complement levels are also useful in the differential diagnosis of glomerulonephritis: C3 and C4 levels are usually

TABLE 1 Classification of vasculitic neuropathy.

Primary systemic vasculitides			Secondary systemic vasculitides		Nonsystemic/localized vasculitis	
Predominantly small-vessel vasculitis	**Predominantly medium-vessel vasculitis**	**Predominantly large-vessel vasculitis**			**Nonsystemic vasculitic neuropathy**	
Microscopic polyangiitis[a]	Polyarteritis nodosa	Giant cell arteritis	CTD	Rheumatoid arthritis	Nonsystemic vasculitic neuropathy	Nondiabetic radiculoplexus neuropathy
Eosinophilic granulomatosis with polyangiitis (CCS)[a]				SLE		Wartenberg's migrant sensory neuritis
Granulomatosis with polyangiitis (WG)[a]				Sjögren's syndrome	Diabetic radiculoplexus neuropathy	
Essential mixed non-HCV cryoglobulinemia				Systemic sclerosis	Localized cutaneous/neuropathic vasculitis	Wartenberg's migrant sensory neuritis
IgA vasculitis (HSP)				Dermatomyositis		Others
Hypocomplementemic urticarial (anti-C1q) vasculitis				MCTD		
			Sarcoidosis			
			Behcet's disease			
			Cogan's syndrome			
			Infection			
			Drugs			
			Malignancy			
			Inflammatory bowel disease			

CCS, Churg-Strauss syndrome; CTD, connectivite tissue disease; HCV, hepatitis C virus; HSP, Henoch-Schönlein purpura; MCTD, mixed connective tissue disease; SLE, systemic lupus erythematosus; WG, Wegener's granulomatosis.
[a] Vasculitis associated with antineutrophil cytoplasmic antibodies (ANCA).
Adapted from Collins et al., 2010.

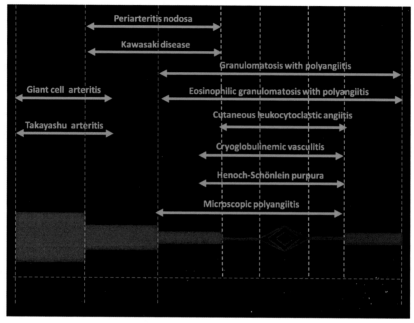

FIG. 1 Schematic distribution of the various forms of primary vasculitis as a function of the caliber of the affected vessels. Large artery refers to the aorta and the largest branches directed toward major body regions (e.g., to the extremities and the head and neck); medium-sized artery refers to the main visceral arteries (e.g., renal, hepatic, coronary, and mesenteric arteries), and small artery refers to the distal intraparenchymal arterial radicals that connect with arterioles. *(Adapted from Jennette et al., 1994).*

decreased in lupus nephritis, cryoglobulinaemia, or endocarditis, but are typically normal in many vasculitic syndromes.[46]

Diagnostic tests to confirm suspicions of vasculitis are based on tissue biopsy: temporal artery biopsy (TAB) (if suspicion of GCA), skin biopsy (in patients with cutaneous involvement), nerve/muscle biopsy (in case of neuromuscular symptoms), renal biopsy (in patients with multisystem disease and rising creatinine, in the setting of proteinuria of unexplained etiology, or in the presence of cellular casts in the urine), nasal/sinus biopsy (if suspicion of GPA or eosinophilic GPA), or even lung biopsy (in case of pulmonary abnormalities).[46] Vascular imaging (angiography, magnetic resonance imaging, ultrasound, computed tomography, PET scanning) may also be helpful to orientate the diagnosis and management of the disease.[46]

Vasculitic peripheral neuropathies: Clinical and electrophysiological features

Vasculitic peripheral neuropathy (VPN) is rare in comparison to other causes with peripheral neuropathy, such as diabetes mellitus. Its annual incidence is estimated to be 0.6–1.2 per 100,000 people.[47] However, among all the manifestations of vasculitis, PNS involvement is a frequent symptom: it occurs in up to 70% of the systemic necrotizing vasculitides,[45] but is rare in other forms of vasculitides such as GCA and predominantly cutaneous vasculitides.[1] The most frequent causes of VPN are PAN (VPN in 50%–70% of the cases), EGPA (VPN in 64% of the cases), cryoglobulinemia (VPN in 50% of the cases), and GPA (VPN in 25% of the cases).[45]

Since the first described cases of systemic necrotized vasculitis at the end of the 19th century, classic textbook teaching has been that VPN usually appears as a "mononeuritis multiplex" (MM, or multiple mononeuropathy) associated with PAN, less commonly with rheumatoid arthritis (RA) or systemic lupus erythematosus (SLE).[48–51] However, VPN is not always linked to a connective tissue disease, and some patients with necrotizing vasculitis and PNS involvement may present with a distal symmetrical sensorimotor polyneuropathy.[52] The classic MM pattern is secondary to lesions in larger vessels (leading to the whole nerve trunk infarction), whereas distal symmetric polyneuropathy is due to a more diffuse peripheral nerve ischemia (multiple ischemic small lesions affecting longer nerves). Between these two patterns, there is an overlap with asymmetric polyneuropathy resulting from the confluence of patchy discrete infarctions of small vessels in many individual peripheral nerves.[45] The classical MM pattern presents as an acute or subacute painful sensorimotor deficit (with numbness) in the territory of a single nerve, followed by similar attacks involving other nerves (multifocal pattern). Various nerves may be affected, with the most common being the ulnar nerve in the upper limbs (35%) as well as the peroneal (90%) and tibial (38%) nerves in the lower limbs; other peripheral nerves may also be involved, such as the median (26%), radial (12%), femoral (6%), or sciatic (3%) nerves,[48, 53, 54] although cranial nerve involvement is rare.[55] Finally, most patients with VPN present with slowly progressive asymmetrical polyneuropathy (36%–85%) or MM pattern (13%–45%), rather than distal symmetric polyneuropathy (2%–25%).[52, 53, 56–62] VPN usually occurs in the sixth through eighth decades,[53, 62] with a mean age at 59.[55]

Electrodiagnostic studies, if sufficiently extensive, almost always reveal evidence of a primary axonal, sensorimotor (predominantly sensory in 10%) peripheral neuropathy, mostly multifocal. On needle electromyogram (EMG) examination, decreased recruitment of motor unit potentials (MUP) and fibrillation potentials are found in up to 90% of the clinically weak muscles (generally in a distally accentuated, but without a clear length-dependent pattern), with long-duration MUP in 50% of the cases.[55] Nerve conduction studies (NCS) usually show an inability to evoke sensory nerve action potentials (SNAP) in the affected nerves, but also sometimes in nerves without clinical symptoms;[52] this sensory involvement may be the only abnormality of NCS in some rare cases.[63] Pure motor presentation is extremely rare, as are indolent forms.[55, 64] Compound muscle action potentials (CMAPs) are less affected overall, except for a frequent inability to evoke a response upon stimulation, especially in the peroneal nerve.[52] Distal latencies may be normal mildly prolonged, conduction velocities mildly reduced, and F-wave or H-reflex latencies normal or mildly prolonged. Partial motor conduction blocks (CB) are rarely seen,[65] but transient "pseudo CB" (axon noncontinuity CB) may occur in 10%–25% of patients, especially if NCS is performed in the acute phase of vasculitis (within 9 days after the onset of symptoms).[66, 67] Pseudo CB is more reflective of focal axonal damage than a demyelinating process.[53, 63] Although 9% of patients with VPN present a mix of axonal and demyelinating electrophysiological features, predominant signs of demyelination have to lead to the search for a differential diagnosis.[55]

The first consensus recommendation on the classification, diagnosis, and treatment of VPN was established in 2010 by the Peripheral Nerve Society Guideline Group. The presence of ANCAs and a high level of ESR (ESR ≥ 100 mm/h) were considered exclusion criteria for nonsystemic vasculitic peripheral neuropathy (NSVPN).[68] Based on these first consensus criteria, new diagnostic criteria for VPN were developed by the Brighton Collaboration Vasculitic Peripheral Neuropathy Working Group in 2015, adding that the existence of any form of vasculitis other than nerve or muscle is exclusion criteria for NSVPN; there are three levels of definition for VPN (Table 2).[69] The diagnosis of VPN

TABLE 2 Brighton collaboration case definition of vasculitic neuropathy.

Level 1 definition (gold standard)

- Biopsy of peripheral nerve meets criteria for histo-pathologically definite vasculitis

Level 2 definition

- Clinical features are suggestive of vasculitic neuropathy[a]
  AND
- Histo-pathological support for the existence of vasculitis: biopsy of peripheral nerve meets criteria for histo-pathologically probable vasculitis
  OR
- Diagnosis of systemic vasculitis confirmed by biopsy
  OR
- Biopsy of skin or muscle meets criteria for histo-pathologically definite vasculitis

Level 3 definition (minimum acceptable evidence)

- Biopsy of peripheral nerve or muscle not done or does not meet criteria for definite or probable vasculitis
  AND
- Clinical features are suggestive of vasculitic neuropathy.[a]

[a] According to the Brighton definition of vasculitic neuropathy, clinical features that are suggestive of vasculitic neuropathy are: (a) electrodiagnostic or clinical examination evidence of peripheral neuropathy and (b) a clinical presentation that is typical for vasculitic neuropathy (multifocal or asymmetric, involving sensory or sensory-motor nerves, lower limb-predominant, painful, and with one or more acute attacks).
Adapted from Hadden et al., 2017.

is generally easy to suspect in a patient with a combination of painful MM or asymmetric sensorimotor polyneuropathy, suggestive extraneurological symptoms (especially with weight loss), and inflammatory biological anomalies. However, in some cases, vasculitis may be less typical as the forms are restricted to the PNS, an old concept described by Kernohan and Woltman,[51] but clearly established as a distinct clinicopathologic entity in the 1980s as NSVPN.[52, 53] Finally, the detection of a characteristic microscopic lesion (skin, kidney, etc.) is mandatory to confirm the diagnosis of vasculitis. In many cases, therefore, a nerve (NB) or nerve/muscle biopsy (NMB) is required to confirm the diagnosis (with or without the clinical features of neuropathy) by showing some specific pathological signs.

Vasculitic peripheral neuropathies: Pathological features

Since the end of the 19th century, many cases of patients with peripheral nerve involvement and vasculitis were reported, sometimes with pathological confirmation (NB),[70–75] some cases were also reported as "infarct in nerves" by Kernohan and Woltman in 1938.[51] As described in the CHCC 2012 and PNS 2010, the histological criteria to classify vasculitis neuropathies are based on the size of the affected vessels, and according to systemic or isolated organ damage: systemic vasculitic peripheral neuropathy (SVPN) or affecting only the peripheral nerves (single-organ nonsystemic vasculitic peripheral neuropathies, NSVPN). The overall sensitivity of a nerve or nerve-plus-muscle biopsy for definite vasculitis is between 50% and 60%. Systemic vasculitides are also classified according to the size of the affected vessels; however, the vessels, when they are intraparenchymal, are regarded as small vessels. Thus, all vessels in peripheral nerves, including the largest arteries, are categorized as small vessels. It is important to realize that medium- and large-vessel vasculitides can also affect small arteries and large arterioles in nerves.[76] As proposed by Gwathmey et al., VPN can therefore be classified in a dichotomous way: nerve large arteriole vasculitis and nerve microvasculitis.[76]

A good reason to perform NB in this treatable peripheral neuropathy is that peripheral nerves are commonly involved (even in the systemic form of the disease), the probability of this diagnosis being higher when sural nerve conduction is abnormal.[77, 78] NB is particularly indicated if obtaining other tissues for diagnosis is not feasible or warranted. In such cases, the most informative nerves are the sural, superficial fibular, and superficial radial nerves, depending on the affected territories.[45] Although taking a nerve sample from a clinically affected nerve is an accepted general rule, NB may have the same diagnostic yield on a clinically unaffected nerve, provided the NCS demonstrates subclinical involvement.[79] Although the sural nerve usually appears as a good site for NB,[45] the superficial fibular nerve is sometimes preferred because it allows simultaneously performing a nerve biopsy (fibular superficial nerve) and muscle biopsy (*peroneus brevis* muscle).[80–82] The diagnostic value of a muscle biopsy (MB) is lower than that of NB in vasculitis, but combined NMB may be helpful by increasing the number of medium-sized arterioles and/or small vessels available for examination,[80, 82–84] therefore increasing the positive diagnosis of vasculitis by 6%–27%.[80, 85] If only MB is available, it is preferable to biopsy a symptomatic muscle or a muscle that shows fibrillation and positive sharp waves on the needle EMG study.[77] Sometimes, vasculitic lesions on the peripheral nerve are focal, only observed on certain slides. So, if the diagnosis of VPN is strongly suspected but not confirmed after the initial microscopic examination, it is mandatory to serially cut the whole peripheral nerve and muscle samples for a second pathological study.[86]

Peripheral nerve trunks are supplied by extrinsic (epineurial vessels and regional arteries) and intrinsic (longitudinal microvessels within the fascicules) plexi of microvessels, collectively termed "vasa nervorum," and resistant to ischemia due to an efficient anastomotic blood supply.[87] Vasculitis is defined as the immunological inflammation of a blood vessel, with consequent destruction of the vascular wall and tissue ischemia. Vasculitic neuropathy is the consequence of ischemic damage due to the occlusion of blood vessels associated with an inflammatory process in the vessel walls of the vasa nervorum. As small-sized arteries and arterioles, vasa nervorum are a common target of systemic vasculitis, especially arterioles of the epineurium (diameter: 20–300 μm)[88] and epineurial capillaries (diameter: 10–20 μm).[89] The endoneurial capillaries, larger and widely spaced (especially in the central region of nerve fascicules), represent a point of vulnerability, explaining the typical pathological findings of the centro-fascicular axon loss observed in ischemic neuropathies;[88] however, for unexplained reasons, epineurial arterioles are the preferential targets in most VPN.[53, 57, 82, 83, 85, 90–92]

In large nerve arteriole, pathological changes occur in the epineurial and perineurial vessels (75–300 μm of diameter).[76] The early neuropathological feature of VPN is the presence of perivascular infiltrates of inflammatory mononuclear cells (Fig. 2A), which are not specific.[88] Such features may also be observed in various types of inflammatory neuropathies where they are usually predominant findings. More specific pathological features are signs of active necrotizing vasculitis, corresponding to the acute hallmark changes observed in VPN. These are intramural and perivascular infiltrates (Fig. 2B) of mixed inflammatory cells (mononuclear cells, polymorphonuclear leukocytes, eosinophils), leukocytoclasia and sometimes granulomas, dissolution of the internal elastic membrane, edema or thickening of the adventitia, fibrinoid necrosis of the media, and occlusion of the lumen of involved vessels (Fig. 2C).[78, 93] Hemorrhage and deposits of hemosiderin (Fig. 2D) into the surrounding tissue can also be observed. Usually, lymphocytes are predominant in the vessel walls and perivascular area, with marked eosinophilic infiltration being suggestive of EGPA.[91, 94] In vessels <40 μm in diameter (arterioles without internal elastic lamina, capillaries, and venules), there is inflammation of the vessel walls with fragmentation and necrosis of the tunica media.[95, 96] For inflammatory

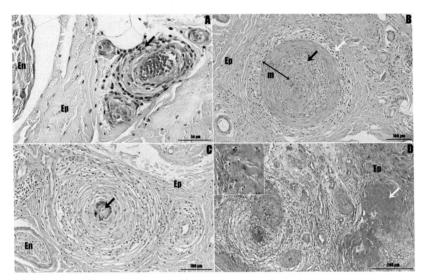

FIG. 2   Nerve biopsy, paraffin embedded section, hematein eosin, optical microscopy (Ep: epineurium; En: endoneurium). (A) Perivascular infiltrate of inflammatory mononuclear cells *(black arrow)* which are not specific in a case of necrotizing vasculitis (observed on another section). (B) Intramural *(black arrow)* into the media (m) and perivascular *(white arrow)* infiltrates of mixed inflammatory cells in necrotizing vasculitis associated with neurolymphomatosis. (C) Fibrinoid necrosis of the media (*), and occlusion of the lumen *(black arrow)* of involved vessels in necrotizing vasculitis associated with neurolymphomatosis. (D) Hemorrhage *(white arrow)* and deposits of hemosiderin (frame) in a necrotizing vasculitis associated with essential mixed cryoglobulinemia.

infiltrates, an immunohistochemistry on paraffin sections may be useful to distinguish the different types of cells (Fig. 3). It should encompass at least LCA (CD45RO, pan-leukocyte), CD3 (pan-T cells), and CD8 (cytotoxic T cells), and sometimes CD4 (T helper), CD20 (B cells), and smooth muscle antigen (SMA).[97] In up to 80% of affected patients, direct immunofluorescence shows deposits of IgM, fibrinogen, and complement (C3 and/or C5b-9) in epineurial vessel walls.[57, 91, 98, 99]

Chronic neuropathological changes correspond to signs of the so-called inactive vasculitis: concentric fibrous scarring and thickening of the intima and media (Fig. 4A); minimal intramural and perivascular infiltrates of inflammatory cells, lymphocytes, and plasma cells; and splitting and actual overgrowth of the internal elastic membrane.[78] Moreover, arterial occlusion is followed after days or weeks by spontaneous recanalization (Fig. 4B) of the artery.[93]

On average, axonal degeneration secondary to ischemic damage affects 65% of the nerve fibers, but its degree depends on the activity of the vasculitic process.[82] Depending on the severity of VPN, axonal degeneration is characterized by typical signs of ischemic neuropathy: acute asymmetric axonal

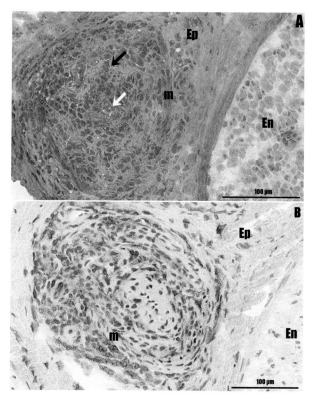

FIG. 3   Nerve biopsy of a necrotizing vasculitis associated to hepatitis C, frozen section, hematein eosin (A) and immunohistochemistry (B), optical microscopy (Ep: epineurium; En: endoneurium). (A) Strong perivascular and intramural infiltrates *(black arrow)* of a small vessel with destruction of the media (m) on the way to occlusion in epineuriumn *(white arrow)*. (B) Anti-CD45 antibody (pan-leukocyte) staining showing infiltrate of mononuclear inflammatory cells (lymphocytes and macrophages).

degeneration between and within fascicles (Fig. 5), axon loss predominated on myelinated fibers larger than 7 μm in diameter, central fascicular degeneration (selective loss of the myelinated fibers of the center of the fascicles), or selective nerve fascicular degeneration (corresponding to the loss of > 50% of nerve fibers only in some fascicules, with other fascicles being intact).[88, 93, 100] With healed vasculitic lesions, the following are observed mimicking arteriosclerotic lesions: perivascular and intramural fibrosis with fragmentation of the internal elastic membrane and narrowing, and occlusion and calcification of the lumen (or recanalization of the previously occluded lumen).[45] Sometimes, these may be associated with other findings suggestive of the presence of remote vasculitis, such as miniature bundles of aberrant regenerating axons[91] or reactive proliferation of capillaries in the epineurium.[101]

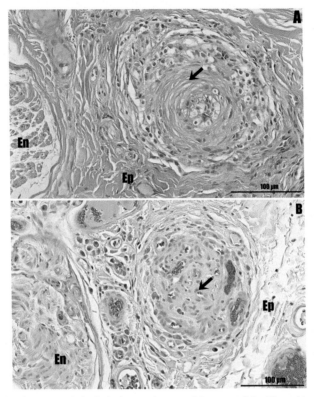

FIG. 4 Chronic neuropathological changes in necrotizing vasculitis. Nerve biopsy, paraffin embedded section, hematein eosin, optical microscopy (Ep: epineurium; En: endoneurium). (A) Concentric fibrous scarring and thickening of the intima and media *(black arrow)* in a necrotizing vasculitis associated with hepatitis C. (B) Spontaneous recanalization *(black arrow)* after days or weeks following occlusion of vessel in a polyarteritis nodosa (PAN).

The diagnosis of VPN is based on criteria (Peripheral Nerve Society guideline) for pathologically "definite" or "probable" vasculitic neuropathy (Table 3).[68] Although NB may establish the vasculitic process, it usually cannot determine the cause of the vasculitis by only analyzing NB. However, NB can give some clues: vasculitic involvement of larger epineurial arterioles (100–250 μm) is typically observed in PAN, GPA, EGPA, and RV;[45] predominant involvement of smaller epineurial arterioles (< 100 μm) is more suggestive of Sjögren's syndrome, SLE, and NSVPN;[102] and the involvement of epineurial veins occurs more commonly in GPA and EGPA.[103] Moreover, NB provides diagnostic guidance according to the type of inflammatory infiltrate: the cellular predominance of inflammatory infiltrate (eosinophils for EGPA), the presence of granulomas (GPA) with or without giant cells (giant cells arteritis), leukocytoclasia, and the type of deposits (IgA in IgA vasculitis).[76]

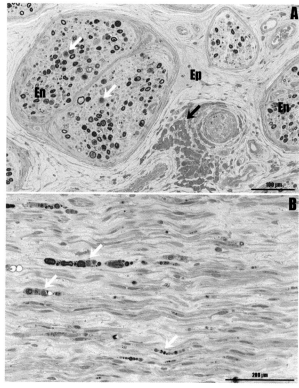

FIG. 5 Nerve biopsy, semithin section, toluidine blue, transversal (A) and longitudinal (B) sections, optical microscopy (Ep: epineurium; En: endoneurium). (A) Heterogeneous and multifocal axonal loss of myelinated fibers associated with ovoids, which are axon and myelin *(white arrow)* debris corresponding to acute axonal lesions in nerve fascicule, perivascular inflammatory cells in epineurium *(black arrow)*. (B) Severe axonal loss associated with acute axonal lesions *(white arrow)*.

TABLE 3 Pathological criteria of vasculitic peripheral neuropathy.

Pathologically definite vasculitis[a]	Pathologically probable vasculitis
I—Active lesions: nerve biopsy showing collection of inflammatory cells in vessel wall AND one or more signs of acute vascular damage 1. Fibrinoid necrosis 2. Loss/disruption of endothelium 3. Loss/fragmentation of internal elastic lamina 4. Loss/fragmentation of smooth muscle cells in media (can be highlighted with antismooth muscle actin staining) 5. Acute thrombosis 6. Vascular/perivascular hemorrhage OR 7. Leukocytoclasia	I—Pathologic criteria for definite vasculitic neuropathy not satisfied AND

Continued

TABLE 3 Pathological criteria of vasculitic peripheral neuropathy—cont'd

Pathologically definite vasculitis[a]	Pathologically probable vasculitis
II—Chronic lesion with signs of healing/repair: nerve biopsy showing collection of mononuclear inflammatory cells in vessel wall AND one or more signs of chronic vascular damage with repair 1. Intimal hyperplasia 2. Fibrosis of media 3. Adventitial/peri-adventitial fibrosis OR 4. Chronic thrombosis with recanalization	II—Presence of predominantly axonal changes AND
III—No evidence of another primary disease process that can mimic vasculitis pathologically: lymphoma, lymphomatoid granulomatosis, or amyloidosis	III—Perivascular inflammation accompanied by signs of active or chronic vascular damage (as defined in the left column) OR —Perivascular/vascular inflammation plus at least one additional class II or III pathologic predictor of definite vasculitic neuropathy[b]: 1. Vascular deposition of complement, IgM, or fibrinogen by direct immunofluorescence 2. Hemosiderin deposits (Perls' stain for iron) 3. Asymmetric nerve fiber loss or degeneration 4. Prominent active axonal degeneration OR 5. Myofiber necrosis, regeneration, or infarcts in peroneus brevis muscle biopsy (not explained by underlying myopathy)

[a] Presence of a chronic lesion does not exclude active vasculitis (vasculitides are usually segmental and multifocal, producing lesions of different ages in the same tissue or end organ).
[b] Additional alterations used by some authorities as supportive of vasculitis but lacking in adequate evidence (more study required):
1. Neovascularization (class II/III evidence suggests that this finding is probably not a predictor of vasculitis).
2. Endoneurial purpura (one negative class II study; one positive class III study).
3. Focal perineurial inflammation, degeneration, thickening (only class IV evidence).
4. Injury neuroma, microfasciculation (only class IV evidence).
5. Swollen axons filled with organelles (one negative but nonconvincing class II study) and other experimentally demonstrated axonal changes of acute ischemia, such as attenuated axons, flattened myelin profiles, tubular profiles, and axonal cytolysis.
Adapted from Collins et al., 2010.

Main characteristics of the various forms of vasculitic peripheral neuropathy

Peripheral nervous system involvement induced by a primary systemic vasculitis

Predominantly small-vessel vasculitis

Microscopic polyangiitis

MPA is an idiopathic autoimmune systemic vasculitis predominantly affecting small-caliber blood vessels. This microscopic form of PAN, first identified in 1923 by Friedreich Wohlwill (1881–1958),[75] was gradually recognized as a new entity distinct from classic PAN and finally classified as a disease since 1985.[104] MPA mainly involves kidneys (rapidly progressive glomerulonephritis), lungs (diffuse alveolar hemorrhage with pulmonary fibrosis), and skin (palpable purpura), but also with gastrointestinal manifestations (abdominal pain). PNS is involved in 37%–72% of patients,[105–107] with necrotizing vasculitis revealed by NB in up to 80% of the cases with a mixed inflammatory infiltrate and sparse immune deposits.[62] Various nerves may be affected (mainly the superficial peroneal and deep peroneal, ulnar, and median nerves), but cranial nerve involvement is rare.[105] It is associated with the presence of perinuclear ANCA in 50%–75% of the cases, but the absence of circulating ANCA does not exclude MPA.[105]

Eosinophilic granulomatosis with polyangiitis

Formerly called Churg-Strauss syndrome, EGPA is a rare systemic disseminated vasculitis affecting small- to medium-sized vessels (including arteries, arterioles, capillaries, veins, and veinules); its estimated annual incidence is approximately 0.11–2.66/1,000,000 people.[108] EGPA is characterized by extravascular granulomas in patients suffering from asthma and tissue eosinophilia. It is associated with the presence of ANCA in 40% of the cases, with specificity to myeloperoxidase (MPO). PNS is involved in about 70% of the cases.[109–113] NB shows a necrotizing vasculitis with mixed infiltrate with eosinophils, granulomas, and sparse immune deposits (Fig. 6A).

Granulomatosis with polyangiitis

Also known as Wegener's granulomatosis, GPA a systemic disorder that is characterized by necrotizing vasculitis of small and medium vessels. Its estimated annual incidence is 8–10/1,000,000 people.[114] GPA is characterized by the triad of necrotizing granuloma of the upper and lower respiratory system, systemic vasculitis, and necrotizing glomerulonephritis; upper respiratory tract involvement, present in 90% of the cases, is usually the first clinical manifestation (sinus pain, epistaxis, etc.).[115] Nervous system involvement is observed in about 33%–50% of the patients; PNS involvement is frequently observed (15%–44%) in GPA, including peripheral neuropathy (mainly MM) and cranial nerve palsy (mostly the second, sixth, and seventh cranial nerves).[116–118] NB shows necrotizing vasculitis, granulomas, collagen necrosis, and sparse immune deposits.

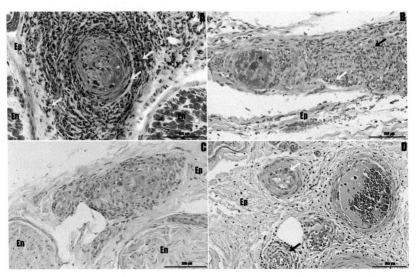

FIG. 6 Nerve biopsy, frozen section (A) and paraffin-embedded section (B–C–D), hematein eosin, optical microscopy (Ep: epineurium; En: endoneurium). (A) Eosinophilic granulomatosis with polyangiitis (EGPA) showing perivascular and intramural infiltrate of mixed inflammatory cells containing polymorphonuclear eosinophils *(white arrows)*. Fibrinoid necrosis (*) and occlusion of the lumen. (B) Leukocytoclastic vasculitis. Intramural infiltrate of mixed inflammatory cells with polymorphonuclear neutrophils *(white arrow)*, some of which degenerate leading to leukocytoclasis *(black arrow)* with nuclear dust (karyorrhexis). Fibrinoid necrosis (*) and occlusion of the lumen. (C) Necrotizing vasculitis associated with rheumatoid arthritis. Perivascular and intramural infiltrate of mixed inflammatory cells. (D) Necrotizing vasculitis associated with neurolymphomatosis. Perivascular infiltrate of inflammatory mononuclear cells that are not specific beside a proliferation of lymphoma cells within the lumina of a small blood vessel.

Essential mixed cryoglobulinemia (non-HCV)

Cryoglobulinemia is a rare condition due to the presence of circulating cryoglobulins; these large cryoproteins correspond to immunoglobulins (Ig) that precipitate below core body temperatures, then dissolve upon rewarming.[119] Cryoglobulinemia may be isolated (essential cryoglobulinemia) or associated with a particular disease (secondary cryoglobulinemia). There are three types of cryoglobulinemia, according to the Ig composition:[120] type I (composed of only one monoclonal Ig, usually IgM, less frequently, IgG, IgA, or light chains); type II (monoclonal IgM with rheumatoid factor activity); and type III (polyclonal IgM with rheumatoid factor activity) cryoglobulinemia. Types II and III cryoglobulinemia are commonly termed mixed cryoglobulinemia.[121] Vasculitis is linked to vessel obstruction by monoclonal cryoglobulin aggregates in type I cryoglobulins and immune complex deposition in types II and III cryoglobulins. It is thus an immune-complex mediated systemic vasculitis involving small- to medium-sized vessels. It is frequently complicated by PNS involvement, and usually characterized by paresthesia of the lower limbs due to a mild sensory peripheral neuropathy; sometimes a more severe sensory or sensorimotor peripheral neuropathy is present.[121] NB is characterized by necrotizing vasculitis (Fig. 2D), microangiopathy, and immune deposits (more frequently IgM).

Henoch-Schönlein purpura

HSP, due to IgA tissue deposits, is the most common vasculitis disorder of childhood, characterized by the association of palpable purpura concentrated in some areas, arthralgia or arthritis, abdominal pain, and glomerulonephritis. PNS involvement is uncommon in HSP, but various clinical phenotypes have been observed: Guillain-Barré syndrome, brachial plexopathy, mononeuropathy (multiple or not), and cranial nerve palsies (mainly facial palsy).[122] NB highlights IgA deposits.

Leukocytoclastic vasculitis

Leukocytoclastic vasculitis (hypersensitivity vasculitis or urticarial vasculitis) concerns the dermal postcapillary venules. This vasculitis is most often idiopathic, but there are some causes such as infections, neoplasms, inflammatory disorders, and drug-induced vasculitis. Clinically, features include palpable purpura, lower extremity location, small vessel involvement, and extracutaneous involvement (such as PNS) in approximately 30% of patients. Microscopically, leukocytoclastic vasculitis is characterized by neutrophil infiltration into small venule vessel walls, which present fibrinoid necrosis and extravasation of red cells. The neutrophils degenerate and are known as leukocytoclasis with nuclear dust (karyorrhexis) (Fig. 6B).[123, 124]

Predominantly medium vessel vasculitis

Polyarteritis nodosa

PAN is a systemic necrotizing vasculitis that predominantly affects medium and small arteries. The most frequent findings are general symptoms in 93%, neurologic manifestations in 79% (mainly MM), renal artery microaneurysms in 62%, skin involvement (livedo reticularis, cutaneous necrosis, and nodules) in 49%, abdominal pain in 35%, and hypertension in 34%.[22] Most cases of PAN are primary systemic vasculitis and the etiopathogenesis of PAN is still not clear,[125] but some cases are triggered by active hepatitis B virus (HBV), a phenomenon known since the 1970s.[126] A necrotizing vasculitis with a mixed inflammatory infiltrate and sparse immune deposits is seen on NB (Fig. 4B).

Predominantly large-vessel vasculitis

Giant cell arteritis

GCA (or temporal arteritis) is the most common idiopathic medium- and large-vessel vasculitis, usually affecting the aorta and its proximal branches; other extraaortic arteries are less frequently affected. The diagnosis criteria for GCA are age > 50, new headache, clinical temporal artery abnormality, an elevated ESR (at least 50 mm/h), and abnormal TAB.[127] TAB typically shows inflammatory infiltrate in all three tunics of the arterial wall with giant cells forming granulomas in the media, particularly at the intima-media border.[103, 128] However, TAB is reported to be negative in approximately 50% of cases.[129] Headache is a frequent symptom in GCA, and optic neuropathy occurs in 10%–12% of patients. PNS involvement is observed in 7% of GCA, usually with cranial nerve palsies (mainly oculomotor nerves).[130] Mononeuropathy has rarely been observed, probably due to the infarction of nutrient vessels of the trunk of a peripheral nerve (usually with normal NB in distal nerves).[131] Another classical neurological manifestation of GCA is the acute brachial radiculo-plexopathy, mainly affecting the fifth and sixth cervical nerve roots (sometimes mistaken with polymyalgia rheumatica if electrodiagnosis is not performed), explained by the frequent involvement of the supraaortic arteries in this disease.[132]

Peripheral nervous system involvement induced by a secondary systemic vasculitis

Connective tissue diseases

Rheumatoid arthritis

RA is a systemic inflammatory disorder affecting primarily the synovial joints as well as extraarticular sites (skin or blood vessels, for example). Vascular inflammation (RV), is mostly asymptomatic, but occasionally may cause severe life-threatening manifestations. RV mainly affects large nerve arterioles, causing either MM or distal symmetric polyneuropathy.[133] It was said to appear in 40%–54% of patients with RV, with epineurial and perineurial necrotizing vasculitis by NB (Fig. 6C).[134] Nowadays, these RV are much less common, probably because of the new and effective drugs that are used at onset.

Systematic lupus erythematosus

SLE is a chronic autoimmune multisystemic disorder with a relapsing-remitting course, characterized by skin and hematological manifestations, polyarthritis, renal involvement, and seritis. PNS involvement occurs in less than 10%–23% of cases, mostly with a symmetric distal polyneuropathy due to the toxic effects of drugs (e.g., thalidomide), infections, and compression. Peripheral neuropathy may also be directly linked to SLE, sometimes with an MM pattern. In such cases, a vasculitic process may be observed (necrotizing vasculitis and lymphocytic infiltrates).[135] In a series of 667 patients with SLE, vasculitis was pathologically confirmed in 46 cases with PNS involvement (MM) in 19 cases.[136]

Sarcoidosis

This multisystem granulomatosis affects the nervous system in 5% of cases. PNS involvement represents 20% of these neurological manifestations, usually focal or multifocal sensorimotor or pure motor neuropathy, although

Guillain-Barré syndrome or symmetric distal polyneuropathy has been reported.[137] NB shows epineurial granulomas and perineurial inflammatory infiltrates with variable axon loss; sometimes necrotizing vasculitis is observed.[137] In such cases, NMB is useful because muscle involvement is frequent in sarcoidosis.[80]

Infection

Viral infections are associated with neuropathy and necrotizing vasculitis in 7% of the cases. Among these, the most commonly described are human immunodeficiency virus (HIV), the hepatitis B and C viruses (with cryoglobulinemia), cytomegalovirus (CMV), and human T cell leukemia/lymphoma virus type 1 (HTLV1).[93]

HIV infection increases the risk of secondary vasculitis such as hepatitis B-associated VPN or even CMV-associated VPN if the CD4 count is <50 cells/μL. HIV VPN probably results from immune complex deposition in the peripheral nerve.[138] In such cases, necrotizing arteritis is usually associated with marked inflammatory infiltrates affecting the endoneurium and capillaries.[93] At the present time, as treatments of HIV infection are started earlier and are more efficient, such neuropathies induced by necrotizing arteritis are becoming less common.[139]

Diffuse infiltrative lymphocytosis syndrome (DILS) is a rare form of neuropathy associated with a systemic host-determined antigen response to HIV. NB shows marked angiocentric CD8 infiltrates without mural necrosis and abundant expression of HIV p24 protein in macrophages.[139]

Drugs

After cutaneous manifestations, renal and PNS involvement (small and medium vessels) are the most frequent consequences (63%) of drug-induced vasculitis.[140] Many drugs are able to induce vasculitis, with or without neuropathy. For example, rituximab, even if it represents a therapeutic option to induce and maintain remission in some patients with vasculitis, may induce systemic reaction and vasculitis (by forming a complex with IgM kappa mixed cryoglobulin), sometimes with an MM pattern.[141] VPN (MM patterns) has also been reported after treatment with minocycline.[142] Other incriminated agents are tumor necrosis factor (TNF) antagonists,[143] propylthiouracil,[144] cocaine/levamisole,[145] hydralazine,[144] montelukast,[146] and statins.[147, 148]

Clinically, the presentation is varied: nonspecific fever, arthralgias, myalgias, and rash to single or multiple organ involvement. The kidney is most commonly involved; rare cases of liver, peripheral, and central nervous system involvement are described.

Withdrawal of the suspected drug is usually efficient, but severe cases may require glucocorticoids and immunosuppressive agents.

Malignancy

As mentioned above, various forms of paraneoplastic neuropathy may be induced by a nonnecrotizing microvasculitis observed on NB.[149] Otherwise, very rare cases of necrotizing vasculitis have been described in association with a malignant hemopathy such as multiple myeloma[150] and malignant lymphoma (Fig. 6D).[151] In such cases, NB is mandatory for the pathological diagnosis and to rule out other etiologies. A coincidental association should also be envisaged.

Peripheral nervous system in nonsystemic vasculitic peripheral neuropathy

NSVPN is confined to peripheral nerves and muscles, but sometimes associated with weight loss (30%) and fever (10%–15%); however, 10% of patients with NSVPN eventually develop systemic vasculitis.[63, 93, 95] As a consequence, NSVPN usually has a less severe prognosis than SVPN because it does not involve life-threatening target organ dysfunction. Almost all patients (96%) with classic NSVPN present a painful peripheral neuropathy, but different clinical phenotypes are observed: MM in 45%, asymmetrical polyneuropathy in 30%, and distal symmetrical polyneuropathy in 25%. NSVPN may be a part of a continuum in the spectrum of systemic necrotizing and inflammatory vascular diseases such as PAN or MPA.[76]

Lumbosacral radiculoplexus neuropathy, diabetic (DLRPN) or not (LRPN), involves roots, plexus, and peripheral nerves. These are typically asymmetrical forms of NSVPN characterized by severe pain and weakness in the proximal part of the lower extremities, eventually affecting the distal part of the lower limbs. DLRPN may occur with mild type 2 diabetes and is associated with autonomic symptoms in half the patients; concomitant upper limb (diabetic cervical radiculoplexus neuropathy) involvement is observed in 10% of the cases as well as diabetic thoracic radiculoplexus neuropathy.[152]

The gold standard for the diagnosis of diabetic NSVPN (painless or not) is NB, showing microvasculitis (epineurial perivascular inflammation in all cases), neovascularization, and multifocal fiber loss. Destruction of vessel wall elements can be rarely observed [153]

We think that combined NMB may be useful when NSVPN is suspected, but studies have shown that the sensitivity of NB alone and NMB is around 50% for both.[154]

Treatment of vasculitic peripheral neuropathy

As a general rule, a thorough neurological evaluation is recommended before starting treatment in vasculitic neuropathy and during follow-up, to precisely assess the neurological status of affected patients and the impact of treatment on the PNS. VPN should be treated according to the guidelines of the underlying disease. It is recommended to promptly institute the appropriate treatment because of a 1-year mortality rate of some untreated systemic vasculitis of around 85%–90%, versus 12%–20% with prompt treatment.[68, 76, 155]

Noninfectious large-vessel vasculitis

The general strategy of treatment in patients with vasculitis relies on short-term induction therapy (always including at least corticosteroids) followed by maintenance treatment. The standard initial induction of most types of vasculitis (systemic or not) is based on corticosteroids. Oral prednisone or prednisolone (1 mg/kg/day) is recommended, sometimes after a high dose of intravenous methylprednisolone (1000 mg daily for 3–5 days) in severe cases (although the superiority of methylprednisolone over oral prednisone has not been proven), then with a dose reduction after 1–2 months (5–10 mg every week). Cyclophosphamide may be used in addition to corticosteroids, usually with pulse therapy (mostly in dosages of 0.6–0.75 g/m^2 every 2–4 weeks). This combination of cyclophosphamide and corticosteroids represents the standard induction therapy in patients with moderate to severe generalized systemic vasculitis (PNA, MPA, GPA, and EGPA). The dose and duration of treatment must be tailored according to severity, prognosis, age, and comorbidities. Usually, once remission has been achieved, after 3–6 months, maintenance therapy is given for at least 18–24 months and careful follow-up is recommended to check for potential relapses. In most patients, methotrexate (20–25 mg/weekly) or azathioprine (1–2 mg/kg/day) replaces cyclophosphamide;[156–158] in patients with GPA, leflunomide is preferred, although a careful neurological evaluation is mandatory in these patients, given the potential neurotoxicity of this drug.[159] The methotrexate-corticosteroid combination may be used for the induction of remission in mild forms of vasculitis (systemic or not), with or without ANCA.[95]

Mycophenolate mofetil has been tried in vasculitis with varying results. Remission was observed in most patients with GPA (with only mild side effects),[160] but with a greater risk of relapse than for azathioprine;[161] its use in VPN is still debated.[162] The chimeric anti-CD20 monoclonal immunoglobulin rituximab (375 mg/m^2, four times every week) is now recommended as a first-line alternative to cyclophosphamide in patients with MPA and GPA, and is effective in cryoglobulinemic vasculitis[163] and AAV.[164]

Finally, intravenous immunoglobulins (IVIg) may represent a suitable alternative when corticosteroids and/or cyclophosphamide are ineffective.[165, 166] Recently in a large study, the clinical benefit of IVIg as adjunctive therapy was confirmed in AAV patients with refractory or relapsing disease.[167]

In case of severe/fulminant AAV or cryoglobulinemic vasculitis, plasma exchange (PLEX) may be tried.[76]

Concerning NSVPN, when the peripheral neuropathy is clinically well controlled and nonrelapsing after steroids only, we decrease the doses of steroids progressively and very slowly during several weeks. During that time, we carefully follow the patient clinically and biologically (by measuring the ESR). If there is a relapse, we keep or increase the steroid doses and introduce rituximab as a second-line treatment. If the patient is still not responding, we discuss the introduction of the other therapeutic modalities as mentioned above. A recent study indicates that the rate of sustained remission for AAV patients, following rituximab or azathioprine, remained superior over 60 months with rituximab, with better overall survival.[168]

Virus-associated vasculitis

In patients with HCV-associated vasculitis, treatment is first based on antiviral molecules such as pegylated interferon-alpha and ribavirin, sometimes supplemented by telaprevir and boceprevir for genotype 1.[169] Rituximab is effective in the presence of cyoglobulinemic vasculitis.[170]

HBV-associated PAN is based on the combination of PLEX and an antiviral agent (after a 2-week course of corticosteroids in the most severe cases). However, in cases of treatment with corticosteroids and immunosuppressants alone, the outcome is poorer than in nonviral vasculitis.[171]

HIV-associated vasculitis is associated with a higher risk of opportunistic infection if corticosteroids or immunosuppressants are used. There is no current consensus on the treatment of HIV-associated vasculitis, but PLEX and antiviral therapy may be helpful.

For LRPN, intravenous methylprednisone (1000 mg, 3 times weekly, then decreased in dose and frequency over 12 weeks) has provided good results for pain in LRPN, diabetic or not.[172] IVIg may also be considered but there is a lack of evidence for its efficacy.[173]

Conclusion

Vasculitic neuropathies represents a heterogeneous group of peripheral neuropathies due to necrotizing vasculitis (either systemic or nonsytemic) of the vasa nervorum, leading to various clinical phenotypes (mononeuropathy multiplex being the most classical one). In some cases, vasculitis may be confined to the peripheral nervous system. Although the electrophysiological, clinical, biological, or radiological signs may be indicative, the diagnosis of vasculitic neuropathy needs to be confirmed by a nerve biopsy, showing a combination of vascular and inflammatory features. The treatment is based on corticosteroids and immunosuppressants, except in virus-associated vasculitis.

References

1. Collins MP, Kissel JT. Neuropathies with systemic vasculitis. In: Dyck PJ, Thomas PK, eds. *Peripheral Neuropathy*. 4th ed.Philadelphia: Elsevier-Saunders; 2005:2335–2404.
2. Collins MP, Dyck PJB. Vasculitides. In: Vallat JM, Weis J, Gray F, Keohane K, eds. *Peripheral Nerve Disorders: Pathology & Genetics*. Oxford: John Wiley & Sons; 2014:175–195.
3. Willan R. Purpura. In: Wilan R, ed. *On Cutaneous Diseases*. Philadelphia: Kimber & Conrad; 1809:342–355.
4. Heberden W. *Commentaries on the History and Cure of Diseases*. 3rd ed. London: T. Payne; 1806.

5. Ollivier (d'Angers) CP. Développement spontané d'ecchymoses cutanées avec oedème aigu sous-cutané, et gastro-entérite. *Arch Gen Med.* 1827;15:206–216.

6. Schönlein JL. *Allgemeine und specielle Pathologie und Therapie. Nach dessen Vorlesungen niedergeschrieben und hrsg. von einigen seiner Zuhörer.* 3rd ed. Herisau: Würzburg; 1837.

7. Matteson E. Historical perspectives of vasculitis. In: *Inflammatory Diseases of Blood Vessels.* 2nd ed.Oxford: Wiley-Blackwell; 2012:161–169.

8. Hunter J. *A Treatise on the Blood, Inflammation, and Gun-Shot Wounds.* London: John Richardson; 1794.

9. Hodgson J. *A Treatise on the Diseases of the Arteries on Veins, Containing the Pathology and Treatment of Aneurysms and Wounded Arteries.* London: Moyes-Street-Garden; 1815.

10. Rokitensky KF. *Handbuch der Pathologischen Anatomie.* Braumiller & Seidel: Wien; 1842.

11. Virchow R. Die Cellularpathologie in ihrer Begründung auf physiologische und pathologische Gewebelehre. In: Virchow R, ed. *Vorlesungen über Pathologie.* Berlin: August Hirschwald; 1858.

12. Matteson EL. Historical perspective on the classification of vasculitis. *Arthritis Care Res.* 2000;13:122–127.

13. Rokitensky KF. *Ueber einige der wichtigsten Krankheiten der Arterien.* Wien: Kaiserlich-Königliche Hof- und Staatsdruckerei; 1852.

14. Crissey JT, Parish LC. Vasculitis: the historical development of the concept. *Clin Dermatol.* 1999;17:493–497.

15. Kussmaul A, Maier R. Ueber eine nicht bisher beschriebene eigenhümliche Arterienerkrankung (Periarteritis Nodosa), die mit Morbus Brightii und rapid fortschreitender allgemeiner Muskellähmung einhergeht. *Deutsch Arch Klin Med.* 1866;1:484–517.

16. Matteson EL. *Polyarteritis Nodosa and Microscopic Polyangiitis. Translation of the Original Articles on Classic Polyarteritis Nodosa by Adolf Kussmaul and Rudolf Maier and Microscopic Polyarteritis Nodosa by Friedrich Wohlwill.* Rochester, MN: Mayo Clinic Press; 1998.

17. Eppinger H. *Pathogenesis (Histogenesis und Aetiologie) der Aneurysmen einschliesslich des Aneurysma equi verminosum. Pathologisch-anatomische Studien.* August Hirschwald: Berlin; 1887.

18. Ferrari E. Ueber Polyarteritis acuta nodosa (sogenannte Periarteritis nodosa), und ihre Beziehungen zur Polymyositis und Polineuritis acuta. *Beitr Pathol Anat Allg Pathol.* 1903;34:350–386.

19. Dickson W. Polyarteritis acuta nodosa and periarteritis nodosa. *J Pathol Bacteriol.* 1908;12:31–57.

20. Tanaka N, Sekimoto K, Naoe S. Kawasaki disease. Relationship with infantile periarteritis nodosa. *Arch Pathol Lab Med.* 1976;100:81–86.

21. Landing BH, Larson EJ. Are infantile periarteritis nodosa with coronary artery involvement and fatal mucocutaneous lymph node syndrome the same? Comparison of 20 patients from North America with patients from Hawaii and Japan. *Pediatrics.* 1977;59:651–662.

22. Pagnoux C, Seror R, Henegar C, et al. Clinical features and outcomes in 348 patients with polyarteritis nodosa: a systematic retrospective study of patients diagnosed between 1963 and 2005 and entered into the French Vasculitis study group database. *Arthritis Rheum.* 2010;62:616–626.

23. Matteson EL. Notes on the history of eponymic idiopathic vasculitis: the diseases of Henoch and Schonlein, Wegener, Churg and Strauss, Horton, Takayasu, Behcet, and Kawasaki. *Arthritis Care Res.* 2000;13:237–245.

24. Faille-Kuyber EH, Kater L, Kooiker CJ, Dorhout Mees EJ. IgA-deposits in cutaneous blood-vessel walls and mesangium in Henoch-Schonlein syndrome. *Lancet.* 1973;1:892–893.

25. Hutchinson J. On a peculiar form of thrombotic arteritis of the aged which is sometimes productive of gangrene. *Arch Surg (Lond).* 1890;1:323–329.

26. Horton BT, Magath TB, Brown GE. Undescribed form of arteritis of temporal vessels. *Proc Staff Meet Mayo Clin.* 1932;7:700–701.

27. Horton BT, Magath TB, Brown GE. Arteritis of the temporal vessels. *Arch Intern Med.* 1934;53:400–409.

28. Horton BT, Magath TB. Arteritis of the temporal vessels: report of 7 cases. *Proc Staff Meet Mayo Clin.* 1937;12:548–553.

29. Takayashu M. Case with unusual changes of the central vessels in the retina. *Acta Soc Ophthalmol Jpn.* 1908;12:554–555.

30. Wegener F. Über generalisierte, septische Gefässerkrankungen. *Verh Dtsch Ges Pathol.* 1936;29:202–210.

31. Wegener F. Über eine eigenartige rhinogene Granulomatose mit besonderer Beteiligung des Arteriensystems und der Nieren. *Beitr Pathol Anat Allg Pathol.* 1939;102:36–68.

32. Klinger H. Grenzformen der Periarteriitis nodosa. *Frankfurt Ztschr Pathol.* 1931;42:455–480.

33. Churg J, Strauss L. Allergic granulomatosis, allergic angiitis, and periarteritis nodosa. *Am J Pathol.* 1951;27:277–294.

34. Kawasaki T. Acute febrile mucocutaneous syndrome with lymphoid involvement with specific desquamation of the fingers and toes in children. *Arerugi.* 1967;16:178–222.

35. Arkin A. A clinical and pathological study of periarteritis nodosa: a report of five cases, one histologically healed. *Am J Pathol.* 1930;6:401–426.

36. Zeek PM. Periarteritis nodosa and other forms of necrotizing angiitis. *N Engl J Med.* 1953;248:764–772.

37. Zeek PM. Periarteritis nodosa; a critical review. *Am J Clin Pathol.* 1952;22:777–790.

38. Gilliam JN, Smiley JD. Cutaneous necrotizing vasculitis and related disorders. *Ann Allergy.* 1976;37:328–339.

39. Hunder GG, Arend WP, Bloch DA, et al. The American College of Rheumatology 1990 criteria for the classification of vasculitis. Introduction. *Arthritis Rheum.* 1990;33:1065–1067.

40. Jennette JC, Falk RJ, Andrassy K, et al. Nomenclature of systemic vasculitides. Proposal of an international consensus conference. *Arthritis Rheum.* 1994;37:187–192.

41. Watts R, Lane S, Hanslik T, et al. Development and validation of a consensus methodology for the classification of the ANCA-associated vasculitides and polyarteritis nodosa for epidemiological studies. *Ann Rheum Dis.* 2007;66:222–227.

42. Jennette JC. Overview of the 2012 revised international Chapel Hill consensus conference nomenclature of vasculitides. *Clin Exp Nephrol.* 2013;17:603–606.

43. Ball GV, Bridges Jr. SL. Nomenclature and classification of vasculitis. In: Ball GV, Fessler BJ, Bridges Jr. SL, eds. *Oxford Textbook of Vasculitis.* 3rd ed.Oxford: Oxford University Press; 2014:3–5.

44. Gonzalez-Gay MA, Garcia-Porrua C. Systemic vasculitis in adults in northwestern Spain, 1988–1997. Clinical and epidemiologic aspects. *Medicine (Baltimore).* 1999;78:292–308.

45. Oh SJ. Vasculitic neuropathy. In: Ball GV, Fessler BJ, Bridges SL Jr., eds. *Oxford Textbook of Vasculitis.* 3rd ed.Oxford: Oxford University Press; 2014:157–177.

46. Fessler BJ. Approach to the diagnosis of vasculitis in adult patients. In: Ball GV, Fessler BJ, Bridges Jr SL, eds. *Oxford Textbook of Vasculitis.* Oxford: Oxford University Press; 2014:275–282.

47. Kieseier BC, Kiefer R, Gold R, Hemmer B, Willison HJ, Hartung HP. Advances in understanding and treatment of immune-mediated disorders of the peripheral nervous system. *Muscle Nerve.* 2004;30:131–156.

48. Chang RW, Bell CL, Hallett M. Clinical characteristics and prognosis of vasculitic mononeuropathy multiplex. *Arch Neurol.* 1984;41:618–621.

49. Conn DL, Dyck PJ. Angiopathic neuropathy in connectivite tissue diseases. In: Thomas PK, Lambert EH, eds. *Peripheral Neuropathy.* Philadelphia: WB Saunders; 1975:1149–1165.

50. Moore PM, Calabrese LH. Neurologic manifestations of systemic vasculitides. *Semin Neurol.* 1994;14:300–306.

51. Kernohan JW, Woltman HW. Periarteritis nodosa: a clinicopathologic study with special reference to nervous system. *Arch NeurPsych.* 1938;39:655–686.

52. Kissel JT, Slivka AP, Warmolts JR, Mendell JR. The clinical spectrum of necrotizing angiopathy of the peripheral nervous system. *Ann Neurol.* 1985;18:251–257.

53. Dyck PJ, Benstead TJ, Conn DL, Stevens JC, Windebank AJ, Low PA. Nonsystemic vasculitic neuropathy. *Brain.* 1987;110(Pt 4):843–853.

54. Kissel JT, Collins MP, Mendell JR. Vasculitic neuropathy. In: Mendell JR, Kissel JT, Cornblath DR, eds. *Diagnosis and Management of Peripheral Nerve Disorders.* Oxford: Oxford University Press; 2001:203–2032.

55. Collins MP, Periquet MI. Non-systemic vasculitic neuropathy. *Curr Opin Neurol.* 2004;17:587–598.

56. Collins MP, Periquet MI, Mendell JR, Sahenk Z, Nagaraja HN, Kissel JT. Nonsystemic vasculitic neuropathy: insights from a clinical cohort. *Neurology.* 2003;61:623–630.

57. Davies L, Spies JM, Pollard JD, McLeod JG. Vasculitis confined to peripheral nerves. *Brain.* 1996;119(Pt 5):1441–1448.

58. Abgrall S, Mouthon L, Cohen P, et al. Localized neurological necrotizing vasculitides. Three cases with isolated mononeuritis multiplex. *J Rheumatol.* 2001;28:631–633.

59. Behari M, Garg R, Dinda AK, Ahuja GK. Peripheral neuropathy due to small vessel vasculitis. *J Assoc Physicians India.* 1995;43:495–497.

60. Panegyres PK, Blumbergs PC, Leong AS, Bourne AJ. Vasculitis of peripheral nerve and skeletal muscle: clinicopathological correlation and immunopathic mechanisms. *J Neurol Sci.* 1990;100:193–202.

61. Chia L, Fernandez A, Lacroix C, Adams D, Plante V, Said G. Contribution of nerve biopsy findings to the diagnosis of disabling neuropathy in the elderly. A retrospective review of 100 consecutive patients. *Brain.* 1996;119(Pt 4):1091–1098.

62. Hattori N, Mori K, Misu K, Koike H, Ichimura M, Sobue G. Mortality and morbidity in peripheral neuropathy associated Churg-Strauss syndrome and microscopic polyangiitis. *J Rheumatol.* 2002;29:1408–1414.

63. Collins MP, Periquet MI. Isolated vasculitis of the peripheral nervous system. *Clin Exp Rheumatol.* 2008;26:S118–S130.

64. Schweikert K, Fuhr P, Probst A, Tolnay M, Renaud S, Steck AJ. Contribution of nerve biopsy to unclassified neuropathy. *Eur Neurol.* 2007;57:86–90.

65. Mohamed A, Davies L, Pollard JD. Conduction block in vasculitic neuropathy. *Muscle Nerve.* 1998;21:1084–1088.

66. McCluskey L, Feinberg D, Cantor C, Bird S. "Pseudo-conduction block" in vasculitic neuropathy. *Muscle Nerve.* 1999;22:1361–1366.

67. Briemberg HR, Levin K, Amato AA. Multifocal conduction block in peripheral nerve vasculitis. *J Clin Neuromuscul Dis.* 2002;3:153–158.

68. Collins MP, Dyck PJ, Gronseth GS, et al. Peripheral Nerve Society Guideline on the classification, diagnosis, investigation, and immunosuppressive therapy of non-systemic vasculitic neuropathy: executive summary. *J Peripher Nerv Syst.* 2010;15:176–184.

69. Hadden RDM, Collins MP, Zivkovic SA, et al. Vasculitic peripheral neuropathy: case definition and guidelines for collection, analysis, and presentation of immunisation safety data. *Vaccine.* 2017;35:1567–1578.

70. Lorenz H. Beitrag zur Kenntnis des multiplen degenerativen Neuritis. *Zeitschr Klin Med.* 1891;18:493–516.

71. Meyer PS. Ueber die klinische Erkenntnis der Periarteriitis nodosa und ihre pathologisch-anatomischen Grundlagen. *Berl Klin Wochenschr.* 1921;58:473–475.
72. Schmincke A. Ueber Neuritis bei Periarteritis nodosa. *Verhandl Deutsch Gesellsch Pathol.* 1921;18:287–293.
73. Marinesco G, Draganesco S. Sur la forme myélo-neuro-myopathique de la maladie de Kussmaul. *Ann Med (Paris).* 1927;22:154–171.
74. Wohlwill F. Fall von Periarteritis nodosa. *Deutsch Med Wochenschr.* 1918;1:366.
75. Wohlwill F. Ueber die nur mikroskopisch erkennbare Form der Periarteritis nodosa. *Virchows Arch Pathol Anat.* 1923;246:377–411.
76. Gwathmey KG, Burns TM, Collins MP, Dyck PJ. Vasculitic neuropathies. *Lancet Neurol.* 2014;13:67–82.
77. Claussen GC, Thomas TD, Goyne C, Vazquez LG, Oh SJ. Diagnostic value of nerve and muscle biopsy in suspected vasculitis cases. *J Clin Neuromuscul Dis.* 2000;1:117–123.
78. Wees SJ, Sunwoo IN, Oh SJ. Sural nerve biopsy in systemic necrotizing vasculitis. *Am J Med.* 1981;71:525–532.
79. Kurt S, Alsharabati M, Lu L, Claussen GC, Oh SJ. Asymptomatic vasculitic neuropathy. *Muscle Nerve.* 2015;52:34–38.
80. Vital C, Vital A, Canron MH, et al. Combined nerve and muscle biopsy in the diagnosis of vasculitic neuropathy. A 16-year retrospective study of 202 cases. *J Peripher Nerv Syst.* 2006;11:20–29.
81. Kissel JT, Mendell JR. Vasculitic neuropathy. *Neurol Clin.* 1992;10:761–781.
82. Said G, Lacroix-Ciaudo C, Fujimura H, Blas C, Faux N. The peripheral neuropathy of necrotizing arteritis: a clinicopathological study. *Ann Neurol.* 1988;23:461–465.
83. Collins MP, Mendell JR, Periquet MI, et al. Superficial peroneal nerve/peroneus brevis muscle biopsy in vasculitic neuropathy. *Neurology.* 2000;55:636–643.
84. Griffin JW. Vasculitic neuropathies. *Rheum Dis Clin North Am.* 2001;27:751–760 [vi].
85. Hawke SH, Davies L, Pamphlett R, Guo YP, Pollard JD, McLeod JG. Vasculitic neuropathy. A clinical and pathological study. *Brain.* 1991;114(Pt 5):2175–2190.
86. Magy L, Vallat JM. Nerve biopsy without muscle sampling: is it enough for diagnosing vasculitis? *J Neurol Neurosurg Psychiatry.* 2008;79:1307.
87. McManis PG, Low PA, Lagerlund TD. Microenvironment of nerve: blood flow and ischemia. In: *Peripheral Neuropathy.* 3rd ed. Philadelphia: W.B. Saunders; 1993:453–475.
88. Dyck PJ, Conn DL, Okazaki H. Necrotizing angiopathic neuropathy. Three-dimensional morphology of fiber degeneration related to sites of occluded vessels. *Mayo Clin Proc.* 1972;47:461–475.
89. Giannini C, Dyck PJ. Ultrastructural morphometric features of human sural nerve endoneurial microvessels. *J Neuropathol Exp Neurol.* 1993;52:361–369.
90. Ohkoshi N, Mizusawa H, Oguni E, Shoji S. Sural nerve biopsy in vasculitic neuropathies: morphometric analysis of the caliber of involved vessels. *J Med.* 1996;27:153–170.
91. Midroni G, Bilbao JM. Vasculitic neuropathy. In: *Biopsy Diagnosis of Peripheral Neuropathy.* 1st ed.Boston: Butterworth-Heinemann; 1995:241–262.
92. Prayson RA, Sedlock DJ. Clinicopathologic study of 43 patients with sural nerve vasculitis. *Hum Pathol.* 2003;34:484–490.
93. Said G, Lacroix C. Primary and secondary vasculitic neuropathy. *J Neurol.* 2005;252:633–641.
94. Oh SJ, Herrera GA, Spalding DM. Eosinophilic vasculitic neuropathy in the Churg-Strauss syndrome. *Arthritis Rheum.* 1986;29:1173–1175.
95. Burns TM, Schaublin GA, Dyck PJ. Vasculitic neuropathies. *Neurol Clin.* 2007;25:89–113.
96. Dyck PJB, Engelstad J, Dyck PJ. Microvasculitis. In: Dyck PJ, Thomas PK, eds. *Peripheral Neuropathy.* 4th ed.Philadelphia: Elsevier-Saunders; 2005:2405–2414.

97. Weis J, Brandner S, Lammens M, Sommer C, Vallat JM. Processing of nerve biopsies: a practical guide for neuropathologists. *Clin Neuropathol.* 2012;31:7–23.

98. Kissel JT, Riethman JL, Omerza J, Rammohan KW, Mendell JR. Peripheral nerve vasculitis: immune characterization of the vascular lesions. *Ann Neurol.* 1989;25:291–297.

99. Collins MP, Periquet-Collins I, Sahenk Z, Kissel JT. Direct immunofluoresence in vasculitic neuropathy: specificity of vascular immune deposits. *Muscle Nerve.* 2010;42:62–69.

100. Harati Y, Niakan E. Clinical significance of selective nerve fascicular degeneration on sural nerve biopsy specimen. *Arch Pathol Lab Med.* 1986;110:195–197.

101. Schröder JM. Proliferation of epineurial capillaries and smooth muscle cells in angiopathic peripheral neuropathy. *Acta Neuropathol.* 1986;72:29–37.

102. Chalk CH, Dyck PJ, Conn DL. Vasculitic neuropathy. In: Dyck PJ, Thomas PK, eds. *Peripheral Neuropathy.* 3rd ed.Philadelphia: W. B. Saunders; 1993:1424–1436.

103. Lie JT. Illustrated histopathologic classification criteria for selected vasculitis syndromes. American College of Rheumatology Subcommittee on classification of Vasculitis. *Arthritis Rheum.* 1990;33:1074–1087.

104. Savage CO, Winearls CG, Evans DJ, Rees AJ, Lockwood CM. Microscopic polyarteritis: presentation, pathology and prognosis. *Q J Med.* 1985;56:467–483.

105. Guillevin L, Durand-Gasselin B, Cevallos R, et al. Microscopic polyangiitis: clinical and laboratory findings in eighty-five patients. *Arthritis Rheum.* 1999;42:421–430.

106. Agard C, Mouthon L, Mahr A, Guillevin L. Microscopic polyangiitis and polyarteritis nodosa: how and when do they start? *Arthritis Rheum.* 2003;49:709–715.

107. Zhang W, Zhou G, Shi Q, Zhang X, Zeng XF, Zhang FC. Clinical analysis of nervous system involvement in ANCA-associated systemic vasculitides. *Clin Exp Rheumatol.* 2009;27:S65–S69.

108. Greco A, Rizzo MI, De Virgilio A, et al. Churg-Strauss syndrome. *Autoimmun Rev.* 2015;14:341–348.

109. Comarmond C, Pagnoux C, Khellaf M, et al. Eosinophilic granulomatosis with polyangiitis (Churg-Strauss): clinical characteristics and long-term followup of the 383 patients enrolled in the French Vasculitis Study Group cohort. *Arthritis Rheum.* 2013;65:270–281.

110. Moosig F, Bremer JP, Hellmich B, et al. A vasculitis centre based management strategy leads to improved outcome in eosinophilic granulomatosis and polyangiitis (Churg-Strauss, EGPA): monocentric experiences in 150 patients. *Ann Rheum Dis.* 2013;72:1011–1017.

111. Uchiyama M, Mitsuhashi Y, Yamazaki M, Tsuboi R. Elderly cases of Churg-Strauss syndrome: case report and review of Japanese cases. *J Dermatol.* 2012;39:76–79.

112. Sinico RA, Di Toma L, Maggiore U, et al. Prevalence and clinical significance of antineutrophil cytoplasmic antibodies in Churg-Strauss syndrome. *Arthritis Rheum.* 2005;52:2926–2935.

113. Keogh KA, Specks U. Churg-Strauss syndrome: clinical presentation, antineutrophil cytoplasmic antibodies, and leukotriene receptor antagonists. *Am J Med.* 2003;115:284–290.

114. Ntatsaki E, Watts RA, Scott DG. Epidemiology of ANCA-associated vasculitis. *Rheum Dis Clin North Am.* 2010;36:447–461.

115. Hoffman GS, Kerr GS, Leavitt RY, et al. Wegener granulomatosis: an analysis of 158 patients. *Ann Intern Med.* 1992;116:488–498.

116. Nishino H, Rubino FA, DeRemee RA, Swanson JW, Parisi JE. Neurological involvement in Wegener's granulomatosis: an analysis of 324 consecutive patients at the Mayo Clinic. *Ann Neurol.* 1993;33:4–9.

117. Collins MP, Periquet MI. Prevalence of vasculitic neuropathy in Wegener granulomatosis. *Arch Neurol.* 2002;59:1333–1334 [author reply 1334].

118. de Groot K, Schmidt DK, Arlt AC, Gross WL, Reinhold-Keller E. Standardized neurologic evaluations of 128 patients with Wegener granulomatosis. *Arch Neurol.* 2001;58:1215–1221.

119. Ferri C, Sebastiani M, Giuggioli D, et al. Mixed cryoglobulinemia: demographic, clinical, and serologic features and survival in 231 patients. *Semin Arthritis Rheum.* 2004;33:355–374.
120. Brouet JC, Clauvel JP, Danon F, Klein M, Seligmann M. Biologic and clinical significance of cryoglobulins. A report of 86 cases. *Am J Med.* 1974;57:775–788.
121. Ferri C, Mascia MT. Cryoglobulinemic vasculitis. *Curr Opin Rheumatol.* 2006;18:54–63.
122. Garzoni L, Vanoni F, Rizzi M, et al. Nervous system dysfunction in Henoch-Schonlein syndrome: systematic review of the literature. *Rheumatology (Oxford).* 2009;48:1524–1529.
123. Bouiller K, Audia S, Devilliers H, et al. Etiologies and prognostic factors of leukocytoclastic vasculitis with skin involvement: a retrospective study in 112 patients. *Medicine (Baltimore).* 2016;95:e4238.
124. Loricera J, Calvo-Rio V, Mata C, et al. Urticarial vasculitis in northern Spain: clinical study of 21 cases. *Medicine (Baltimore).* 2014;93:53–60.
125. Ozen S. The changing face of polyarteritis nodosa and necrotizing vasculitis. *Nat Rev Rheumatol.* 2017;13:381–386.
126. Gocke DJ, Hsu K, Morgan C, Bombardieri S, Lockshin M, Christian CL. Association between polyarteritis and Australia antigen. *Lancet.* 1970;2:1149–1153.
127. Hunder GG, Bloch DA, Michel BA, et al. The American College of Rheumatology 1990 criteria for the classification of giant cell arteritis. *Arthritis Rheum.* 1990;33:1122–1128.
128. Liozon F, Catanzano G. L'artérite temporale de Horton. Etude anatomopathologique en microscopie optique. A propos de 123 biopsies temporales. *Rev Med Interne.* 1982;3: 295–301.
129. Weyand CM, Goronzy JJ. Giant-cell arteritis and polymyalgia rheumatica. *Ann Intern Med.* 2003;139:505–515.
130. Caselli RJ, Hunder GG. Neurologic complications of giant cell (temporal) arteritis. *Semin Neurol.* 1994;14:349–353.
131. Lacoste I, Duval F, Daubigney A, et al. Acute tibial neuropathy in an elderly. *J Clin Neurosci.* 2017;46:58–59.
132. Duval F, Lacoste I, Galli G, et al. Acute brachial radiculoplexopathy and giant cell arteritis. *Neurologist.* 2018;23:23–28.
133. Genta MS, Genta RM, Gabay C. Systemic rheumatoid vasculitis: a review. *Semin Arthritis Rheum.* 2006;36:88–98.
134. Puéchal X, Said G, Hilliquin P, et al. Peripheral neuropathy with necrotizing vasculitis in rheumatoid arthritis. A clinicopathologic and prognostic study of thirty-two patients. *Arthritis Rheum.* 1995;38:1618–1629.
135. Rivière E, Cohen Aubart F, Maisonobe T, et al. Clinicopathological features of multiple mononeuropathy associated with systemic lupus erythematosus: a multicenter study. *J Neurol.* 2017;264:1218–1226.
136. Drenkard C, Villa AR, Reyes E, Abello M, Alarcon-Segovia D. Vasculitis in systemic lupus erythematosus. *Lupus.* 1997;6:235–242.
137. Said G, Lacroix C, Plante-Bordeneuve V, et al. Nerve granulomas and vasculitis in sarcoid peripheral neuropathy: a clinicopathological study of 11 patients. *Brain.* 2002;125:264–275.
138. Calabrese LH. Vasculitis and infection with the human immunodeficiency virus. *Rheum Dis Clin North Am.* 1991;17:131–147.
139. Chimelli L, Vallat JM. Infectious and tropical neuropathies. In: Vallat JM, Weis J, Gray F, Keohane K, eds. *Peripheral Nerve Disorders: Pathology & Genetics.* Oxford: John Wiley & Sons; 2014:196–209.
140. Grau RG. Drug-induced vasculitis: new insights and a changing lineup of suspects. *Curr Rheumatol Rep.* 2015;17:71.

141. Sène D, Ghillani-Dalbin P, Amoura Z, Musset L, Cacoub P. Rituximab may form a complex with IgMkappa mixed cryoglobulin and induce severe systemic reactions in patients with hepatitis C virus-induced vasculitis. *Arthritis Rheum.* 2009;60:3848–3855.

142. Kang MK, Gupta RK, Srinivasan J. Peripheral vasculitic neuropathy associated with minocycline use. *J Clin Neuromuscl Dis.* 2018;19:138–141.

143. Saint Marcoux B, De Bandt M. Vasculitides induced by TNFalpha antagonists: a study in 39 patients in France. *Joint Bone Spine.* 2006;73:710–713.

144. Choi HK, Merkel PA, Walker AM, Niles JL. Drug-associated antineutrophil cytoplasmic antibody-positive vasculitis: prevalence among patients with high titers of antimyeloperoxidase antibodies. *Arthritis Rheum.* 2000;43:405–413.

145. Espinoza LR, Perez Alamino R. Cocaine-induced vasculitis: clinical and immunological spectrum. *Curr Rheumatol Rep.* 2012;14:532–538.

146. Hauser T, Mahr A, Metzler C, et al. The leucotriene receptor antagonist montelukast and the risk of Churg-Strauss syndrome: a case-crossover study. *Thorax.* 2008;63:677–682.

147. Sen D, Rosenstein ED, Kramer N. ANCA-positive vasculitis associated with simvastatin/ezetimibe: expanding the spectrum of statin-induced autoimmunity? *Int J Rheum Dis.* 2010;13:e29–e31.

148. Kalra A, Yokogawa N, Raja H, et al. Hydralazine-induced pulmonary-renal syndrome: a case report. *Am J Ther.* 2012;19:e136–e138.

149. Rudnicki SA, Dalmau J. Paraneoplastic syndromes of the peripheral nerves. *Curr Opin Neurol.* 2005;18:598–603.

150. Hutterer M, Steurer M, Hoftberger R, et al. Polyarteritis nodosa complicating multiple myeloma—a case report and review of the literature. *Clin Neuropathol.* 2014;33:143–151.

151. Duchesne M, Mathis S, Corcia P, et al. Value of nerve biopsy in patients with latent malignant hemopathy and peripheral neuropathy: a case series. *Medicine (Baltimore).* 2015;94:e394.

152. Dyck PJ, Norell JE, Dyck PJ. Microvasculitis and ischemia in diabetic lumbosacral radiculoplexus neuropathy. *Neurology.* 1999;53:2113–2121.

153. Garces-Sanchez M, Laughlin RS, Dyck PJ, Engelstad JK, Norell JE. Painless diabetic motor neuropathy: a variant of diabetic lumbosacral radiculoplexus neuropathy? *Ann Neurol.* 2011;69:1043–1054.

154. Collins MP, Hadden RD. The nonsystemic vasculitic neuropathies. *Nat Rev Neurol.* 2017;13:302–316.

155. Watts RA, Scott DG, Pusey CD, Lockwood CM. Vasculitis-aims of therapy. An overview. *Rheumatology (Oxford).* 2000;39:229–232.

156. Langford CA. Vasculitis. *J Allergy Clin Immunol.* 2010;125:S216–S225.

157. de Groot K, Harper L, Jayne DR, et al. Pulse versus daily oral cyclophosphamide for induction of remission in antineutrophil cytoplasmic antibody-associated vasculitis: a randomized trial. *Ann Intern Med.* 2009;150:670–680.

158. Pagnoux C, Mahr A, Hamidou MA, et al. Azathioprine or methotrexate maintenance for ANCA-associated vasculitis. *N Engl J Med.* 2008;359:2790–2803.

159. Metzler C, Miehle N, Manger K, et al. Elevated relapse rate under oral methotrexate versus leflunomide for maintenance of remission in Wegener's granulomatosis. *Rheumatology (Oxford).* 2007;46:1087–1091.

160. Silva F, Specks U, Kalra S, et al. Mycophenolate mofetil for induction and maintenance of remission in microscopic polyangiitis with mild to moderate renal involvement—a prospective, open-label pilot trial. *Clin J Am Soc Nephrol.* 2010;5:445–453.

161. Hiemstra TF, Walsh M, Mahr A, et al. Mycophenolate mofetil vs azathioprine for remission maintenance in antineutrophil cytoplasmic antibody-associated vasculitis: a randomized controlled trial. *JAMA.* 2010;304:2381–2388.

162. Blaes F. Diagnosis and therapeutic options for peripheral vasculitic neuropathy. *Ther Adv Musculoskelet Dis*. 2015;7:45–55.
163. De Vita S, Quartuccio L, Isola M, et al. A randomized controlled trial of rituximab for the treatment of severe cryoglobulinemic vasculitis. *Arthritis Rheum*. 2012;64:843–853.
164. Stone JH, Merkel PA, Spiera R, et al. Rituximab versus cyclophosphamide for ANCA-associated vasculitis. *N Engl J Med*. 2010;363:221–232.
165. Levy Y, Uziel Y, Zandman GG, et al. Intravenous immunoglobulins in peripheral neuropathy associated with vasculitis. *Ann Rheum Dis*. 2003;62:1221–1223.
166. Levy Y, Uziel Y, Zandman G, et al. Response of vasculitic peripheral neuropathy to intravenous immunoglobulin. *Ann N Y Acad Sci*. 2005;1051:779–786.
167. Crickx E, Machelart I, Lazaro E, et al. Intravenous immunoglobulin as an immunomodulating agent in antineutrophil cytoplasmic antibody-associated vasculitides: a French Nationwide study of ninety-two patients. *Arthritis Rheumatol*. 2016;68:702–712.
168. Terrier B, Pagnoux C, Perrodeau E, et al. Long-term efficacy of remission-maintenance regimens for ANCA-associated vasculitides. *Ann Rheum Dis*. 2018;77:1150–1156.
169. Chiche L, Bataille S, Kaplanski G, Jourde N. The place of immunotherapy in the management of HCV-induced vasculitis: an update. *Clin Dev Immunol*. 2012;2012:315167.
170. Ferri C, Cacoub P, Mazzaro C, et al. Treatment with rituximab in patients with mixed cryoglobulinemia syndrome: results of multicenter cohort study and review of the literature. *Autoimmun Rev*. 2011;11:48–55.
171. Guillevin L, Mahr A, Callard P, et al. Hepatitis B virus-associated polyarteritis nodosa: clinical characteristics, outcome, and impact of treatment in 115 patients. *Medicine (Baltimore)*. 2005;84:313–322.
172. Dyck PJ, Norell JE. Methylprednisolone may improve lumbosacral radiculoplexus neuropathy. *Can J Neurol Sci*. 2001;28:224–227.
173. Tamburin S, Zanette G. Intravenous immunoglobulin for the treatment of diabetic lumbosacral radiculoplexus neuropathy. *Pain Med*. 2009;10:1476–1480.

Chapter 8

Paraneoplastic peripheral neuropathies

Jean-Christophe Antoine

Department of Neurology, University Hospital of Saint-Etienne, Saint-Etienne, France

Introduction

Paraneoplastic peripheral neuropathies are rare inflammatory disorders of the peripheral nervous system (PNS) while clinically overt peripheral neuropathy is frequent in patients with cancer (1.7%–16% of cases).[1,2] The most frequent underlying mechanisms include compression or infiltration by the tumor; the adverse effects of treatments, sometimes months or years after their application; metabolic and nutritional factors; and viral infections favored by the immunodepression induced by the cancer and its treatments.[3]

Following their definition by Boudin in 1961,[4] paraneoplastic peripheral neuropathies are disorders that develop prior to or during a cancer as a remote effect of the tumor that cannot be explained by one of the aforementioned mechanisms. They affect probably < 1% of patients with cancer. As cancer and peripheral neuropathy each affect millions of people worldwide, such a negative definition leaves open the possibility of frequent fortuitous associations so that specific criteria are needed for considering a neuropathy as paraneoplastic.

In addition, the question of paraneoplastic PNS syndromes involves different levels of complexity. The first concerns the inflammatory mechanisms by which cancer affects the PNS. The second level is topographic because any part of the PNS can be affected, including the ventral horns of the spinal cord, the dorsal root ganglia, the autonomic nervous system, nerve roots, plexuses, and the cranial and peripheral nerves. The third level corresponds to the cellular structures that are targeted, the neuron cell body, the axon, or the myelin sheath. Finally, the nature of the cancer is responsible for the fourth and last level of complexity because lymphoma and carcinoma have a different ability to induce paraneoplastic disorders. All of these points have practical consequences for the diagnosis and management of patients.

Dysimmune Neuropathies. https://doi.org/10.1016/B978-0-12-814572-2.00008-X

Classification of paraneoplastic neuropathies

The 2004 recommended criteria of the PNS-Euronetwork consortium for para-neoplastic neurological disorders concern all the categories of paraneoplastic neurological diseases,[5] but can be specifically adapted for neuropathies. Definite paraneoplastic neuropathies include disorders for which a direct pathogenic link between the tumor and the neuropathy is demonstrated, that is: (1) neuropathies associated with onconeural antibodies, (2) well-established paraneoplastic neurological syndromes but no identified antibodies, which corresponds to sero-negative sensory neuronopathies (SNN) and chronic gastrointestinal pseudoobstruction, and (3) neuropathies unequivocally improved by the tumor treatment provided that the neuropathy has no spontaneous tendency to recovery. Any other neuropathy occurring within 2 years of a cancer is a possible paraneoplastic disorder. Here, we will only consider definite paraneoplastic neurological disorders.

The identified mechanisms linking a tumor with a paraneoplastic neurological disorder mostly involve the immune system. With carcinoma, the expression by the tumor of a self-antigen present on the nervous system (therefore called onconeural antigen) leads to a breakdown of immune tolerance and the production of onconeural antibodies.[6] With thymoma, the mechanism probably combines the liberation of defective immune-regulatory cells and the expression of self-antigens by the tumor.[7] Two categories of onconeural antigens are now distinguished: intracellular and cell surface antigens.[8] With paraneoplastic neuropathies, HuD and CRMP5 are the main intracellular antigens while Caspr2 is an axonal membrane antigen. Another characteristic is that with antibodies directed toward intracellular antigens, a tumor is present in > 90% of cases while it is inconstant when the antigen is on the cell surface. Finally, antibodies toward CRMP5 or Caspr 2 occur with both carcinoma and thymoma.

With lymphoma, the tumor itself produces factors that are responsible for the neuropathy. Usually, this factor is a monoclonal component. Monoclonal IgM can behave as antibodies reacting with a membrane antigen such as myelin-associated glycoprotein (MAG) or gangliosides. These antibodies are likely responsible for the neuropathy and more frequently occur with monoclonal gammopathy of unknown significance rather than with Waldenström's disease or other lymphomas.[9] In other cases, the physicochemical properties of the M component lead to the formation of amyloid deposits (AL amyloidosis) or cryoglobulinemia. Finally, with POEMS syndrome, the pathogenic factor is not the monoclonal component but probably cytokines produced by the tumor. These disorders, which are described in other chapters of this book, will not be discussed here. However, there also exist paraneoplastic neuropathies with lymphoma that are clearly inflammatory and are not linked to the presence of a monoclonal component. Table 1 summarizes the different forms of definite paraneoplastic neuropathies.

TABLE 1 The different forms of definite parneoplastic peripheral neuropathies.

Neuropathy	Cancer	Number of reported cases	Antibodies	Other criteria for definite paraneoplastic	Comments
Neuronopathies					
Sensory neuronopathy	SCLC 80% -HL and other carcinoma	>500	Hu, CV2/CRMP5 Abs, other onconeural		10% without Abs
Lower motor neuron disease	SCLC-HL-carcinoma	<20 cases	Hu Abs with SCLC only	Some improved with tumor treatment	Rare cases Ma2 Abs
Mixed sensory and motor	SCLC-70%	>200	Hu		According to presentation, may be confused with different forms of axonal sensory-motor neuropathy
Autonomic neuropathy	SCLC 70% -HL and other carcinoma	SCLC <200 -other <10	Hu Abs, (ganglionic AChR)	Some with HL improved with immunotherapy	Frequently associated with SSN and anti-Hu Abs
Sensory-motor neuropathies					
Axonal	Carcinoma and HL	Rare	Usually none	Some improved with tumor treatment	Rare cases with Yo or Ma2 Abs
Axonal and demyelinating	SCLC, thymoma	<50 with CV2/CRMP5 Abs	CV2/CRMP5 Abs		Frequently associated with CNS involvement with CV2/CRMP5 Abs

Continued

TABLE 1 The different forms of definite parneoplastic peripheral neuropathies—cont'd

Neuropathy	Cancer	Number of reported cases	Antibodies	Other criteria for definite paraneoplastic	Comments
Demyelinating (CIDP)	Carcinoma and NHL	<50	Rarely CV2/CRMP5 Abs	Some improved with tumor treatment	With NHL neurolymphomatosis is the differential diagnosis
Vasculitic neuropathy	SCLC, NHL: type I cryoglobulinemia, other carcinoma	<50	Rarely Hu Abs	Some improved with tumor treatment	
Neuromyotonia	Thymoma (SCLC, NHL) 30%	<100	Caspr2, Netrin 1 receptorAbs		Insomnia, delirium with Morvan syndrome. Myasthenia gravis frequent

CIDP, chronic inflammatory demyelinating polyneuropathy; SCLC, small cell lung cancer; HL, Hodgkin's lymphoma; NHL, non-Hodgkin's lymphoma; Abs, antibodies; SSN, sensory neuronopathies; CNS, central nervous system.

Paraneoplastic peripheral neuropathies with carcinoma or thymoma

Subacute sensory neuronopathy (SSN)

SNN was described by Denny-Brown in 1948[10] and was the first peripheral nervous system disorder that was associated with an autoantibody,[11] later identified as the anti-Hu antibody.[12] The pathological hallmark is the destruction of sensory neurons in dorsal root ganglia with the secondary degeneration of their peripheral and central process, the proliferation of glial cells of the neuron capsule forming Nageotte's nodules, and mononuclear cell infiltration.[11,13,14] Inflammatory cells are only present during the early phase of the disease and disappear later. SNN is the most frequent and predominant component of a more complex inflammatory disorder called paraneoplastic encephalomyelitis, which affects the DRG, spinal cord, brain, and autonomous nervous system, explaining that SSN can occur alone or in association with other neurological manifestations.[14,15] Paraneoplastic encephalomyelitis, which was described long before the identification of onconeural antibodies, can now be almost equated with the anti-Hu syndrome.

SSN is the most frequent paraneoplastic neurological syndrome, representing 24% of cases in the series of about 1000 paraneoplastic patients of the PNS Euronetwork group.[16] The onset is subacute or rapidly progressive, but indolent and protracted courses over several months may occur.[17] Sensory loss is frequently multifocal or asymmetrical, and as a rule, involves the upper limbs in a nonlength-dependent distribution. The face, chest, or trunk can also be concerned.[18] Although large and small sensory neurons are simultaneously affected, in some cases, lesions predominate on one type of neuron, resulting in a mostly ataxic or painful small fiber neuropathy.[19] Some patients develop pseudoathetoid abnormal movements in limb extremities due to loss of proprioception. The autonomous nervous system is involved in 20%–24% of patients and manifests as gastrointestinal dysmotility, orthostatic hypotension, arrhythmia, or urinary dysfunction.[15] Patients may also develop minor symptoms of spinal cord involvement or limbic encephalitis such as temporal epilepsy, so that pure SNN is relatively rare.[15]

If paraneoplastic SNN is reputedly a severe disorder leaving patients unable to stand or to develop purposeful activities with their hands, an important proportion only have moderate to minor symptoms. In the PNS Euronetwork database, 63% of the patients have a Rankin's score equal to 1 or 2 (unpublished data). The limited sensory manifestations frequently have a multifocal and patchy distribution, which may lead to the diagnosis of sensory mononeuritis multiplex.

The electrodiagnostic hallmark of SNN is a severe and diffuse alteration of sensory nerve action potentials. Motor conduction velocities are typically normal but mild alterations are frequent,[16,20,21] consisting of the reduction of the amplitude of compound motor action potentials (CMAP), a mild reduction of conduction velocities, or neurogenic changes on needle examination,[20,21] which may lead to an inappropriate diagnosis if the clinical presentation is not correctly evaluated. These changes result from the subclinical involvement of lower motor neurons in the spinal cord, but also from the extension of the inflammatory reaction into the roots and the peripheral nerve (see below). The CSF usually shows elevated protein concentration, pleocytosis, and oligoclonal bands.[14] In 70%–80% of cases, SSN occurs with small cell lung cancer (SCLC). Most patients have anti-Hu antibodies. Antiamphyphisin or CV2/CRMP5 antibodies occur in 5%–10% of cases with or without anti-Hu antibodies, and in 10%–16% of patients, onconeural antibodies are not found. These patients usually have another type of tumor, including breast cancer or Hodgkin's disease.[22]

Diagnosis may be difficult in the first stages of the disease or in seronegative patients. To avoid this, a simple and sensitive score has been proposed that has good sensitivity and specificity for SNN diagnosis (Table 2).[23] In our French series, paraneosplatic SSN represents about 20% of all the SNN cases[18] so that a diagnostic strategy is necessary to identify them early.[24] A search for onconeural antibody should be done in every case and when negative, patients with rapid evolution must be investigated for cancer, particularly when pain, abnormal CSF, and mild motor nerve conduction abnormalities are present.

TABLE 2 Simple diagnostic score for the diagnosis of sensory neuronopathy.

Diagnostic criteria of sensory neuronopathy (a sumscore above 6.5 makes the diagnisis of sensory neuronopathy probale)	
In a patient with a clinically pure sensory neuropathy, a diagnosis of sensory neuronopathy (SNN) is considered possible if the total score is > 6.5 points	
1. Ataxia in the lower or upper limbs at onset or full development of the neuropathy	½ 3.1
2. Asymmetrical distribution of sensory loss at onset or full development of the neuropathy	½ 1.7
3. Sensory loss not restricted to the lower limbs at full development	½ 2.0
4. At least one SAP absent or three SAP < 30% of the lower limit of normal in the upper limbs, not explained by entrapment neuropathy	½ 2.8
5. Less than two nerves with abnormal motor NCS in the lower limbs[a]	½ 3.1

[a] Abnormal if CMAP or MCV\95% of LLN, distal latencies > 110% of LLN or F waves latency > 110% of LLN.
SAP, sensory action potential; CMAP, compound motor action potential; NCS, nerve conduction study; MCV, motor conduction velocities; LLN, lower limit of normal.
Adapted from Antoine JC, Robert-Varvat F, Maisonobe T, et al. Testing the validity of a set of diagnostic criteria for sensory neuronopathies: a francophone collaborative study. J Neurol 2014;261(11):2093–2100.

Sensory-motor neuronopathy

This disorder, which represents 12% of PNS,[16] is due to the combination of sensory and motor neuron involvement in the setting of paraneoplastic encephalomyelitis, and as a rule occurs with anti-Hu antibodies. Lower motor neuron involvement induces motor deficit, amyotrophy, and fasciculations.[15] The clinical presentation varies with the respective extension of lesions in the sensory and motor system, their spatial rostro-caudal distribution, and their evolution. Extensive and acute cases can be misdiagnosed as axonal Guillain-Barré syndrome while other cases may be considered polyradiculitis or a mononeuritis multiplex. Diagnosis may be made difficult by the fact that a nerve biopsy in patients with the anti-Hu syndrome may show vasculitis or inflammatory cell infiltrates.[21,25] Demyelinating changes have been reported in one case.[26]

Pure motor neuron diseases

Amyotrophic lateral sclerosis is not a paraneoplastic disorder.[27] Pure lower motor neuron disease is very rare with onconeural antibodies. It has been reported and confirmed by autopsy in a few patients with anti-Hu antibodies.[28,29] If the pyramidal tract is involved in the spinal cord, the presentation may mimic amyotrophic lateral sclerosis. More frequently, mild sensory changes are present clinically and electrophysiologically. Some patients develop lower motor neuron disease as a second and delayed paraneoplastic disorder.[30] The reported cases have anti-Hu or CV2/CRMP5 antibodies and the second disorder corresponds to a relapse of the cancer or the development of a new one. A particular disorder has been reported in patients with anti-Ma2 antibodies, consisting of lower motor neuron involvement in the cervical spinal cord with snake eyes-like changes on MRI.[31]

Pure autonomic neuronopathy

Pure paraneoplastic autonomic neuropathy is rare. The most frequent is digestive pseudoobstruction due to the destruction of neurons in the enteric plexuses.[15,32] Patients present with nausea, vomiting, persistent constipation, weight loss, and abdominal distention. Imaging studies demonstrate dilated intestinal loops without evidence of obstruction. In most of the cases, an anti-Hu antibody is present, explaining that SSN or sensory motor neuronopathy frequently develops after a few weeks or months.

Subacute pandysautonomia, also called autoimmune autonomic neuropathy, affects the sympathetic and parasympathetic autonomous system and combines orthostatic hypotension, urinary retention, abnormal pupillary reaction, a fixed heart rate, and digestive dysmotility.[33] It is rarely paraneoplastic, except when it is associated with the involvement of another part of the nervous system.[34] Antiganglionic acetylcholine receptor antibodies occur in about 20% of patients with acute or subacute pandysautonomia.[35] They have been detected in some patients with paraneoplastic autonomic involvement, but are not specific to a paraneoplastic origin of the disorder.[36]

Peripheral neuropathies

Peripheral neuropathies with anti-CV2/CRMP5 antibodies

Neuropathy occurs in 60%–80% of patients with anti-CV2/CRMP5 antibodies.[37,38] It is frequently the presenting symptom and the evolution is subacute. The clinical pattern is mostly sensory-motor with variations, according to the two published series.[37,38] In one of them, pain and the asymmetrical distribution of the disorder suggestive of polyradiculoneuropathy are the main features while in the other, it is the predominance of lower limb involvement. A few patients fulfill the criteria of sensory neuronopathies. The electrodiagnostic exploration shows axonal features with a reduction of sensory and motor action potentials and neurogenic changes on needle examination. However, a mild slowing of conduction velocities may occur,[38,39] and in one case, the pattern was clearly demyelinating.[40] The CSF is usually inflammatory and a nerve biopsy shows axonal loss and in some patients demyelination and remyelination with mild inflammatory changes.[39] Such variability in the clinical pattern may be explained by the distribution of the antigen in the peripheral nervous system because CRMP5 is expressed in sensory neurons, axons, and Schwann cells, particularly nonmyelinating Schwann cells (Fig. 1).[39,41]

The simultaneous involvement of the cerebellum, spinal cord, optic nerve, or retina is frequent and some patients also have Lambert Eaton myasthenic syndrome. It is also frequent that patients with anti-CV2/CRMP5 antibodies harbor anti-Hu antibodies; in this case, the clinical presentation is a mixture of the two. SCLC and more rarely thymoma are the usual tumors. Interestingly, two published series independently found that the prognosis of SCLC was better in patients with anti-CV2/CRMP5 antibodies than those with anti-Hu antibodies,[37,38]

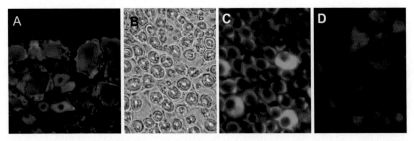

FIG. 1 Expression of CRMP5 in rat dorsal root ganglion (A) and sciatic nerve (B–D). Immunohistochemistry with an anti-CRMPR antibody. (A) In the dorsal root ganglion, CRMP5 is expressed in the cytoplasm of large and small sensory neurons and their satellite cells. (B–D) Same field of a sciatic nerve. A: bright field showing myelinated fibers. B: Schwann cells reveled with an anti-S100 antibody. C: expression of CRMP5. The protein is expressed in the cytoplasm of myelinating and nonmyelinating Schwann cells.

suggesting that the expression of CRMP5 by the tumor may modify either the antitumoral immune response or the cancer proliferation and diffusion.

Neuropathy with other onconeural antibodies

Neuropathy occurs only occasionally with other onconeural antibodies. Anecdotal cases of sensory neuropathy have been reported with anti-Yo antibodies,[42] mononeuritis multiplex[43] and myeloradiculopathy with Ma2 antibodies,[44] and sensorimotor neuropathy mimicking plexopathy with antiamphiphysin antibodies.[45] Immunoreactivities against ßIV spectrin,[46] gangliosides,[47,48] or inositol 1,4,5-trisphosphate receptor type 1[49] reported in the setting of cancer and neuropathy need confirmation.

Peripheral neuropathies improving with tumor treatment

A variety of neuropathies have been reported as paraneoplastic with carcinoma, but with no detectable onconeural antibodies, including motor neuron disease, plexopathy, sensory neuropathy, Guillain-Barré syndrome, CIDP, vasculitic neuropathies, and autonomic neuropathies.[50] Most of them are only possible paraneoplastic disorders, according to the aforementioned classification. However, rare cases of lower motor neuron disease,[51] nerve vasculitis,[52] or CIDP[53] that improved with tumor treatment can be considered definite paraneoplastic neuropathies. At the difference of the disorders seen previously that are massively associated with lung cancer, here the tumor does not affect a specific organ. Among these tumors, melanoma has been associated with neuropathies and antiganglioside antibodies. In one case, the neuropathy fulfilled the criteria of CIDP and the antibodies reacted with GM2.[47] In another case, the neurological disorder combined axonal motor neuropathy and ophthalmoplegia with anti-GQ1b antibodies.[54] Interestingly, in the first case it was demonstrated that the tumor expressed GM2 while in the second, the neuropathy appeared after immunization with a tumor antigen, arguing that theses neuropathies depended on a cross-immunological reaction between the melanoma and the PNS.

Neuromyotonia

Acquired neuromyotonia, peripheral nerve hyperexcitablity (PNH), and Isaacs' syndrome are different designations of a disorder marked by abnormal muscle activities, cramps, stiffness, twitching, spasms, and abnormal relaxation.[55–57] Weakness, paraesthesiae, and hyperhidrosis also occur. Neuromyotonia, sleep disruption, mood changes, and hallucinations characterize Morvan syndrome.[58] Diagnosis relies on the recording of fibrillation and fasciculation potentials; myokimia organized in doublets, triplets, or multiplets; and myokimic, neuromyotonic, and posteffort or poststimulation discharges.[57] Neuromyotonia occurs with thymoma in 15%–20% of cases and rarely with SCLC or lymphoma.[56] Thymoma incidence is higher in the case of Morvan syndrome, explaining that myasthenia gravis is particularly frequent in this disorder.[56,59] Some patients may also develop small fiber neuropathy.[60] PNH has been associated with anticontactin-associated protein-2 (Caspr2), a membrane protein of the juxta-paranodal region.[61] As Caspr2 antibodies also occur with limbic encephalitis, their role in PNH remains unclear. In one study, anti-Caspr2 antibodies were detected in the serum with PNH while they were mostly detected in the CSF with limbic encephalitis;[59] in another study, they mostly occurred with Morvan syndrome and thymoma.[62] With Caspr2 antibodies, Netrin 1 receptor antibodies can predict thymoma in patients with PNH and myasthenia gravis.[62] As Caspr2 antibodies are usually absent in isolated neuromyotonia, other antibodies are probably responsible for the disorder.[62]

Paraneoplastic neuropathies with lymphoma

If we except neuropathies associated with monoclonal gammopathy, para-neoplastic neuropathies occurring with lymphoma are particularly rare. With Hodgkin's disease, several cases of histologically proven SNN have been re-ported[22,63] while cases of neuropathy improving with the tumor treatment in-clude a single observation of pure motor radiculopathy[64] and sensory axonal polyneuropathy.[65] None of these patients have onconeural antibodies. One pa-tient with sensory-motor neuropathy, inflammatory CSF, and Hodgkin's dis-ease harbored an antibody reacting with the PNS, but the neuropathy did not responded to the tumor treatment.[66] Other peripheral nervous system disorders have been associated with Hodgkin's disease, but their link with the lymphoma is unclear, in particular because they can appear when the tumor has been in complete remission for several years. Thus, Schold et al.[67] reported a subacute lower motor neuron disorder that may improve spontaneously, suggesting that there was no motor neuron degeneration. However, in the pathologically studied cases, motor neuron loss was observed. Several of these patients received radio-therapy so that a secondary effect of the treatment cannot be ruled out.[68] Several cases of Guillain-Barré syndrome have also been reported in patients with Hodgkin's disease[69] but again, the link between the two disorders is unclear, even if the incidence of tumor in Guillain-Barré syndrome is possibly slightly increased.[70] The same conclusion applies to cases of vasculitic neuropathies.[71]

With non-Hodgkin's lymphomas, the main concern is to differentiate para-neoplastic neuropathies from neoplastic infiltration. The frequent predomi-nance of neurolymphomatosis in the proximal regions of the PNS makes this identification frequently difficult.[72] In a recent series of 32 cases, only five could be considered paraneoplastic (three chronic inflammatory demyelinating poly-neuropathies [CIDP], one SNN, and one nerve vasculitis) while in the others, neurolymphomatosis was demonstrated or highly suspected, including in cases fulfilling the EFNS-PNS criteria of CIDP or with peripheral nerve vasculitis.[73] Repeated and thorough investigations using PET-scanner imaging, immuno-histochemistry, and retrograde polymerase chain reaction to demonstrate the monoclonal nature of the cell infiltrate on tissue biopsy play a major role in the diagnostic process, but sometimes only an autopsy allows a final conclusion.[74] As a whole, demyelinating neuropathy followed by nerve vasculitis is the most frequent pattern of paraneoplastic neuropathies with non-Hodgkin's lymphoma, and the best therapeutic results are obtained when combining immunomodulating treatments and chemotherapy.[75] A wide range of neuropathies has been reported in the setting of Waldenström's disease[76,77] or myeloma.[78] Most of them depend on the presence of a monoclonal component while others involve unclear mechanisms.

Pathophysiology

Most of our knowledge on the pathophysiology of paraneoplastic peripheral neuropathies comes from the anti-Hu syndrome. Similar mechanisms probably apply to the other onconeural antigens, but all the definite paraneoplastic peripheral neuropathies probably cannot be explained in a single way.

HuD, the target of anti-Hu antibodies, is a neuronal-specific mRNA binding protein.[79] In mature neurons (Fig. 1D), it is located in the nucleus, mitochondria, and the Golgi apparatus, where it enables mRNA interactions with subcellular organelles and regulates their localization.[80] HuD is also expressed in a normal nonmutated form by most SCLCs,[81] so that its recognition in the tumor by the immune system probably leads to the development of the neurological disorder. This hypothesis has recently been supported by an experimental model of crossed immunity against an artificial antigen shared by a tumor and the nervous system under the control of CD8 and CD4 T-cells.[82] The high degree of natural immune tolerance against HuD[83] probably explains why only a very few patients develop a paraneoplastic disorder.

In neural tissue (Fig. 2A–C),[13,84–87] inflammatory cells mostly consist of T-cells. CD8 + cytotoxic T-cells come in close contact with sensory neurons while CD4 + helper cells and macrophages gather in the interstitial space. Cytotoxic T-cells express perforin or TIA-1, the agents of cellular toxicity. At the same time, sensory neurons and their satellite cells overexpress major histocompatibility complex classes I and II molecules and adhesion molecules such as ICAM-1, which are essential for the recognition by and the adhesion of T-cells. The absence of production of Fas, Fasligand, C9neo, and activated caspase-3 indicates that cell death results from cytotoxicity and not from apoptosis.[86] Circulating[88] and neural tissue[89] CD8 + T-lymphocytes display a restricted oligoclonal repertoire of their TCR genes, indicating that they are specifically directed toward one or few antigens. If circulating, CD4 +, probably Th1 cells, has been shown to react with HuD.[90] Results are conflicting concerning CD8 + T-cells.[91,92]

On the other hand, IgG1 and the 3 anti-Hu antibody are present around sensory neurons.[85,93] Although these antibodies are able to activate the complement and natural killer (NK), complement deposits and NK cells are scarce or absent in lesions, which does not support the hypothesis of an antibody-dependent

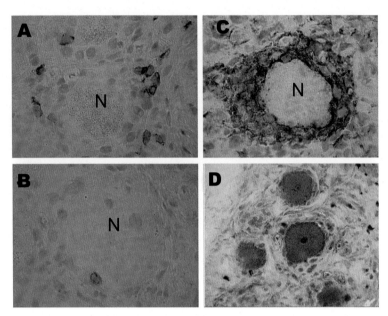

FIG. 2 Dorsal root ganglion of a patient with sensory neuropathy and anti-Hu antibodies. Immunohischemical analysis. (A) CD4+ helper T-cells surround a sensory neuron (N). (B) A cytotoxic T-cell expressing perforine is in close contact with the sensory neuron (N) cytoplasmic membrane. (C) Overexpression of MHC II molecules by the sensory neurons (N) and surrounding satellite cells. (D) Expression of the HuD protein in the nucleus and cytoplasm of sensory neurons.

cytotoxicity.[85] Conversely, anti-Hu antibodies have been shown to induce neuron lysis in vitro in the presence of complement,[94] but this was not confirmed when using SCLC cell lines.[95] The particular weakness of the blood-nerve barrier in the dorsal root and autonomic ganglia[96] may facilitate the access of antibodies—and T-cells as well—to this structure and explain why SNN and dysautonomia are so frequent in patients with anti-Hu antibodies. The transfer of the disease by antibodies would be an important argument in favor of their role, but immunization of rodents with HuD led to the production of a high titer of antibodies, IgG deposits in the brain, and no development of neuronal lesions and clinical manifestation.[97] Taken as a whole, these results suggest that T-cells are probably the main effector of the immune process while antibody production, although very useful for the diagnosis of patients, is probably a bystanding phenomenon.

CRMP5 is also expressed in most SCLCs while in the thymus and thymoma, a peptide shared by all the CRMP family members is produced, suggesting that the process leading to autoimmunization is not the same with the two tumors.[98] Anti-Caspr2 antibodies, which are mostly IgG4 antibodies, may theoretically have access to their target in the paranodal regions and interfere with their functioning.[99] However, their pathogenic role has not been demonstrated yet as in one experiment, anti-Caspr2 antibodies were not able to reach the paranodal region after intraneural injection.[100]

The search for a cancer in patients with peripheral neuropathy

In > 80% of cases, the paraneoplastic neurological disorder precedes by months or years the discovery of the cancer or its relapse. There are two main circumstances in which a search for cancer is necessary. The first is when a well-established paraneoplastic disorder is diagnosed. This includes SSN, digestive pseudoobstruction, neuromyotonia, and the presence of a well-characterized onconeural antibody. As paraneoplastic SNN can be seronegative, the search for a tumor must be performed if the evolution is acute or subacute and the CSF inflammatory. The question of a paraneoplastic disorder may arise in patients treated with platinum salts for SCLC and who develop SNN. Some clinical features distinguish toxic from paraneoplastic SNN, in particular platinum salt-induced SNN has a symmetrical distribution and almost spare small fibers.[101,102] A search for onconeural antibodies may help to distinguish the two disorders, but only high titers are indicative of a paraneoplastic origin.[5]

The second circumstance is when the peripheral neuropathy occurs with the involvement of the central or autonomic nervous system. A subacute and severely deteriorating evolution is frequent with paraneoplastic disorders. Therefore, peripheral neuropathies with an unusual, rapid, and severe course or that don't respond to expected effective treatments should be considered suspect, inasmuch as the CSF is inflammatory. These patients may or may not have onconeural antibodies. Although there is no validated recommendation for the management of seronegative patients, it may be preferable to search for an underlying tumor when the neuropathy follows one of these patterns. Apart from these circumstances, axonal distal polyneuropathy or CIDP does not deserve a systematic search for a malignancy, except when a monoclonal gammopathy is detected. The question remains open for nerve vasculitis, for which there exist several reports mentioning an association with lymphoma or carcinoma (see above).

The strategy in the search for the responsible cancer depends heavily on the paraneoplastic disorders and the associated antibodies.[103] In patients with SSN and/or onconeural antibodies, SCLC must be suspected first. The tumor is frequently limited to metastatic lymph nodes that may escape detection by a CT scan or lung fibroscopy. An FDG-PET scanner (Fig. 3) is then recommended. However, it should be kept in mind that while the method is highly sensitive, it is also unspecific.[104] Mediastinal lymph nodes may be difficult to reach for biopsy and each case must be carefully discussed with a trained lung specialist or thoracic surgeon.[103] When a first careful workup is negative, it is recommended to renew it after 3–6 months and then every 6 months for a period of at least 4 years.[103] When searching for the underlying tumor, it is not rare to find a

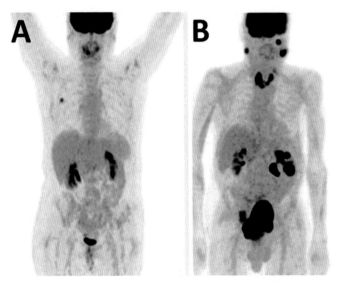

FIG. 3 FDG-PET scanner. (A) Small infraclinical carcinoma of the right breast of a female patient with very mild sensory neuronopathy, oligoclonal cerebrospinal fluid, and no onconeural antibody. (B) Pelvic infiltration of a small cell prostate cancer with cervical lymph node metastasis in a patient with an amyotrophic lateral sclerosis-like syndrome and inflammatory cerebrospinal fluid.

malignancy that is at odds with the expected cancer (e.g., a colon cancer with an anti-Hu antibody). If expression of the onconeural antigen by the tumor is not demonstrated, SCLC must be still suspected.[15] A search for lymphoma would also need an FDG-PET scanner and a search for a circulating, bone marrow, or intraneural monoclonal B-cell proliferation.

Treatment

Owing to the rarity of these disorders, quality controlled studies are difficult to conduct and most of the evidence relies on uncontrolled studies or expert opinion. It is recognized that tumor treatment is the best way to stabilize and sometimes improve the patient.[15,105] This is a crucial point because in patients with onconeural antibodies, the inflammatory phase of the disorder lasts some weeks to a few months, even though autoantibodies persist in the serum. At the same time, irreversible neuron damage occurs and as a result, the therapeutic widow in SNN is probably below 3 months,[106] stressing the need for early diagnosis of the disorder and of the cancer.

Immunomodulatory treatments including prednisolone, intravenous immunoglobulins (IVIg),[107,108] plasma exchanges,[109] cyclophosphamide,[110] tacrolimus,[111] and rituximab[112] in monotherapy or in combination[113,114] have been tested in disorders associated with onconeural antibodies. Their efficacy is not clearly proven although some patients improve, particularly those with early treatment and minor or mild disability. With onconeural antibodies, our Reference Center treats patients with high-dose steroids and/or IVIg. Cyclophosphamide can be used as a second-line treatment when the cancer is not detected or the patient deteriorates despite cancer treatment. Clearly, controlled studies are necessary with drugs that can rapidly block the access of immune cells to the nervous system, such as natalizumab.

Symptomatic treatments are also recommended.[115] Drugs that have shown efficacy for neuropathic pain such as amitriptyline, duloxetine, venlafaxine, gabapentin, or pregabalin may be given in SNN as a first-line treatment while tramadol and opioids may be used as the second line.[116] In PNH, antiepileptic drugs and particularly carbamazepine may reduce muscle overactivity.[117] As Lambert-Eaton may occur in patients with anti-Hu or CV2/CRMP5 antibodies and is a treatable disorder, a search for potentiation must systematically be performed in patients with these antibodies when the CMAP amplitude is reduced.

References

1. Croft PB, Wilkinson M. The incidence of carcinomatous neuromyopathy in patients with various types of carcinoma. *Brain*. 1965;88(3):427–434.
2. Currie S, Henson RA, Morgan HG, Poole AJ. The incidence of the nonmetastatic neurological syndromes of obscure origin in the reticuloses. *Brain*. 1970;93(3):629–640.
3. Antoine JC, Camdessanche JP. Peripheral nervous system involvement in patients with cancer. *Lancet Neurol*. 2007;6(1):75–86.
4. Boudin G. Neuropathie péripéhrique dégénérative et myélome. *Bull Soc méd Hôp Paris*. 1961;77.
5. Graus F, Delattre JY, Antoine JC, et al. Recommended diagnostic criteria for paraneoplastic neurological syndromes. *J Neurol Neurosurg Psychiatry*. 2004;75(8):1135–1140.
6. Graus F, Dalmau J. Paraneoplastic neurological syndromes. *Curr Opin Neurol*. 2012;25(6):795–801.
7. Shelly S, Agmon-Levin N, Altman A, Shoenfeld Y. Thymoma and autoimmunity. *Cell Mol Immunol*. 2011;8(3):199–202.
8. Didelot A, Honnorat J. Paraneoplastic disorders of the central and peripheral nervous systems. *Handb Clin Neurol*. 2014;121:1159–1179.
9. Svahn J, Petiot P, Antoine JC, et al. Anti-MAG antibodies in 202 patients: clinicopathological and therapeutic features. *J Neurol Neurosurg Psychiatry*. 2017.
10. Denny-Brown D. Primary sensory neuropathy with muscular changes associated with carcinoma. *J Neurol Neurosurg Psychiatry*. 1948;11(2):73–87.
11. Croft PB, Henson RA, Urich H, Wilkinson PC. Sensory neuropathy with bronchial carcinoma: a study of four cases showing serological abnormalities. *Brain*. 1965;88(3):501–514.
12. Graus F, Cordon-Cardo C, Posner JB. Neuronal antinuclear antibody in sensory neuronopathy from lung cancer. *Neurology*. 1985;35(4):538–543.
13. Graus F, Ribalta T, Campo E, Monforte R, Urbano A, Rozman C. Immunohistochemical analysis of the immune reaction in the nervous system in paraneoplastic encephalomyelitis. *Neurology*. 1990;40(2):219–222.
14. Dalmau J, Graus F, Rosenblum MK, Posner JB. Anti-Hu-associated paraneoplastic encephalomyelitis/sensory neuronopathy. A clinical study of 71 patients. *Medicine (Baltimore)*. 1992;71(2):59–72.

15. Graus F, Keime-Guibert F, Rene R, et al. Anti-Hu-associated paraneoplastic encephalomyelitis: analysis of 200 patients. *Brain*. 2001;124(Pt 6):1138–1148.
16. Giometto B, Grisold W, Vitaliani R, Graus F, Honnorat J, Bertolini G. Paraneoplastic neurologic syndrome in the PNS Euronetwork database: a European study from 20 centers. *Arch Neurol*. 2010;67(3):330–335.
17. Graus F, Bonaventura I, Uchuya M, et al. Indolent anti-Hu-associated paraneoplastic sensory neuropathy. *Neurology*. 1994;44(12):2258–2261.
18. Antoine JC, Robert-Varvat F, Maisonobe T, et al. Testing the validity of a set of diagnostic criteria for sensory neuronopathies: a francophone collaborative study. *J Neurol*. 2014;261(11):2093–2100.
19. Oki Y, Koike H, Iijima M, et al. Ataxic vs painful form of paraneoplastic neuropathy. *Neurology*. 2007;69(6):564–572.
20. Camdessanche JP, Antoine JC, Honnorat J, et al. Paraneoplastic peripheral neuropathy associated with anti-Hu antibodies. A clinical and electrophysiological study of 20 patients. *Brain*. 2002;125(Pt 1):166–175.
21. Oh SJ, Gurtekin Y, Dropcho EJ, King P, Claussen GC. Anti-Hu antibody neuropathy: a clinical, electrophysiological, and pathological study. *Clin Neurophysiol*. 2005;116(1):28–34.
22. Horwich MS, Cho L, Porro RS, Posner JB. Subacute sensory neuropathy: a remote effect of carcinoma. *Ann Neurol*. 1977;2(1):7–19.
23. Camdessanche JP, Jousserand G, Ferraud K, et al. The pattern and diagnostic criteria of sensory neuronopathy: a case-control study. *Brain*. 2009;132(Pt 7):1723–1733.
24. Camdessanche JP, Jousserand G, Franques J, et al. A clinical pattern-based etiological diagnostic strategy for sensory neuronopathies: a French collaborative study. *J Peripher Nerv Syst*. 2012;17(3):331–340.
25. Younger DS, Dalmau J, Inghirami G, Sherman WH, Hays AP. Anti-Hu-associated peripheral nerve and muscle microvasculitis. *Neurology*. 1994;44(1):181–183.
26. Antoine JC, Mosnier JF, Honnorat J, et al. Paraneoplastic demyelinating neuropathy, subacute sensory neuropathy, and anti-Hu antibodies: clinicopathological study of an autopsy case. *Muscle Nerve*. 1998;21(7):850–857.
27. Corcia P, Gordon PH, Camdessanche JP. Is there a paraneoplastic ALS? *Amyotroph Lateral Scler Frontotemporal Degener*. 2015;16(3–4):252–257.
28. Forsyth PA, Dalmau J, Graus F, Cwik V, Rosenblum MK, Posner JB. Motor neuron syndromes in cancer patients. *Ann Neurol*. 1997;41(6):722–730.
29. Verma A, Berger JR, Snodgrass S, Petito C. Motor neuron disease: a paraneoplastic process associated with anti-hu antibody and small-cell lung carcinoma. *Ann Neurol*. 1996;40(1):112–116.
30. Ducray F, Graus F, Vigliani MC, et al. Delayed onset of a second paraneoplastic neurological syndrome in eight patients. *J Neurol Neurosurg Psychiatry*. 2010;81(8):937–939.
31. Waragai M, Chiba A, Uchibori A, Fukushima T, Anno M, Tanaka K. Anti-Ma2 associated paraneoplastic neurological syndrome presenting as encephalitis and progressive muscular atrophy. *J Neurol Neurosurg Psychiatry*. 2006;77(1):111–113.
32. Condom E, Vidal A, Rota R, Graus F, Dalmau J, Ferrer I. Paraneoplastic intestinal pseudoobstruction associated with high titres of Hu autoantibodies. *Virchows Arch A Pathol Anat Histopathol*. 1993;423(6):507–511.
33. Koike H, Hashimoto R, Tomita M, et al. The spectrum of clinicopathological features in pure autonomic neuropathy. *J Neurol*. 2012.
34. Koike H, Watanabe H, Sobue G. The spectrum of immune-mediated autonomic neuropathies: insights from the clinicopathological features. *J Neurol Neurosurg Psychiatry*. 2012.

35. Vernino S, Low PA, Fealey RD, Stewart JD, Farrugia G, Lennon VA. Autoantibodies to ganglionic acetylcholine receptors in autoimmune autonomic neuropathies. *N Engl J Med.* 2000;343(12):847–855.

36. Vernino S, Adamski J, Kryzer TJ, Fealey RD, Lennon VA. Neuronal nicotinic ACh receptor antibody in subacute autonomic neuropathy and cancer-related syndromes. *Neurology.* 1998;50(6):1806–1813.

37. Dubey D, Lennon VA, Gadoth A, et al. Autoimmune CRMP5 neuropathy phenotype and outcome defined from 105 cases. *Neurology.* 2018;90(2):e103–e110.

38. Honnorat J, Cartalat-Carel S, Ricard D, et al. Onco-neural antibodies and tumour type determine survival and neurological symptoms in paraneoplastic neurological syndromes with Hu or CV2/CRMP5 antibodies. *J Neurol Neurosurg Psychiatry.* 2009;80(4):412–416.

39. Antoine JC, Honnorat J, Camdessanche JP, et al. Paraneoplastic anti-CV2 antibodies react with peripheral nerve and are associated with a mixed axonal and demyelinating peripheral neuropathy. *Ann Neurol.* 2001;49(2):214–221.

40. Samarasekera S, Rajabally YA. Demyelinating neuropathy with anti-CRMP5 antibodies predating diagnosis of breast carcinoma: favorable outcome after cancer therapy. *Muscle Nerve.* 2011;43(5):764–766.

41. Camdessanche JP, Ferraud K, Boutahar N, et al. The collapsin response mediator protein 5 onconeural protein is expressed in Schwann cells under axonal signals and regulates axon-Schwann cell interactions. *J Neuropathol Exp Neurol.* 2012;71(4):298–311.

42. Taieb G, Renard D, Deverdal M, Honnorat J, Labauge P, Castelnovo G. Pure monomelic sensory neuronopathy associated with anti-yo antibodies. *Muscle Nerve.* 2012;45(2):297–298.

43. Ayrignac X, Castelnovo G, Landrault E, et al. Ma2 antibody and multiple mononeuropathies. *Rev Neurol (Paris).* 2008;164(6–7):608–611.

44. Murphy SM, Khan U, Alifrangis C, et al. Anti Ma2-associated myeloradiculopathy: expanding the phenotype of anti-Ma2 associated paraneoplastic syndromes. *J Neurol Neurosurg Psychiatry.* 2012;83(2):232–233.

45. Coppens T, Van den Bergh P, Duprez TJ, Jeanjean A, De Ridder F, Sindic CJ. Paraneoplastic rhombencephalitis and brachial plexopathy in two cases of amphiphysin auto-immunity. *Eur Neurol.* 2006;55(2):80–83.

46. Berghs S, Ferracci F, Maksimova E, et al. Autoimmunity to beta IV spectrin in paraneoplastic lower motor neuron syndrome. *Proc Natl Acad Sci U S A.* 2001;98(12):6945–6950.

47. Weiss MD, Luciano CA, Semino-Mora C, Dalakas MC, Quarles RH. Molecular mimicry in chronic inflammatory demyelinating polyneuropathy and melanoma. *Neurology.* 1998;51(6):1738–1741.

48. Antoine JC, Camdessanché JP, Ferraud K, Caudie C. Antiganglioside antibodies in paraneoplastic peripheral neuropathies. *J Neurol Neurosurg Psychiatry.* 2004;75:1765–1767.

49. Jarius S, Ringelstein M, Haas J, et al. Inositol 1,4,5-trisphosphate receptor type 1 autoantibodies in paraneoplastic and nonparaneoplastic peripheral neuropathy. *J Neuroinflammation.* 2016;13(1):278.

50. Graus F, Dalmau J. Paraneoplastic neuropathies. *Curr Opin Neurol.* 2013;26(5):489–495.

51. Evans BK, Fagan C, Arnold T, Dropcho EJ, Oh SJ. Paraneoplastic motor neuron disease and renal cell carcinoma: improvement after nephrectomy. *Neurology.* 1990;40(6):960–962.

52. Oh SJ, Slaughter R, Harrell L. Paraneoplastic vasculitic neuropathy: a treatable neuropathy. *Muscle Nerve.* 1991;14(2):152–156.

53. Antoine JC, Mosnier JF, Lapras J, et al. Chronic inflammatory demyelinating polyneuropathy associated with carcinoma. *J Neurol Neurosurg Psychiatry.* 1996;60(2):188–190.

54. Kloos L, Sillevis Smitt P, Ang CW, Kruit W, Stoter G. Paraneoplastic ophthalmoplegia and subacute motor axonal neuropathy associated with anti-GQ1b antibodies in a patient with malignant melanoma. *J Neurol Neurosurg Psychiatry*. 2003;74(4):507–509.

55. Sinha S, Newsom-Davis J, Mills K, Byrne N, Lang B, Vincent A. Autoimmune aetiology for acquired neuromyotonia (Isaacs' syndrome). *Lancet*. 1991;338(8759):75–77.

56. Maddison P, Mills KR, Newsom-Davis J. Clinical electrophysiological characterization of the acquired neuromyotonia phenotype of autoimmune peripheral nerve hyperexcitability. *Muscle Nerve*. 2006.

57. Hart IK, Maddison P, Newsom-Davis J, Vincent A, Mills KR. Phenotypic variants of autoimmune peripheral nerve hyperexcitability. *Brain*. 2002;125(Pt 8):1887–1895.

58. Irani SR, Pettingill P, Kleopa KA, et al. Morvan syndrome: clinical and serological observations in 29 cases. *Ann Neurol*. 2012;72(2):241–255.

59. Joubert B, Saint-Martin M, Noraz N, et al. Characterization of a subtype of autoimmune encephalitis with anti-contactin-associated protein-like 2 antibodies in the cerebrospinal fluid, prominent limbic symptoms, and seizures. *JAMA Neurol*. 2016;73(9):1115–1124.

60. Laurencin C, Andre-Obadia N, Camdessanche JP, et al. Peripheral small fiber dysfunction and neuropathic pain in patients with Morvan syndrome. *Neurology*. 2015;85(23):2076–2078.

61. Lancaster E, Huijbers MG, Bar V, et al. Investigations of caspr2, an autoantigen of encephalitis and neuromyotonia. *Ann Neurol*. 2011;69(2):303–311.

62. Torres-Vega E, Mancheno N, Cebrian-Silla A, et al. Netrin-1 receptor antibodies in thymoma-associated neuromyotonia with myasthenia gravis. *Neurology*. 2017;88(13):1235–1242.

63. Case Records of the Massachusetts General Hospital. Weekly Clinicopathological Exercises. Case 8-1990. A 45-year-old woman with Hodgkin's disease and a neurologic disorder. *N Engl J Med*. 1990;322(8):531–543.

64. Flanagan EP, Sandroni P, Pittock SJ, Inwards DJ, Jones Jr LK. Paraneoplastic lower motor neuronopathy associated with Hodgkin lymphoma. *Muscle Nerve*. 2012;46(5):823–827.

65. Plante-Bordeneuve V, Baudrimont M, Gorin NC, Gherardi RK. Subacute sensory neuropathy associated with Hodgkin's disease. *J Neurol Sci*. 1994;121(2):155–158.

66. Blacs F, Strittmatter M, Schwamhorn J, et al. Antineuronal antibody-associated paraneoplastic neuropathy in Hodgkin's disease. *Eur J Neurol*. 1998;5(1):109–112.

67. Schold SC, Cho ES, Somasundaram M, Posner JB. Subacute motor neuronopathy: a remote effect of lymphoma. *Ann Neurol*. 1979;5(3):271–287.

68. de Greve JL, Bruyland M, de Keyser J, Storme G, Ebinger G. Lower motor neuron disease in a patient with Hodgkin's disease treated with radiotherapy. *Clin Neurol Neurosurg*. 1984;86(1):43–46.

69. Lisak RP, Mitchell M, Zweiman B, Orrechio E, Asbury AK. Guillain-Barre syndrome and Hodgkin's disease: three cases with immunological studies. *Ann Neurol*. 1977;1(1):72–78.

70. Vigliani MC, Magistrello M, Polo P, Mutani R, Chio A. Risk of cancer in patients with Guillain-Barre syndrome (GBS). A population-based study. *J Neurol*. 2004;251(3):321–326.

71. Vincent D, Dubas F, Hauw JJ, et al. Nerve and muscle microvasculitis in peripheral neuropathy: a remote effect of cancer? *J Neurol Neurosurg Psychiatry*. 1986;49(9):1007–1010.

72. Vallat JM, De Mascarel HA, Bordessoule D, et al. NonHodgkin malignant lymphomas and peripheral neuropathies—13 cases. *Brain*. 1995;118(Pt 5):1233–1245.

73. Tomita M, Koike H, Kawagashira Y, et al. Clinicopathological features of neuropathy associated with lymphoma. *Brain*. 2013;136(Pt 8):2563–2578.

74. Baehring JM, Damek D, Martin EC, Betensky RA, Hochberg FH. Neurolymphomatosis. *Neuro Oncol*. 2003;5(2):104–115.

75. Viala K, Behin A, Maisonobe T, et al. Neuropathy in lymphoma: a relationship between the pattern of neuropathy, type of lymphoma and prognosis? *J Neurol Neurosurg Psychiatry.* 2007.

76. Viala K, Stojkovic T, Doncker AV, et al. Heterogeneous spectrum of neuropathies in Waldenstrom's macroglobulinemia: a diagnostic strategy to optimize their management. *J Peripher Nerv Syst.* 2012;17(1):90–101.

77. Levine T, Pestronk A, Florence J, et al. Peripheral neuropathies in Waldenstrom's macroglobulinaemia. *J Neurol Neurosurg Psychiatry.* 2006;77(2):224–228.

78. Kelly Jr JJ, Kyle RA, Miles JM, O'Brien PC, Dyck PJ. The spectrum of peripheral neuropathy in myeloma. *Neurology.* 1981;31(1):24–31.

79. Szabo A, Dalmau J, Manley G, et al. HuD, a paraneoplastic encephalomyelitis antigen, contains RNA-binding domains and is homologous to Elav and sex-lethal. *Cell.* 1991;67(2):325–333.

80. Fornaro M, Raimondo S, Lee JM, Giacobini-Robecchi MG. Neuron-specific Hu proteins subcellular localization in primary sensory neurons. *Ann Anat.* 2007;189(3):223–228.

81. Carpentier AF, Voltz R, DesChamps T, Posner JB, Dalmau J, Rosenfeld MR. Absence of HuD gene mutations in paraneoplastic small cell lung cancer tissue. *Neurology.* 1998;50(6):1919.

82. Gebauer C, Pignolet B, Yshii L, Maure E, Bauer J, Liblau R. CD4 + and CD8 + T cells are both needed to induce paraneoplastic neurological disease in a mouse model. *Oncoimmunology.* 2017;6(2):e1260212.

83. DeLuca I, Blachere NE, Santomasso B, Darnell RB. Tolerance to the neuron-specific paraneoplastic HuD antigen. *PLoS One.* 2009;4(6):e5739.

84. Wanschitz J, Hainfellner JA, Kristoferitsch W, Drlicek M, Budka H. Ganglionitis in paraneoplastic subacute sensory neuronopathy: a morphologic study. *Neurology.* 1997;49(4):1156–1159.

85. Jean WC, Dalmau J, Ho A, Posner JB. Analysis of the IgG subclass distribution and inflammatory infiltrates in patients with anti-Hu-associated paraneoplastic encephalomyelitis. *Neurology.* 1994;44(1):140–147.

86. Bernal F, Graus F, Pifarre A, Saiz A, Benyahia B, Ribalta T. Immunohistochemical analysis of anti-Hu-associated paraneoplastic encephalomyelitis. *Acta Neuropathol (Berl).* 2002;103(5):509–515.

87. Kuntzer T, Antoine JC, Steck AJ. Clinical features and pathophysiological basis of sensory neuronopathies (ganglionopathies). *Muscle Nerve.* 2004;30(3):255–268.

88. Plonquet A, Gherardi RK, Creange A, et al. Oligoclonal T-cells in blood and target tissues of patients with anti-Hu syndrome. *J Neuroimmunol.* 2002;122(1–2):100–105.

89. Voltz R, Dalmau J, Posner JB, Rosenfeld MR. T-cell receptor analysis in anti-Hu associated paraneoplastic encephalomyelitis. *Neurology.* 1998;51(4):1146–1150.

90. Benyahia B, Liblau R, Merle-Beral H, Tourani JM, Dalmau J, Delattre JY. Cell-mediated autoimmunity in paraneoplastic neurological syndromes with anti-Hu antibodies. *Ann Neurol.* 1999;45(2):162–167.

91. de Beukelaar JW, Verjans GM, van Norden Y, et al. No evidence for circulating HuD-specific CD8 + T cells in patients with paraneoplastic neurological syndromes and Hu antibodies. *Cancer Immunol Immunother.* 2007;56(9):1501–1506.

92. Tanaka M, Maruyama Y, Sugie M, Motizuki H, Kamakura K, Tanaka K. Cytotoxic T cell activity against peptides of Hu protein in anti-Hu syndrome. *J Neurol Sci.* 2002;201(1–2):9–12.

93. Dalmau J, Furneaux HM, Rosenblum MK, Graus F, Posner JB. Detection of the anti-Hu antibody in specific regions of the nervous system and tumor from patients with paraneoplastic encephalomyelitis/sensory neuronopathy. *Neurology.* 1991;41(11):1757–1764.

94. Greenlee JE, Parks TN, Jaeckle KA. Type IIa ('anti-Hu') antineuronal antibodies produce destruction of rat cerebellar granule neurons in vitro. *Neurology.* 1993;43(10):2049–2054.

95. Verschuuren JJ, Dalmau J, Hoard R, Posner JB. Paraneoplastic anti-Hu serum: studies on human tumor cell lines. *J Neuroimmunol*. 1997;79(2):202–210.
96. Allen DT, Kiernan JA. Permeation of proteins from the blood into peripheral nerves and ganglia. *Neuroscience*. 1994;59(3):755–764.
97. Sillevis Smitt PA, Manley GT, Posner JB. Immunization with the paraneoplastic encephalomyelitis antigen HuD does not cause neurologic disease in mice. *Neurology*. 1995;45(10):1873–1878.
98. Camdessanche JP, Lassabliere F, Meyronnet D, et al. Expression of the onconeural CV2/CRMP5 antigen in thymus and thymoma. *J Neuroimmunol*. 2006;174(1–2):168–173.
99. Huijbers MG, Querol LA, Niks EH, et al. The expanding field of IgG4-mediated neurological autoimmune disorders. *Eur J Neurol*. 2015;22(8):1151–1161.
100. Manso C, Querol L, Mekaouche M, Illa I, Devaux JJ. Contactin-1 IgG4 antibodies cause paranode dismantling and conduction defects. *Brain*. 2016;139(Pt 6):1700–1712.
101. Quasthoff S, Hartung HP. Chemotherapy-induced peripheral neuropathy. *J Neurol*. 2002;249(1):9–17.
102. Thompson SW, Davis LE, Kornfeld M, Hilgers RD, Standefer JC. Cisplatin neuropathy. Clinical, electrophysiologic, morphologic, and toxicologic studies. *Cancer*. 1984;54(7):1269–1275.
103. Titulaer MJ, Soffietti R, Dalmau J, et al. Screening for tumours in paraneoplastic syndromes: report of an EFNS task force. *Eur J Neurol*. 2011;18(1):19–e13.
104. Younes-Mhenni S, Janier MF, Cinotti L, et al. FDG-PET improves tumour detection in patients with paraneoplastic neurological syndromes. *Brain*. 2004;127(Pt 10):2331–2338.
105. Keime-Guibert F, Graus F, Broet P, et al. Clinical outcome of patients with anti-Hu-associated encephalomyelitis after treatment of the tumor. *Neurology*. 1999;53(8):1719–1723.
106. Antoine JC, Robert-Varvat F, Maisonobe T, et al. Identifying a therapeutic window in acute and subacute inflammatory sensory neuronopathies. *J Neurol Sci*. 2016;361:187–191.
107. Uchuya M, Graus F, Vega F, Rene R, Delattre JY. Intravenous immunoglobulin treatment in paraneoplastic neurological syndromes with antineuronal autoantibodies. *J Neurol Neurosurg Psychiatry*. 1996;60(4):388–392.
108. Berzero G, Karantoni E, Dehais C, et al. Early intravenous immunoglobulin treatment in paraneoplastic neurological syndromes with onconeural antibodies. *J Neurol Neurosurg Psychiatry*. 2018;89(7):789–792.
109. Graus F, Vega F, Delattre JY, et al. Plasmapheresis and antineoplastic treatment in CNS paraneoplastic syndromes with antineuronal autoantibodies. *Neurology*. 1992;42(3 Pt 1):536–540.
110. Stark E, Wurster U, Patzold U, Sailer M, Haas J. Immunological and clinical response to immunosuppressive treatment in paraneoplastic cerebellar degeneration. *Arch Neurol*. 1995;52(8):814–818.
111. Albert ML, Austin LM, Darnell RB. Detection and treatment of activated T cells in the cerebrospinal fluid of patients with paraneoplastic cerebellar degeneration. *Ann Neurol*. 2000;47(1):9–17.
112. Shams'ili S, de Beukelaar J, Gratama JW, et al. An uncontrolled trial of rituximab for antibody associated paraneoplastic neurological syndromes. *J Neurol*. 2006;253(1):16–20.
113. Keime-Guibert F, Graus F, Fleury A, et al. Treatment of paraneoplastic neurological syndromes with antineuronal antibodies (anti-Hu, anti-Yo) with a combination of immunoglobulins, cyclophosphamide, and methylprednisolone. *J Neurol Neurosurg Psychiatry*. 2000;68(4):479–482.
114. Vernino S, O'Neill BP, Marks RS, O'Fallon JR, Kimmel DW. Immunomodulatory treatment trial for paraneoplastic neurological disorders. *Neuro Oncol*. 2004;6(1):55–62.

115. Vedeler CA, Antoine JC, Giometto B, et al. Management of paraneoplastic neurological syndromes: report of an EFNS task force. *Eur J Neurol.* 2006;13(7):682–690.
116. Attal N, Cruccu G, Baron R, et al. EFNS guidelines on the pharmacological treatment of neuropathic pain: 2010 revision. *Eur J Neurol.* 2010;17(9):1113–e1188.
117. Skeie GO, Apostolski S, Evoli A, et al. Guidelines for treatment of autoimmune neuromuscular transmission disorders. *Eur J Neurol.* 2010;17(7):893–902.

Chapter 9

Cervical and lumbosacral radiculoplexus neuropathies

Pariwat Thaisetthawatkul[a], P. James B. Dyck[b]

[a]*Department of Neurological Sciences, University of Nebraska Medical Center, Omaha, NE, United States,* [b]*Department of Neurology, Mayo Clinic College of Medicine, Rochester, MN, United States*

Introduction

The nerve plexuses are proximal segments of peripheral nerves emerging from the foramina of the spine with interchanging and intertwining nerves from different spinal levels that then form individual nerves more distally. There are two major nerve plexuses: the brachial and lumbosacral plexus. The brachial plexus emerges from the cervical spine and the lumbosacral plexus emerges from the lumbosacral spine. Many disorders that can afflict peripheral nerves can affect the brachial and lumbosacral plexuses causing brachial and lumbosacral plexopathies, respectively. The diagnosis of plexopathies can be challenging and the clinical syndrome can be difficult to recognize because of the complexity of the anatomical arrangement of the nerve plexuses. This chapter outlines details of the anatomy and many neurological disorders that may involve the nerve plexuses as well as their diagnostic approaches and management. This chapter provides a comprehensive review of brachial and lumbosacral plexopathies but will focus mainly on immune-mediated or inflammatory causes, the cervical and lumbosacral radiculoplexus neuropathies.

Brachial plexopathy

Anatomy

The brachial plexus (BP) is derived from the lateral extension of C5-T1 nerve roots, with some contribution from C4 and T2 roots. BP consists of five main components from proximal to distal: roots, trunks, divisions, cords, and individual distal nerves. At the root levels, there are four branches: the nerves to the scalene and longus colli muscles (C5-8), the long thoracic nerve supplying the serratus anterior muscle (C5-7), a portion of the phrenic nerve supplying the diaphragm (C5), and a portion of the dorsal scapular nerve supplying the rhomboids and levator scapulae (C5). Sympathetic supply to

Dysimmune Neuropathies. https://doi.org/10.1016/B978-0-12-814572-2.00009-1

199

the head and neck branches out of the C8-T1 roots (white rami communicantes). The anterior rami of the C5 and C6 roots join and become the upper trunk. The C7 roots continues as the middle trunk. The C8 and T 1 join and become the lower trunk. These trunks emerge into the triangular area between the anterior and middle scalene muscles.[1] At the trunk level, there are two main branches: the suprascapular nerve supplying the supraspinatus and infraspinatus and the nerve to the subclavius. The trunks then give off the anterior and posterior divisions at the space between the clavicle and the first rib.[1] The divisions have no branches and provide nerve supply to two main different muscle groups in the upper extremity: the anterior division to the flexor muscle group and the posterior division to the extensor muscle group.[2] The anterior divisions of the upper and middle trunks form the lateral cord. The anterior division of the lower trunk continues as the medial cord. All the posterior divisions from the upper, middle, and lower trunks form the posterior cord. These cords are named according to their anatomical relationship to the axillary artery, which is adjacent to these cords in the axilla.[2] The lateral cord gives off the musculocutaneous and the lateral head of the median nerve. The medial cord gives off the ulnar and the medial head of the median nerve. The posterior cord gives off the radial and the axillary nerves.[3] BP may take one complete level cranially (fourth cervical root) and less contribution from the first thoracic root (prefixation) or one complete level caudally (second thoracic root) and less contribution from the fifth cervical root (postfixation).[3] The prevalence of prefixed BP varies from 10 to 65% and postfixed BP from 2% to 70%.[4]

Clinical features, pathogenesis, and management

Disorders of BP or brachial plexopathy can be divided into two major categories: disorders that affect BP regionally and diffusely.[5] Regional causes for brachial plexopathy are usually site-specific and often affect BP in a particular region. These can be divided into supraclavicular and infraclavicular brachial plexopathies.[5] Supraclavicular plexopathies affect predominantly the upper plexus including the upper trunk, but can also involve the lower trunk. Upper plexopathies are usually caused by traction from stretch injury, burner syndrome, rucksack paralysis, and postoperative brachial plexopathy.[5] Lower plexopathies are usually caused by thoracic outlet syndrome, postmedian sternotomy plexopathy, or Pancoast syndrome. Infraclavicular plexopathies usually affect the three cords and vary according to which cord is involved, such as plexopathy related to axillary lymph node irradiation, high radial nerve injury from using a crutch (crutch palsy), or axillary nerve injury from a fracture of the humerus. The diffuse involvement of BP is usually not specific for a particular region. This includes CRPN (neuralgic amyotrophy), hereditary neuralgic amyotrophy, radiation-induced brachial plexopathy, and neoplastic brachial plexopathy.

Site-specific brachial plexopathy

Stretch injury of the upper BP

A stretch injury of the upper trunk and roots occurs when the neck and shoulder are forced apart violently, when an adducted limb is pulled downward forcefully, or when a blow or weight depresses the shoulder. However, if forceful traction is applied to the upper limb, it is the lower trunk that is mostly at risk. The pathology of stretch injury varies according to the magnitude of force, the severity of the deformation, and the rapidity with which the trauma affects the deformation.[3] It includes neurapraxia, disruption in the nerve trunk, or, less commonly, root avulsion.[6] The most common cause is motorcycle accidents.[3,7] The other causes include industrial accidents, football, and other sports such as skiing or mountain/rock climbing.[8,9] The management of a BP stretch injury includes observation, particularly for neurapraxic lesions, or surgical intervention, usually performed about 3–4 months after injury with severe deficits if there is no recovery.[9] Surgery performed after 6 months is not recommended due to poor results.[9] The procedures include neurolysis, the placement of nerve grafts, or neurotization.[6,9] Root avulsion, the most severe form of stretch injury, responds poorly to any surgical intervention and is contraindicated for surgery.[10] In this category, pain management and occupational therapy remain vital.[9]

Burner syndrome

Burner or stinger syndrome is a syndrome resulting from injuries to either the upper cervical nerve roots or the upper trunk of BP.[11] It is commonly seen in contact sports, particularly football, causing forceful deviation of the head and posterior movement of the shoulder. It increases the distance between the head and the shoulder and causes traction injury.[11] The other sports that causes this syndrome include wrestling, rugby, basketball, boxing, and weight lifting.[9,11] An athlete experiences transient, short-lived paresthesia or burning pain shooting from the shoulder to the hand lasting only seconds or minutes. The athlete may shake the shoulder to relieve the symptoms.[11] Neck pain is usually not seen. Neurologic examination is usually normal but mild weakness or even muscle atrophy supplied by the C5-6 roots can be observed in a more severe case with repeated episodes. The anatomical localization for burner syndrome remains controversial. An electrodiagnostic study is usually normal but, in some cases, fibrillations can be seen in muscles supplied by C5 and C6 roots but not in paraspinal muscles.[12] Radiologic evidence of cervical disk disease or cervical foraminal narrowing could be seen in up to 90% of cases in one study, but the cause and effect may not be convincingly proved.[13] The management of burner syndrome is physical therapy to improve the range of motion and muscle strength. Tackling techniques should be reviewed and protective devices such as cervical collars, neck rolls, custom cervical orthosis, and shoulder pads should be used properly.[11]

Rucksack paralysis

Rucksack paralysis is reported to be caused by compression on the upper trunk by a backpack or rucksack that has shoulder straps that hold the weight on both shoulders. However, many of these cases are likely due to inflammatory brachial plexopathy that predominantly involves the upper trunk of BP. The symptoms consist of gradual onset of weakness and numbness without pain in the shoulder girdle muscles, particularly on the nondominant side but bilateral involvement is also possible. On examination, there is muscle weakness and atrophy in the deltoid, biceps, supra- and infraspinatus, and triceps muscles. This entity can be seen in both military[14] and nonmilitary persons, and even in children.[15] The risk factors include the weight of the rucksack (usually over 40 pounds), use in a difficult terrain, and duration of use. A previous injury to the bony structures in the shoulder such as a fracture of the clavicle can predispose a wearer to this condition.[14] Sufficient recovery of function is expected in most cases after the cessation of wear and physical/occupational therapy. A relapse of the symptoms may occur when the rucksack is used again, even with reduced weight.[14]

Postoperative brachial plexopathy

Brachial plexopathy can be seen in the postoperative period. Surgery, particularly under general anesthesia, can predispose a patient to have brachial plexopathy by stretching the brachial plexus from the malpositioning of the extremity on the operating table.[9] This will present in two different ways that likely have two different mechanisms: direct trauma, compression, or stretch to the nerve versus a delayed presentation that likely is inflammatory or immune-mediated. In the abrupt onset, the patient is unconscious and muscle relaxants are administered. The onset is usually immediate as soon as the patient wakes up from general anesthesia. The immediate onset distinguishes this type of postoperative brachial plexopathy from postoperative CRPN, where the onset is usually a few days after surgery. A patient experiences weakness and/or numbness in the shoulder, the fingers, or the medial part of the upper extremity, depending on what part of the brachial plexus is involved. Pain symptoms are usually mild or not present in contrast to CRPN, where pain is usually severe and persistent.[16] The surgery could be close to or at a distance from BP. The fact that the onset is delayed and spatially removed from where the surgery was performed led one of the authors (PJBD) to perform a study where nerves from the involved nerve distribution in such patients were biopsied and inflammatory infiltrates were found. The findings were suggestive of an inflammatory/immune mechanism of the neuropathy. Many of these patients were treated with immunotherapy and they usually improved. These findings led us to call this condition "postsurgical inflammatory neuropathy."[17] One type of surgery that is particularly associated with postoperative brachial plexopathy is median sternotomy for cardiac surgery or a transplant.[18] In this surgery, the sternum will be split open and each side is retracted laterally. This can result in the clavicle being pulled down and the first rib being pulled upward, injuring the medial cord between them.[19] The incidence of BP injury related to median sternotomy is about 0.5%–15% and BP injury has become the most common neurological complication after median sternotomy.[20–23] Brachial plexopathy associated with this surgery typically involves the medial cord, resulting in weakness and numbness in the muscles supplied by the C8-T1 roots.[24] Electrophysiological studies, however, show predominantly C8 rather than T1 involvement (i.e., more severe deficits in the ulnar motor and sensory nerves than the median motor or the medial antebrachial sensory nerves).[25] The prognosis is usually good with a median time to recover of 10 weeks; most patients have a full recovery.[24] Brachial plexopathy related to noncardiac surgery affects the upper and middle trunks more often.[24] The risk factors for this type of brachial plexopathy include use of the Trendelenburg position, abduction of the upper limb to > 90 degrees, restraint of the upper limb in an abduction, external rotation and extension position, and the lateral flexion and rotation of the head to the opposite side.[9] A patient usually experiences weakness and numbness over muscles supplied by the upper and middle trunks. This type of brachial plexopathy usually has a more prolonged recovery period and incomplete recovery.[24] Although compression and stretch injury likely account for many of these cases, many others are likely due to an inflammatory attack triggered by the stress of the surgery and are really examples of postsurgical inflammatory neuropathy.

Thoracic outlet syndrome

Thoracic outlet syndrome (TOS) particularly affects the lower trunk of the brachial plexus (C8 and T1 roots). Anatomically, the thoracic outlet is defined as the opening of the rib cage bound by the first rib, the first thoracic vertebral body, and the manubrium of the sternum. C8 and T1 roots join to become the lower trunk of the brachial plexus inside the thoracic cage, but the T1 root has to ascend and angulate superiorly as it joins the C8 root from below to clear itself from the firm posterior border of Sibson's fascia, which attaches the C7 transverse process to the first rib.[3] This anatomy subjects the T1 root and the lower trunk to stretch and pressure when there is anatomical variation in this region. The subclavian artery also follows the same course and is hooked over the first rib behind the anterior scalene muscle. The diameter of the subclavian artery is reduced when it crosses the muscle.[3] Anatomical variations in this small region therefore affect the neurovascular structures and cause the symptoms and signs of TOS. The symptoms of TOS consist of either vascular or neural symptoms or both. Neurological symptoms and signs that arise from the lesion affecting the neural structures are called true neurogenic TOS.[26] True neurogenic TOS results from stretching, angulation, or pressure on the lower trunk of the brachial plexus, causing motor and/or sensory symptoms. The most common cause of true neurogenic TOS is the fibrous brand that extends from the first rib to a

C7 cervical rib or the persistent rudimentary of the C7 transverse process.[27] The fibrous brand pushes the lower trunk from below and stretches and angulates the T1 more than the C8 component of the lower trunk,[26] causing neurologic injury. The other causes of TOS include hypertrophy of the anterior scalene muscle, the scalenus minimus wedging the lower trunk with the anterior scalene muscle, and the sharp-edged tendons of the anterior and middle scalene muscles that can angulate, rub, and traumatize the neurovascular structures.[3] Most cases of true neurogenic TOS are female.[26] Common clinical presentation is chronic wasting and weakness of the hand muscles, particularly the median-innervated intrinsic hand muscles associated with varying numbness in the distribution of C8-T1 roots causing difficulty with the hand grip.[27] The clinical features are those of predominantly T1 > C8 root injury (median-innervated hand muscles have a predominantly T1 supply). Atrophy and weakness in the ulnar-innervated hand muscles are much less common. The numbness is seen mostly along the forearm in the distribution of the medial antebrachial sensory nerve, which has mainly a T1 supply.[27] An electrodiagnostic study reveals chronic reinnervation and reduced amplitudes (axon loss) in the median-innervated hand muscle such as abductor pollicis brevis in > 90%, but less so in ulnar-innervated hand muscles.[27] Sensory responses from recordings at the medial antebrachial sensory nerve are abnormal to > 90% while the recording from the ulnar sensory nerve at the fifth digit (predominantly C8) was abnormal in about 70%.[27] Fibrillations are seen in only about 30% of the muscles affected due to the chronicity and the slowness of the pathological process.[27] A plain radiograph of the cervical spine can identify a cervical rib or other bony abnormalities, but a fibrous band is radiolucent and needs high-resolution MR neurography[28] or high-resolution ultrasound[29] to visualize it. It has been estimated that there are only about 1/5000 individuals with a cervical rib and true neurogenic TOS.[26] The presence of a cervical rib with nonspecific hand or upper extremity symptoms without confirmed electrodiagnostic abnormalities therefore does not establish the diagnosis of true neurogenic TOS. Associated vascular injury causing thrombus formation, effort-related claudication, aneurysm formation and poststenotic dilatation, digital ulceration, abrupt onset of limb ischemia, pallor, extremity coolness, the absence of distal radial pulsation, embolization to the vertebral or carotid artery, and tissue necrosis may be seen when the subclavian artery is involved in TOS.[30] Venous TOS is rare but seen more commonly in young men with symptoms in the dominant limb with prolonged, vigorous repetitive activities from sports or manual work causing constriction of the thoracic outlet (i.e., hyperabduction and extension of the upper extremity). The symptoms consist of acute swelling of the upper extremity associated with cyanosis and pain.[30] An evaluation for vascular structures when clinically indicated includes ultrasonographic studies, CT angiography, and conventional arteriography in the case of arterial involvement or venous ultrasonography and an MRI with MR venography in the case of venous involvement.[30] The management of true neurogenic TOS is a surgical resection of the band and/or other bony abnormalities.[26]

In most cases, the sensory symptoms of pain and paresthesia improve after surgery but motor symptoms (i.e., weakness and atrophy) do not improve significantly.[26] Arterial injury, if identified, requires prompt surgical intervention to restore distal circulation.[26] This include surgical decompression, repair of the aneurysm, and subclavian reconstruction (i.e., bypass graft). Venous thrombosis requires intravenous thrombolysis followed by decompressive surgery if residual thrombus remains, then followed by long-term anticoagulation.

Pancoast tumor

Pancoast syndrome describes the neurological symptoms and signs caused by a tumor, usually lung cancer, at the apex of the lung encasing the subclavian artery, infiltrating the pleura, the lower trunk of the brachial plexus, the stellate sympathetic ganglion, and the first or second rib.[31,32] The characteristic symptom is pain in the shoulder area, radiating up on the neck and head to the scapular area or to the medial aspect of the arm and forearm.[33–35] The pain could be misdiagnosed as a rotator cuff injury or arthritic condition. Horner's syndrome is variably present from 14% to 83%.[35] It can be associated with anhidrosis ipsilaterally and facial flushing and hyperhidrosis contralaterally.[35] Weakness and paresthesia in the ipsilateral arm and hand are frequently seen, predominantly in C8 and T1 distribution, causing hand weakness, atrophy, and sensory symptoms at the fourth and fifth digits. If the tumor extends into the intervertebral foramina and involves the vertebral body, a spinal cord compression may occur.[36] These symptoms usually come on slowly and progress over many months. Electrophysiological testing usually shows involvement of the median and ulnar motor studies and the ulnar sensory studies without involvement of the median sensory studies characteristic of the lesion at the lower trunk.[37] Needle EMG usually shows fibrillation potentials and neurogenic changes in the motor units in the C8 and T1 median and ulnar innervated muscles.[36] A chest x-ray shows apical cap thickening ($>5\,mm$), an apical mass, or bone destruction.[38] An MRI is superior to a CT scan as it not only clearly shows the mass at the apex but also the involvement of the brachial plexus, the subclavian artery, and the vertebral body.[38] The most common cause of Pancoast syndrome is nonsmall cell lung carcinoma (squamous cell carcinoma or adenocarcinoma) in about 70%.[39] Small cell carcinoma comprises a very small number of patients.[40] The other malignancies causing Pancoast syndrome include lymphoma, myeloma, and metastatic cancer from the thyroid gland or larynx.[35] Very rarely, benign conditions such as tuberculosis, fungal infection, pulmonary amyloidoma, or a hydatid cyst can cause Pancoast syndrome.[35,41] The most sensitive diagnostic tool for histopathology is percutaneous transthoracic needle biopsy, either by the posterior or cervical approach and guided by ultrasound or a CT scan.[42] This procedure can yield positive result in 95% of cases while fiberoptic bronchoscopy has about 30%–40% positive rates.[35] The treatment of a Pancoast tumor is currently neoadjuvant chemoradiation therapy followed by surgical resection.[43]

This is achieved by using cisplatin-based chemotherapy followed by R0 resection and a complete lobectomy with mediastinal lymph node resection.[43] The treatment approach could give 2-year survival and 5-year survival up to 90% and 50%, respectively.[43]

Site-nonspecific brachial plexopathy

Cervical radiculoplexus neuropathy (CRPN) or neuralgic amyotrophy

In 1948, Parsonage and Turner wrote in the Lancet on neuralgic amyotrophy, describing "the shoulder-girdle syndrome" among 136 patients.[44] The clinical picture consisted of the sudden onset of pain, arising in the shoulder and radiating to the outer side of the upper arm followed by flaccid paralysis of the muscles in the shoulder girdle and a patch of numbness over the outer side of the arm. They noted spontaneous recovery of the motor weakness in about 6 months in most cases.[44] It is now known that neuralgic amyotrophy can be caused by the diffuse involvement of BP, regions within BP, or multiple BP-derived nerves. It has also been called many other names, including brachial plexus neuropathy,[45] Parsonage Turner syndrome,[46] inflammatory brachial plexopathy,[47] or most recently, CRPN.[48] The clinical syndrome is well recognized and typically consists of the sudden onset of severe pain in 80%–90%.[45,46] The pain usually emerges in a few hours and often awakens the patient at night (60%).[46] Most patients describe typical neuropathic pain: sharp, stabbing, and throbbing pain, although deep aching, gnawing pain, or muscle soreness are less commonly reported and are elicited by movement or pressure on the affected limb.[45,46] These types of pain are often mistaken for orthopedic or musculoskeletal conditions.[45] Pain is usually localized to the shoulder but can also be felt in the interscapular area, trapezius ridge, upper arm, forearm or hand.[45] Hand dominance has no relationship with the side of the attack.[46] The duration of pain varies from several hours to a few weeks.[45] A smaller number of patients could have pain lasting longer than 2 months.[46] In the majority of patients, muscle weakness starts within the first 2 weeks, usually when the pain subsides.[46] The weakness is confined to the shoulder girdle in about half the patients and the remaining patients have weakness in either single or multiple individual nerves, including the median (anterior interosseous), radial (posterior interosseous), axillary, long thoracic, and suprascapular nerves[45] or the lower brachial plexus. In the case of phrenic nerve involvement, difficulty with breathing may develop due to unilateral diaphragmatic or bilateral diaphragmatic weakness, particularly when the patient is lying down.[49] Some studies suggest that multiple individual nerve involvement rather than involvement of the brachial plexus itself could be more common than previously appreciated.[50,51] However, in different cases, the syndrome can have variable involvement of nerves, plexus, and roots, making the term radiculoplexus neuropathy appropriate. The attack is unilateral in about 60% of cases while bilateral cases remain asymmetrical in the majority of cases.[45] The most common muscles affected are the spinati, deltoid, serratus anterior, and rhomboid muscles.[45,46] Mild to profound atrophy is commonly seen in up to 80% of cases.[45] Sensory symptoms are usually described as hypoesthesia or paresthesia. These are usually felt in the distribution of the nerves involved, most commonly seen at the lateral shoulder or upper arm.[46] The incidence of CRPN has been estimated to be about 1–3/100,000 per year and can be seen more commonly in males (male-to-female ratio=2:1) with a mean age of about 40.[52] CRPN has been rarely reported in children with similar clinical manifestation and male-to-female incidence ratio.[53] In a review of CRPN in children, there were two peaks of age at onset.[54] The younger peak (<8 weeks of age) was associated with osteomyelitis/septic arthritis of the humerus while among the older peak (between 9 and 12 years of age), more than half the cases were associated with a preceding upper respiratory tract or other viral infection.[54] In adult CRPN, on the contrary, only 25% have a history of upper respiratory tract infection[45] and another 25% have had a prior surgery, pregnancy and puerperium, vaccination, or trauma.[46] Overall, about 50% of adult CRPN patients report no preceding event. CRPN has been reported to occur in diabetic patients with a somewhat different presentation than in nondiabetic patients. In diabetics, there is more lower trunk brachial plexus and more bilateral limb involvement than in nondiabetic CRPN. Furthermore, in half the cases of diabetic CRPN, there was another body region involved (often lower limb or thoracic); this widespread involvement is uncommon for nondiabetic CRPN.[48] For these reasons, it seems reasonable to classify the diabetic CRPN, diabetic thoracic radiculopathies, and the diabetic LRPN together in one category of diabetic radiculoplexus neuropathy. Electrodiagnostic studies are the mainstay diagnostic workup for CRPN. The studies can confirm the presence of brachial plexus neuropathy or multiple individual nerve lesions, although it may be hard to differentiate between these if the findings are widespread. Sensory studies are important to identify the nerves and the level of the brachial plexus involved (reduced or absent sensory potentials mean the nerve damage is at or distal to the dorsal root ganglion). Motor studies assess the severity of motor nerve involvement, and needle electromyography delineates the extent of involvement of the process while also helping to localize the damage to the nerve, plexus, and root level or a combination.[55] Routine blood and CSF tests usually yield negative or nonspecific findings, but can be considered if there is suspicion of a specific cause of CRPN[52] such as hepatitis E, which has been reported in Europe and associated with bilateral asymmetrical CRPN.[56] A chest x-ray is not helpful in identifying lesions at the brachial plexus, but may help showing diaphragmatic paralysis with uni- or bilateral elevation of the hemidiaphragm in the case of phrenic nerve involvement. Advanced neuroimaging techniques such as magnetic resonance neurography (MRN) with a 3.0T scanner with fat and blood suppression in a two- or three-dimensional T2 W or TSE with Dixon reconstruction have been shown to give a clear delineation of the brachial plexus nerves.[57,58]

MRN of the brachial plexus has been shown to correlate well with electrodiagnostic test results and has an impact on clinical decision-making.[59] The abnormalities in MRN for CRPN include increased T2 signal intensity with fat suppression, focal or diffuse enlargement of the nerve trunks, enhancement of the nerves, and an elevated T2 signal in the muscles suggestive of denervation.[60] MRN also has an advantage of superior visualization of individual brachial plexus nerves in CRPN.[61] Ultrasound can be helpful in showing lesions in individual plexus nerves, including enlargement, focal constriction, torsion, and fascicular entwinement,[62] but its use has been limited.[52] The pathogenesis of CRPN has been shown in nondiabetic[47] and diabetic[48] CRPN to be due to an inflammatory attack and microvasculitis. Upper limb sensory nerve biopsies show findings of ischemic injury (axonal degeneration, multifocal fiber loss, focal perineurial thickening, injury neuromas), epineurial perivascular inflammation, hemosiderin deposits, and microvasculitis in the majority of CRPN patients biopsied.[48] CRPN treatment includes pain management, physical therapy, and rehabilitation.[52] Due to CRPN's pathogenesis of inflammatory/microvasculitis, some authors recommend administering corticosteroids either orally or intravenously for a varying period of time, if the patient is seen early after onset.[47,48] However, there has been no controlled study to prove its efficacy and it is unclear if corticosteroids change the natural course of CRPN. The prognosis of CRPN is that of spontaneous improvement and recovery even without immunotherapy, usually within the first month after the attack.[45] CRPN is usually not a progressive neurologic condition and about 60% recover in 1 year[45] and by 3 years, 90% have recovered.[52] However, in some cases, it could take up to 8 years to recover.[45] Unilateral cases do better than bilateral cases and upper plexus lesions do better than lower plexus lesions.[45] The recurrence of diabetic CRPN has been reported to be 21%[48] whereas the recurrence of typical CRPN was reported in a wide range from <5%[45] to about 26%.[46]

Hereditary neuralgic amyotrophy (HNA)

HNA is a hereditary form of neuralgic amyotrophy. The symptoms are similar to CRPN with acute onset of severe pain followed by weakness and/or atrophy in one or both arms, as described before. In HNA, the attack tends to recur: more than five attacks in 23% of cases and rare cases had up to 13 attacks.[46] The time between the first attack and recurrence varies but could be up to 6 years.[46] There are some differences between HNA and CRPN. First, the recurrence rate in HNA is much higher than CRPN (75% versus 26%).[46] Second, the age of onset in HNA is usually in the second or third decade while CRPN usually has the first attack in the fourth decade.[46] Third, HNA has more involvement of the nerves outside BP than CRPN.[46] Associated lumbosacral plexopathy could be seen in about 30% of cases of HNA (as in the case in diabetic CRPN). HNA has two clinical patterns: classic relapsing-remitting (acute onset of pain followed by motor weakness with full recovery) and chronic undulating (gradual onset of pain and weakness with pain symptoms persisting between attacks and incomplete recovery).[63] In the latter type, neurological deficits usually accumulate over time. There are craniofacial and cutaneous features that are frequently seen in the HNA phenotype. These include short interpapillary and intercanthal distance (ocular hypotelorism), cleft palate, pronounced skin folds around the neck and arms, and cutis verticis gyrate.[64] The attacks are often precipitated by pregnancy, immunization, preceding viral or bacterial infections, surgery, and vigorous use of the upper extremities.[65] HNA is an autosomal dominant disease that in some cases is caused by mutation in the SEPT9 gene on chromosome 17q25, which codes for the septin 9 protein[66] and is the only gene in which mutation is known to cause HNA.[65] In the United States, the frequency of SEPT9 mutation-related HNA has been reported to be about 85%, but less so in other countries.[65] The pathogenesis of attacks in at least some cases of HNA appears to be an inflammatory/immune-mediated process.[67] In those cases, upper limb sensory nerve biopsies showed prominent perivascular inflammatory infiltrates with vessel wall disruption and extensive axonal degeneration without tomaculous change.[67] Because of the possible pathogenesis of inflammation, the use of corticosteroids to abort the attacks has been suggested and, in some cases, seems to be effective.[65] The prophylactic use of corticosteroids to prevent HNA attacks during surgery or in the postpartum period has been shown to be effective.[68]

Radiation-induced brachial plexopathy (RIBP)

RIBP is a rare complication of radiotherapy (RT) that occurs in surviving cancer patients, particularly patients with breast cancer receiving RT to the axillary-supraclavicular lymph nodes.[69] The time of RT to onset of symptoms varies from several months to decades.[70] In some cases, the onset was 30 years after RT.[71] RIBP is a difficult diagnosis to make, as patients have had previous diagnoses of cancer. Separating recurrent cancer from radiation injury can be difficult and necessitates an extensive investigation of the brachial plexopathy that may include a biopsy. The risk factors of RIBP include the RT dose, duration, treatment technique, and concomitant use of chemotherapy.[71] Concomitant surgery, advanced age, obesity, diabetes mellitus, and alcohol consumption are also considered risk factors.[70] The symptoms consist of the gradual onset of paresthesia and dysesthesia, progressing to hypoesthesia and anesthesia eventually over many months. Motor weakness starts much later, then progresses slowly but relentlessly to atrophy and fasciculations in the upper limb.[69,70] Pain is usually mild to moderate and is less commonly seen[69,70] in contrast to neoplastic brachial plexopathy, in which the pain can be severe. Topographical involvement depends on the part of BP involved. Overlying atrophic skin changes can be observed as well as subcutaneous fibrosis of the axillary, lymphedema of the arm or supraclavicular regions, and osteonecrosis of the clavicle, all of which result from RT.[69,70] An electrodiagnostic study reveals reduced amplitudes in both motor and sensory studies, proximal conduction blocks in the motor studies, and often myokymic discharges and fasciculations in needle electro-myography.[72] Although myokymia usually does mean there is radiation injury, it does not exclude the possibility of recurrent cancer. We have seen cases in which the affected person suffers from both radiation and recurrent cancer. An MRI of the BP shows hypersignal intensity in T2 W images with gadolinium enhancement of BP.[73,74] A PET scan of BP can help in excluding neoplastic infiltration, which may show an intense hypermetabolic zone in BP.[70] However, in some less aggressive tumors, the PET scan may be negative. Consequently, in some difficult cases, a nerve biopsy from BP is required to diagnose the cause. The pathogenesis of RIBP is microvascular damage related to local chronic inflammation, the proliferation of fibroblasts and an extracellular matrix, leading to eventual dense fibrosis and the loss of parenchymal cells.[70] All these take several years to develop. RIBP is not reversible or curable and management is symptomatic, including pain management, physical therapy, managing or removal of comorbidities such as diabetes mellitus and alcohol use, and avoiding trauma in the area.[69,70]

Neoplastic brachial plexopathy

Apart from the Pancoast tumor mentioned above, neoplasm involving BP is usually a metastatic tumor from the lung or breast,[75] coming to the regional lymph node or by direct extension. The other tumors that metastasize to BP include primary head and neck neoplasm, melanoma, non-Hodgkin's lymphoma, Burkitt lymphoma, renal cell carcinoma, and testicular cancer.[76] Pain is the most common symptom, usually radicular in quality. It involves the medial arm and forearm, as the lower BP is most commonly involved (75%).[76] Pain is usually accompanied by muscle weakness and atrophy in the same distribution. Horner syndrome is observed in about 25%–50%[76] and could suggest an epidural tumor. The involvement could be patchy and diffuse. MRI is the imaging of choice for neoplasm in BP[75,76] showing T2 hyperintensity and enhancement. An FDG-PET can provide supporting evidence for the diagnosis by showing an intense focal uptake in the plexus nerves or in the regional lymph nodes.[75,76] The diagnosis can be confirmed by a biopsy of the involved plexus or other tissue that shows imaging abnormalities. The plexus biopsy procedure, however, can be considered only in some specialized centers that can perform such a procedure. Prognosis is usually poor with persistent pain and weakness. The treatment of neoplasm in BP is radiotherapy.[75,76]

Lumbosacral plexopathy

Anatomy

The lumbosacral plexus (LP) is derived from the anterior rami of the L1-S4 nerve roots. The LP consists of the upper (L1-L4) and the lower (L4-S4) plexus. Similar to BP, prefixed and postfixed LP can be seen. The LP supplies motor and sensory functions of the ipsilateral low limb and pelvis. The LP is located within the psoas muscles and emerges into the pelvis at the lateral edge of the muscle. The major nerves that branch off the upper LP include the iliohypogastric nerve (T12-L1), the ilioinguinal nerve (L1), the genitofemoral nerve (L1-L2), the lateral femoral cutaneous nerve (L2-L3), the femoral nerve (L2-L4), and the obturator nerve (L2-L4). The major nerves from the lower LP include the superior gluteal nerve (L4-S1), the inferior gluteal nerve (L5-S2), the sciatic nerve (L4-S3), the posterior femoral cutaneous nerve (S1-S3), and the pudendal nerve (S1-S4).

Clinical features, pathogenesis, and management

Lumbosacral plexopathy is caused by malignancy or mass, infection, trauma, radiation therapy for pelvic malignancy, hematoma, vascular lesion, and inflammation/microvasculitis (lumbosacral radiculoplexus neuropathy: LSRPN).[77] Unlike brachial plexopathy, lumbosacral plexopathy is often more diffuse, although many cases will present as predominantly upper lumbar plexopathies (L2-L4) whereas others will present as lower lumbosacral plexopathies (L5-S1). Frequently in lumbosacral plexopathies, there is involvement of the lumbosacral roots, plexus, and nerves altogether, hence the term LSRPN. The symptoms and clinical signs depend on the extent of involvement and the anatomical localization of the pathology.

Neoplastic lumbosacral plexopathy

Neoplasm is an important and common cause of nontraumatic lumbosacral plexopathy.[77] The LP can be invaded by cancers from adjacent pelvic organs such as the colon, cervix, ovaries, and urinary bladder due to its close proximity.[77] Metastasis from the lungs, breast, and lymphoma can also affect regional lymph nodes and the LP. An enlarged retroperitoneal lymph node from metastasis can also compress the LP. Some tumors such as prostrate,[78] bladder,[79] rectal, and cervical cancers[80] can spread perineurally to the LP. In these cases, the tumor cells grow within the perineurial lining of the nerves. Most cases of neoplastic lumbosacral plexopathy are unilateral, but bilateral cases are seen in 25%,[76] usually in a setting of more extensive metastasis.[77] Pain is the most common symptom in neoplastic lumbosacral plexopathy, usually located at the low back, buttock, thigh, or hip. The pain is exacerbated by lying down but relieved by getting up and walking. Patients who have malignant involvement in the iliopsoas muscle tend to flex their legs and hips to relieve the pain (malignant psoas syndrome).[81] Once the pain starts, motor weakness and sensory loss develop slowly over time. A rectal mass may indicate malignancy as a cause for lumbosacral plexopathy.[77] The diagnosis of malignancy of the LP may be suggested by an MRI of the pelvis.[76] To demonstrate the LP in the pelvic area, high-resolution 3T MR neurography often provides an excellent depiction.[82] FDG-PET imaging is helpful in demonstrating the intense uptake in the pelvic area.[75] The most definite way to confirm the diagnosis of malignant involvement is with a lumbosacral plexus nerve biopsy, but the lumbosacral plexus is a deep structure and often hard to approach surgically. Nonetheless, it may be justifiable when no other means for a diagnosis is available. The biopsy procedure, however, can be considered only in some specialized centers that can perform such a procedure. Neurolymphomatosis (peripheral nerve lymphoma) can present as a lumbosacral plexopathy. It is important to make this diagnosis as conventional chromotherapy des not cross the blood-nerve barrier and a high dose of methotrexate followed by autologous stem cell transplantation may be required.[83] The management of neoplastic lumbosacral plexopathy is similar to neoplastic brachial plexopathy and depends on the type of malignancy involved. Apart from malignancy, a benign tumor or other cause of the mass can involve the LP. Primary nerve sheath tumors such as neurofibromas and intraneural perineurioma[84] can affect the LP. Perineurioma often affects young people and presents with insidious focal motor weakness in a predominantly sciatic nerve distribution.[84] The symptoms are predominantly motor with mild sensory symptoms. It is slowly progressive, and surgical removal of the tumor does not help to improve the symptoms and should be avoided.[84] Amyloidoma is a rare mass lesion that can affect the LP, causing slowly progressive focal weakness and sensory symptoms; it may be seen without systemic amyloidosis.[85] It is associated with light chain but not hereditary amyloidosis.

Infection

Lumbosacral plexopathy caused by infection gives symptoms similar to neoplasm, but there are usually systemic symptoms such as fever, malaise, point of tenderness, weight loss, and night sweats.[77] Infection usually arises from the adjacent organs such as the gastrointestinal, urinary, and lumbar spine.[86] Tuberculosis can cause a local abscess in the psoas muscle affecting the LP (Pott disease).[87] A perirectal abscess can cause lumbosacral plexopathy in HIV patients.[88] Lumbosacral plexopathy in HIV patients may be caused by diffuse infiltrative lymphomatosis syndrome (DILS).[89] DILS is a hyperimmune reaction against HIV characterized by excessive proliferation of CD8 T cells and infiltration of CD8 T cell into organs. It can cause acute painful lumbosacral plexopathy.[89] This condition improves with antiretroviral therapy. In infection-induced lumbosacral plexopathy, neuroimaging studies may reveal findings suggestive of infection, such as local gas and abscess accumulation or the destruction of bone and intervertebral discs.[86] Diagnostic and therapeutic percutaneous drainage of the abscess can be considered under neuroimaging studies.[86]

Traumatic lumbosacral plexopathy

The LP suffers much less commonly from trauma compared to BP.[90] The reason is that the LP is located in a protective bony environment of the pelvic brim and in the retroperitoneal space with minimal mobility.[77] Traumatic lumbosacral plexopathy is usually seen with severe, high-velocity trauma to the pelvis and is usually associated with pelvic fracture.[90] A high-velocity trauma causing hip dislocation or hip fracture can also cause lumbosacral plexopathy, usually most severely involving the sciatic nerve, particularly in the peroneal division.[91] An open traumatic lumbosacral plexopathy can also be caused by a gunshot wound. The symptoms of traumatic lumbosacral plexopathy are usually pain, limited mobility due to trauma and swelling of the surrounding tissues, motor weakness, and sensory loss depending on the anatomical involvement of the LP. In traumatic lumbosacral plexopathy, the common peroneal nerve is most commonly involved, followed by the gluteal nerve, the tibial nerve, and the obturator nerve.[92] Trauma to adjacent organs in the pelvis, such as genitourinary, gastrointestinal, and vascular structures, is usually seen.[92] Another common traumatic lumbosacral plexopathy is seen in the postpartum period, particularly in a mother with a short stature and a large newborn.[93] This usually presents with a postpartum foot drop and is caused by compression on the LP by the head of the newborn at the pelvic brim.[93] Recovery is usually complete in months.

Radiation-induced lumbosacral plexopathy (RILP)

Similar to RIBP, RILP can be seen after radiotherapy to pelvic cancers such as cervical or ovarian cancer in women and prostrate or testicular cancer in men, and colon cancers in both genders.[77] Radiotherapy to the pelvic lymph nodes in Hodgkin's disease can also cause RILP. The pathogenesis of RILP is similar to RIBP, as discussed before. The symptoms of RILP are insidious and progressive, with mild pain or painless, motor weakness, and atrophy as well as sensory loss in the legs, unilaterally or asymmetrically bilaterally developing after radiotherapy for several months or years.[75] There can be symptoms related to damage from radiation to the local organs such as the urinary bladder, the rectum, or a vertebral compression fracture from radiation-induced osteonecrosis. Similar to RIBP, the risk factors of RILP are a large total radiation dose, a large dose per fraction, a radiation area including a large part of the nerve fibers, a hot-spot high dose, the concomitant use of chemotherapy, and underlying peripheral neuropathy.[69] Electrodiagnostic tests in RILP show myokymic discharges in about 60% of cases.[76] The presence of myokymia, however, cannot exclude the coexisting recurrence of cancer in the irradiated nerves. An MRI of the LP in RILP may show increased signal intensity in T2 W images but no enhancement in the nerves, in contrast to neoplastic lumbosacral plexopathy.[76] Similar to RIBP, the treatment is supportive and symptomatic.

Hematoma and vascular lesions in the pelvis

The LP can be compressed by hematoma or vascular lesions in the pelvis. A retroperitoneal hematoma in the psoas muscle can cause compartment syndrome, compressing the LP within its mass.[90] A retroperitoneal hematoma causing lumbosacral plexopathy can be caused by hemophilia, taking anticoagulants, hematologic malignancy, or trauma.[77] Several vascular lesions in the pelvis have been reported to cause lumbosacral plexopathy. These include an unruptured aneurysm of the common iliac artery,[94] occlusion of the lower aorta and common iliac artery causing ischemic bilateral lumbosacral plexopathy,[95] rupture of the common iliac artery aneurysm causing a hematoma compressing the LP,[96] ischemic injury causing lumbosacral plexopathy from intravascular stents or bypass grafts during aorto-iliac procedures,[97] and a hematoma from an internal iliac pseudoaneurysm caused by trauma compressing the LP.[98] A lumbosacral plexopathy caused by these vascular lesions and a hematoma share common symptoms of acute onset of local back or flank pain associated with motor weakness and sensory loss in the ipsilateral lower extremity.[77]

Lumbosacral radiculoplexus neuropathy (LRPN)

LRPN is probably the most common type of lumbosacral plexopathy and is caused by an inflammatory attack or microvasculitis affecting the plexus nerves, the lumbosacral nerve roots, and/or the individual nerves supplying the lower extremities, causing ischemic injury to the nerves as evidenced from nerve biopsies obtained from these patients.[77] The symptoms are typically acute or subacute onset of pain in the back, buttock, thigh, leg, or foot that usually begins focally and unilaterally. This is followed by weakness and sensory loss that also begins focally in the back, buttock, thigh, leg, or foot, but that evolve to become more widespread and bilateral. With time, it usually will become an asymmetrical disorder affecting the proximal and distal segments of the lower extremities bilaterally. There are several types of pain that include contact allodynia where a light touch (clothing or bedding) causes extreme pain; burning, sharp, stabbing, electrical pain; and severe deep, aching, and hurting pain. All these symptoms are often associated with weight loss that can be to a large extent. There are many subtypes for this entity, including diabetic LRPN, nondiabetic LRPN, postsurgical LRPN, painless diabetic LRPN, and some cases of intrapartum LRPN.[77] Diabetic LRPN has been called diabetic amyotrophy,[99] Bruns Garland syndrome,[100] diabetic polyradiculopathy,[101] proximal diabetic neuropathy,[102] and many other names with varying hypotheses on the cause. Diabetic LRPN usually occurs in type 2 diabetic patients who have good control of blood glucose and weight loss at the onset of their neuropathy.[103] Diabetic LRPN tends to occur sooner after the diagnosis of diabetes mellitus than diabetic polyneuropathy.[103] The onset of symptoms is usually characterized by severe pain (tightness, lancinating, burning, or skin hypersensitivity) starting in the thigh and then spreading to involve the entire lower extremity.[103] It can involve unilateral or bilateral but asymmetrical lower extremities. Soon after the onset of pain, patients develop motor weakness and sensory loss affecting the proximal and/or distal segments of the lower extremities, by which time the pain symptoms begin to subside. The motor weakness is usually severe and many patients are not able to walk by the time they see their physicians. Many of these cases actually end up in wheelchairs. In some cases, diabetic thoracic radiculopathy or diabetic cervical radiculoplexus neuropathy occurs concomitantly with diabetic LRPN.[103] Electrodiagnostic studies are helpful in confirming the involvement of the plexus, roots, and individual nerves.[77] The electrophysiologic definition for lumbosacral plexopathy is the involvement of muscles from at least two lumbosacral root levels and at least two peripheral nerves.[77] Nerve conduction studies usually show decreased amplitudes of the motor and sensory responses in an asymmetrical manner with normal or mildly reduced conduction velocities. Needle electromyography usually shows fibrillation potentials and neurogenic motor units in the muscles involved. Of note is that in LRPN, needle electromyography in the paraspinal muscles can be abnormal in contrast to pure lumbosacral plexopathy. In LRPN cases with typical symptoms and signs, a sensory nerve biopsy may not be needed for diagnostic purposes, but if performed, it usually shows evidence of inflammation and ischemic injury of the nerve (multifocal fiber loss, perineurial thickening, necrosis of the perineurium, injury neuroma, and neovascularization) (Fig. 1).[103] Multiple perivascular inflammatory infiltrates are commonly seen in association with hemosiderin deposits and disruption by the inflammatory cells of the wall of small arterioles, venules, and capillaries, suggesting microvasculitis (Fig. 2).[103] Axonal degeneration and increased empty nerve strands are the most common abnormalities in teased fiber preparation.[103] Diabetic LRPN is clearly distinguished from a more common diabetic sensorimotor polyneuropathy in that the latter occurs in a more insidious onset; has length-dependent and symmetrical involvement; is predominantly sensory without significant motor weakness; and it occurs late in the course of diabetes mellitus, usually in the setting of weight gain and poorly controlled blood glucose.[77] Another form of diabetic LRPN has also been described in a group of diabetic patients who have no pain and a slower and progressive symmetrical motor weakness over weeks to months with bilateral foot drop and proximal weakness in many cases.[104] Because of the insidious motor-predominant, painless, symmetrical, and proximal and distal distribution that these cases present with, some experts postulated that this syndrome represented diabetic chronic inflammatory demyelinating polyradiculoneuropathy (CIDP). In this group of patients, pathologic studies from a nerve biopsy show similar findings of inflammation, microvasculitis, and ischemic injury (and not inflammatory demyelination), suggesting that this painless, motor-predominant diabetic neuropathy is really a variant of diabetic LRPN and not diabetic CIDP.[104] Nondiabetic LRPN has similar symptoms, natural history, course, and pathological findings from a nerve biopsy to diabetic LRPN.[105,106] Nondiabetic LRPN causes acute and subacute pain, motor weakness, and sensory loss in the lower extremities bilaterally and asymmetrically or is unilaterally associated with weight loss in middle-aged nondiabetic patients.[106] Sensory nerve biopsies in nondiabetic LRPN cases have similar findings as diabetic LRPN cases,

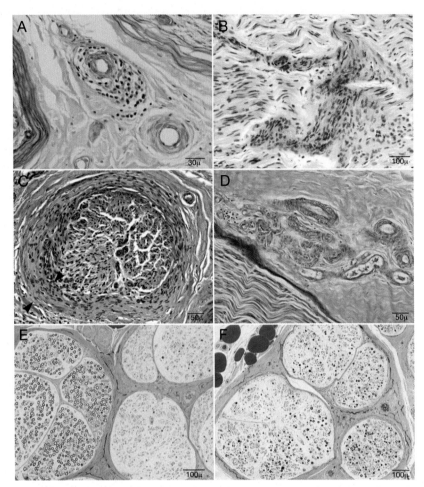

FIG. 1 Representative photomicrographs of sural nerve biopsies (A–D paraffin and E–F epoxy) of patients with LRPN in postsurgical inflammatory neuropathy. (A) Nerve cross-section stained with luxol fast blue and periodic acid-Schiff showing a small perivascular epineurial inflammatory collection. (B) Longitudinal section showing hemosiderin-laden macrophages (evidence of prior bleeding) in the perineurium (stained with Turnbull blue stain). (C) Cross-section of nerve fascicle showing thickening of the perineurium (between *arrowheads*) (stained with hematoxylin and eosin). (D) Longitudinal section showing neovascularization (LFB/PAS). (E) Epoxy cross-section showing multifocal fiber loss among fascicles (fascicles on right have few fibers) (methylene blue). (F) Epoxy cross-section showing intrafascicular multifocal fiber loss (methylene blue).*(From Rattananan W, Thaisetthawatkul P, Dyck PJ. Postsurgical inflammatory neuropathy: a report of five cases. J Neurol Sci. 2014;337(1–2):137–40.)*

showing inflammatory infiltrates and microvasculitis associated with ischemic nerve injury suggesting the same pathogenesis.[105] Nerve tissues from both diabetic and nondiabetic LRPN show upregulation of inflammatory mediators such as intercellular adhesion molecule-1, tumor necrosis factor-α, interleukin-6, and nuclear factor κB.[107] The natural history and outcome of LRPN is similar

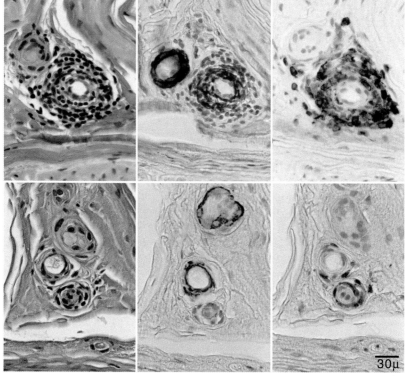

FIG. 2 Serial skip paraffin sections of a microvessel from the sural nerve of a patient with diabetic LRPN. The *upper row* shows the region of microvasculitis and the *lower row* shows the region distal to it. The sections in the *left column* are stained with hematoxylin-eosin, the sections in the *middle column* are reacted to antihuman smooth muscle actin, and the sections in the *right column* are reacted with leucocyte common antigen (CD45). The smooth muscle or the tunica media in the region of microvasculitis is separated by mononuclear cells. These changes of microvasculitis are seen in diabetic LRPN, nondiabetic LRPN, and postsurgical inflammatory neuropathy.*(From Dyck PJB. Radiculoplexus neuropathies: diabetic and nondiabetic varieties. In: Dyck PJ, Thomas PK, eds. Peripheral Neuropathy. 4th ed. Philadelphia: Elsevier Saunders; 2005:1993–2015.)*

between diabetic LRPN and nondiabetic LRPN in that in most cases, motor functions improve and pain subsides, even though the recovery is not complete and motor weakness remains the most troublesome long-term symptom in the majority of patients.[106] Uncommonly, a patient with LRPN has a complete recovery. Rare patients with nondiabetic LRPN may develop diabetes mellitus afterward, although most do not.[106] The management of LRPN remains symptomatic, focusing mainly on pain management, physical therapy, and the use of assistive devices.[108] The use of immunotherapy, particularly corticosteroids in nondiabetic LRPN, has been trialed in an open study with the rationale of inflammatory/microvasculitic pathogenesis from nerve biopsies; it showed significant improvement in pain and neurologic deficits.[109] However, a multicenter double-blind controlled study of intravenous methylprednisolone in diabetic

LRPN did not show significant improvement in the primary end point (time to improve in neuropathy impairment score by four points) compared to a placebo, but it did show improvement in neuropathic symptoms, especially pain and positive neuropathic symptoms in the group receiving methylprednisolone.[110]

Postsurgical inflammatory neuropathy

Lumbar plexopathy can occur in the postoperative period as a result of direct trauma to the LP from the surgical or anesthetic procedures or an inflammatory process causing LRPN, the so-called "postsurgical inflammatory neuropathy."[17] The notion of an inflammatory neuropathy occurring following a surgical procedure is not new, and has been recorded since 1968.[111] Postoperative LRPN occurs after hip surgery, intraabdominal surgery, dental procedures, cardiac bypass surgery, or minor procedures such as circumcision.[17] Postoperative LRPN after hip surgery can occur ipsilateral[112] or less commonly contralateral[17] to the surgical site; it can also have bilateral involvement. The symptoms and courses of postoperative LRPN are similar to the other forms of LRPN mentioned above. Postoperative LRPN differs from traumatic postoperative lumbosacral plexopathy in that the first entity tends to occur not immediately after surgery and continues to progress or worsen after the onset, whereas the latter usually has the onset of symptoms right after surgery with maximum deficits and continues to be stable or has improvement after the onset.[113] The recognition of these two clinical entities is very important as management is totally different. The pathogenesis of postsurgical inflammatory neuropathy causing LRPN is similar to the other forms of LRPN in that a nerve biopsy shows inflammation, microvasculitis, and ischemic nerve injury (Fig. 1).[17,112,113] Therefore, a sensory nerve biopsy is helpful in differentiating postsurgical inflammatory LRPN from traumatic postoperative lumbosacral plexopathy.

In conclusion, brachial and lumbosacral plexopathies are important causes of pain, weakness, and numbness, and they produce a great amount of suffering. There are many different underlying causes to plexopathies, some of which are treatable. Careful evaluation of these cases using clinical history and examination, laboratory and electrophysiological testing, imaging, and the judicious use of nerve biopsies is very helpful in sorting out the underlying causes and providing the best treatment for those affected.

References

1. Ferrante MA, Tsao BE. Brachial plexopathies. In: Katirji B, Kaminski HJ, Ruff RL, eds. *Neuromuscular Disorders in Clinical Practice*. New York: Springer; 2014:1029–1062.
2. Ferrante MA. Brachial plexopathies. *Continuum*. 2014;20:1323–1342.
3. Sunderland S. *Nerve and Nerve Injuries*. 2nd ed. New York: Churchill Livingstone; 1978.
4. Pellerin M, Kimball Z, Tubbs RS, et al. The prefixed and postfixed brachial plexus: a review with surgical implications. *Surg Radiol Anat*. 2010;32:251–260.

5. Ferrante MA. Brachial plexopathies: classification, causes, and consequences. *Muscle Nerve.* 2004;30:547–568.

6. Bertelli JA, Ghizoni MF, Soldado F. Patterns of brachial plexus stretch palsy in a prospective series of 565 surgically treated patients. *J Hand Surg Am.* 2017;42:443–446.

7. Dubuisson AS, Kline DG. Brachial plexus injury: a survey of 100 consecutive cases from a single service. *Neurosurgery.* 2002;51:673–682.

8. Daly CA, Payne SH, Seiler JG. Severe brachial plexus injuries in American football. *Orthopedics.* 2016;39:e1188–e1192.

9. Wilbourn A. Brachial plexus lesions. In: Dyck PJ, Thomas OK, eds. *Peripheral Neuropathy.* 4th ed. Philadelphia: Elsevier Saunders; 2005:1339–1373.

10. Dubuisson A, Kline DG. Indications for peripheral nerve and brachial plexus surgery. *Neurol Clin.* 1992;10:935–951.

11. Feinberg JH. Burners and stingers. *Phys Med Rehabil Clin N Am.* 2000;11:771–784.

12. Wilbourn AJ. Electrodiagnostic testing of neurologic injuries in athletes. *Clin Sports Med.* 1990;9:229–245.

13. Levitz CL, Reilly PJ, Torg JS. The pathomechanics of chronic, recurrent cervical nerve root neurapraxia. The chronic burner syndrome. *Am J Sports Med.* 1997;25:73–76.

14. Daube JR. Rucksack paralysis. *JAMA.* 1969;208:2447–2452.

15. Rothner AD, Wilbourn A, Mercer RD. Rucksack palsy. *Pediatrics.* 1975;56:822–824.

16. Eggers KA, Asai T. Postoperative brachial plexus neuropathy after total knee replacement under spinal anaesthesia. *Br J Anaesth.* 1995;75:642–644.

17. Staff NP, Engelstad J, Klein CJ, et al. Post-surgical inflammatory neuropathy. *Brain.* 2010;133:2866–2880.

18. Healey S, O'Neill B, Bilal H, Waterworth P. Does retraction of the sternum during median sternotomy result in brachial plexus injuries? *Interact Cardiovasc Thorac Surg.* 2013;17:151–157.

19. Seyfer AE, Grammer NY, Bogumill GP, Provost JM, Chandry U. Upper extremity neuropathies after cardiac surgery. *J Hand Surg Am.* 1985;10:16–19.

20. Morin JE, Long R, Elleker MG, Eisen AA, Wynands E, Ralphs-Thibodeau S. Upper extremity neuropathies following median sternotomy. *Ann Thorac Surg.* 1982;34:181–185.

21. Lederman RJ, Breuer AC, Hanson MR, et al. Peripheral nervous system complications of coronary artery bypass graft surgery. *Ann Neurol.* 1982;12:297–301.

22. Tomlinson DL, Hirsch IA, Kodali SV, Slogoff S. Protecting the brachial plexus during median sternotomy. *J Thorac Cardiovasc Surg.* 1987;94:297–301.

23. Vander Salm TJ, Cutler BS, Okike ON. Brachial plexus injury following median sternotomy. Part II. *J Thorac Cardiovasc Surg.* 1982;83:914–917.

24. Ben-David B, Stahl S. Prognosis of intraoperative brachial plexus injury: a review of 22 cases. *Br J Anaesth.* 1997;79:440–445.

25. Levin KH, Wilbourn AJ, Maggiano HJ. Cervical rib and median sternotomy-related brachial plexopathies: a reassessment. *Neurology.* 1998;50:1407–1413.

26. Ferrante MA, Ferrante ND. The thoracic outlet syndromes: Part 1. Overview of the thoracic outlet syndromes and review of true neurogenic thoracic outlet syndrome. *Muscle Nerve.* 2017;55:782–793.

27. Tsao BE, Ferrante MA, Wilbourn AJ, Shields RW. Electrodiagnostic features of true neurogenic thoracic outlet syndrome. *Muscle Nerve.* 2014;49:724–727.

28. Baumer P, Kele H, Kretschmer T, et al. Thoracic outlet syndrome in 3T MR neurography-fibrous bands causing discernible lesions of the lower brachial plexus. *Eur Radiol.* 2014;24:756–761.

29. Simon NG, Ralph JW, Chin C, Kliot M. Sonographic diagnosis of true neurogenic thoracic outlet syndrome. *Neurology.* 2013;81:1965.
30. Ferrante MA, Ferrante ND. The thoracic outlet syndromes: Part 2. The arterial, venous, neurovascular, and disputed thoracic outlet syndromes. *Muscle Nerve.* 2017;56:663–673.
31. Pancoast HK. Superior sulcus tumor. *JAMA.* 1932;99:1391–1396.
32. Pancoast HK. Importance of careful roentgen-ray investigations of apical chest tumors. *JAMA.* 1924;83:1407–1411.
33. Mayo P, Long GA, Tanedo P. Pancoast tumor; diagnosis and treatment. *J Lancet.* 1961;81:282–284.
34. Paulson DL. Carcinomas in the superior pulmonary sulcus. *J Thorac Cardiovasc Surg.* 1975;70:1095–1104.
35. Arcasoy SM, Jett JR. Superior pulmonary sulcus tumors and Pancoast's syndrome. *N Engl J Med.* 1997;337:1370–1376.
36. Gandhi S, Walsh GL, Komaki R, et al. A multidisciplinary surgical approach to superior sulcus tumors with vertebral invasion. *Ann Thorac Surg.* 1999;68:1778–1784.
37. Kishan AU, Syed S, Fiorito-Torres F, Thakore-James M. Shoulder pain and isolated brachial plexopathy. *BMJ Case Rep.* 2012;28:2012.
38. Takasugi JE, Rapoport S, Shaw C. Superior sulcus tumors: the role of imaging. *J Thorac Imaging.* 1989;4:41–48.
39. Solli P, Casiraghi M, Brambilla D, Maisonneuve P, Spaggiari L. Surgical treatment of superior sulcus tumors: a 15-year single-center experience. *Semin Thorac Cardiovasc Surg.* 2017;29:79–88.
40. Johnson DH, Hainsworth JD, Greco FA. Pancoast's syndrome and small cell lung cancer. *Chest.* 1982;82:602–606.
41. Rabiou S, Issoufou I, Belliraj L, et al. Pancoast syndrome revealing a hydatid cyst of the lung. *QJM.* 2016;109:337–338.
42. Walls WJ, Thornbury JR, Naylor B. Pulmonary needle aspiration biopsy in the diagnosis of Pancoast tumors. *Radiology.* 1974;111:99–102.
43. Kratz JR, Woodard G, Jablons DM. Management of lung cancer invading the superior sulcus. *Thorac Surg Clin.* 2017;27:149–157.
44. Parsonage MJ, Turner JW. Neuralgic amyotrophy; the shoulder-girdle syndrome. *Lancet.* 1948;1:973–978.
45. Tsairis P, Dyck PJ, Mulder DW. Natural history of brachial plexus neuropathy. Report on 99 patients. *Arch Neurol.* 1972;27:109–117.
46. van Alfen N, van Engelen BG. The clinical spectrum of neuralgic amyotrophy in 246 cases. *Brain.* 2006;129:438–450.
47. Suarez GA, Giannini C, Bosch EP, et al. Immune brachial plexus neuropathy: suggestive evidence for an inflammatory-immune pathogenesis. *Neurology.* 1996;46:559–561.
48. Massie R, Mauermann ML, Staff NP, et al. Diabetic cervical radiculoplexus neuropathy: a distinct syndrome expanding the spectrum of diabetic radiculoplexus neuropathies. *Brain.* 2012;135:3074–3088.
49. Garcia-Santibanez R, Zaidman CM, Russell T, Bucelli RC. Serial diaphragm ultrasound studies in neuralgic amyotrophy with bilateral phrenic neuropathies. *Muscle Nerve.* 2017;56:E168–E170.
50. England JD, Sumner AJ. Neuralgic amyotrophy: an increasingly diverse entity. *Muscle Nerve.* 1987;10:60–68.
51. Ferrante MA, Wilbourn AJ. Lesion distribution among 281 patients with sporadic neuralgic amyotrophy. *Muscle Nerve.* 2017;55:858–861.

52. van Eijk JJ, Groothuis JT, Van Alfen N. Neuralgic amyotrophy: an update on diagnosis, pathophysiology, and treatment. *Muscle Nerve.* 2016;53:337–350.
53. Al-Ghamdi F, Ghosh PS. Neuralgic amyotrophy in children. *Muscle Nerve.* 2018;57:932–936.
54. C1 H, Skov L. Idiopathic neuralgic amyotrophy in children. Case report, 4 year follow up and review of the literature. *Eur J Paediatr Neurol.* 2010;14:467–473.
55. Ferrante MA. Electrodiagnostic assessment of the brachial plexus. *Neurol Clin.* 2012;30: 551–580.
56. van Eijk JJJ, Dalton HR, Ripellino P, et al. Clinical phenotype and outcome of hepatitis E virus-associated neuralgic amyotrophy. *Neurology.* 2017;89:909–917.
57. Wang X, Harrison C, Mariappan YK, et al. MR Neurography of brachial plexus at 3.0 T with robust fat and blood suppression. *Radiology.* 2017;283:538–546.
58. Chhabra A, Madhuranthakam AJ, Andreisek G. Magnetic resonance neurography: current perspectives and literature review. *Eur Radiol.* 2018;28:698–707.
59. Fisher S, Wadhwa V, Manthuruthil C, Cheng J, Chhabra A. Clinical impact of magnetic resonance neurography in patients with brachial plexus neuropathies. *Br J Radiol.* 2016;89(1067):20160503.
60. Andreisek G, Chhabra A. MR neurography: pitfalls in imaging and interpretation. *Semin Musculoskelet Radiol.* 2015;19:94–102.
61. Sneag DB, Rancy SK, Wolfe SW, et al. Brachial plexitis or neuritis? MRI features of lesion distribution in Parsonage-Turner syndrome. *Muscle Nerve.* 2018;58(3):359–366. https://doi.org/10.1002/mus.26108.
62. Arányi Z, Csillik A, Dévay K, et al. Ultrasonographic identification of nerve pathology in neuralgic amyotrophy: enlargement, constriction, fascicular entwinement, and torsion. *Muscle Nerve.* 2015;52:503–511.
63. van Alfen N, van Engelen BG, Reinders JW, Kremer H, Gabreëls FJ. The natural history of hereditary neuralgic amyotrophy in the Dutch population: two distinct types? *Brain.* 2000;123:718–723.
64. Jeannet PY, Watts GD, Bird TD, Chance PF. Craniofacial and cutaneous findings expand the phenotype of hereditary neuralgic amyotrophy. *Neurology.* 2001;57:1963–1968.
65. van Alfen N, Hannibal MC, Chance PF, van Engelen BGM. Hereditary neuralgic amyotrophy. In: Adam MP, Ardinger HH, Pagon RA, Wallace SE, LJH B, Stephens K, Amemiya A, eds. *GeneReviews® [Internet].* Seattle, WA: University of Washington, Seattle; 1993-2018.
66. Kuhlenbäumer G, Hannibal MC, Nelis E, et al. Mutations in SEPT9 cause hereditary neuralgic amyotrophy. *Nat Genet.* 2005;37:1044–1046.
67. Klein CJ, Dyck PJ, Friedenberg SM, Burns TM, Windebank AJ, Dyck PJ. Inflammation and neuropathic attacks in hereditary brachial plexus neuropathy. *J Neurol Neurosurg Psychiatry.* 2002;73:45–50.
68. Klein CJ, Barbara DW, Sprung J, Dyck PJ, Weingarten TN. Surgical and postpartum hereditary brachial plexus attacks and prophylactic immunotherapy. *Muscle Nerve.* 2013;47:23–27.
69. Delanian S, Lefaix JL, Pradat PF. Radiation-induced neuropathy in cancer survivors. *Radiother Oncol.* 2012;105:273–282.
70. Pradat PF, Delanian S. Late radiation injury to peripheral nerves. *Handb Clin Neurol.* 2013;115:743–758.
71. Schierle C, Winograd JM. Radiation-induced brachial plexopathy: review. Complication without a cure. *J Reconstr Microsurg.* 2004;20:149–152.
72. Lederman RJ, Wilbourn AJ. Brachial plexopathy: recurrent cancer or radiation? *Neurology.* 1984;34:1331–1335.

73. Bowen BC, Verma A, Brandon AH, Fiedler JA. Radiation-induced brachial plexopathy: MR and clinical findings. *AJNR Am J Neuroradiol.* 1996;17:1932–1936.

74. Wouter van Es H, Engelen AM, Witkamp TD, Ramos LM, Feldberg MA. Radiation-induced brachial plexopathy: MR imaging. *Skeletal Radiol.* 1997;26:284–288.

75. Jaeckle KA. Neurologic manifestations of neoplastic and radiation-induced plexopathies. *Semin Neurol.* 2010;30:254–262.

76. Gwathmey KG. Plexus and peripheral nerve metastasis. *Handb Clin Neurol.* 2018;149:257–279.

77. Dyck PJ, Thaisetthawatkul P. Lumbosacral plexopathy. *Continuum (Minneap Minn).* 2014;20:1343–1358.

78. Ladha SS, Spinner RJ, Suarez GA, Amrami KK, Dyck PJ. Neoplastic lumbosacral radiculoplexopathy in prostate cancer by direct perineural spread: an unusual entity. *Muscle Nerve.* 2006;34:659–665.

79. Aghion DM, Capek S, Howe BM, et al. Perineural tumor spread of bladder cancer causing lumbosacral plexopathy: an anatomic explanation. *Acta Neurochir.* 2014;156:2331–2336.

80. Capek S, Howe BM, Amrami KK, Spinner RJ. Perineural spread of pelvic malignancies to the lumbosacral plexus and beyond: clinical and imaging patterns. *Neurosurg Focus.* 2015;39:E14.

81. Stevens MJ, Gonet YM. Malignant psoas syndrome: recognition of an oncologic entity. *Australas Radiol.* 1990;34:150–154.

82. Soldatos T, Andreisek G, Thawait GK, et al. High-resolution 3-T MR neurography of the lumbosacral plexus. *Radiographics.* 2013;33:967–987.

83. Ghobrial IM, Buadi F, Spinner RJ, et al. High-dose intravenous methotrexate followed by autologous stem cell transplantation as a potentially effective therapy for neurolymphomatosis. *Cancer.* 2004;100:2403–2407.

84. Mauermann ML, Amrami KK, Kuntz NL, et al. Longitudinal study of intraneural perineurioma – a benign, focal hypertrophic neuropathy of youth. *Brain.* 2009;132:2265–2276.

85. Ladha SS, Dyck PJ, Spinner RJ, et al. Isolated amyloidosis presenting with lumbosacral radiculoplexopathy: description of two cases and pathogenic review. *J Peripher Nerv Syst.* 2006;11:346–352.

86. Planner AC, Donaghy M, Moore NR. Causes of lumbosacral plexopathy. *Clin Radiol.* 2006;61:987–995.

87. Schaller MA, Wicke F, Foerch C, Weidauer S. Central nervous system tuberculosis: etiology, clinical manifestations and neuroradiological features. *Clin Neuroradiol.* 2018;29(1):3–18. https://doi.org/10.1007/s00062-018-0726-9.

88. Holtzman DM, Davis RE, Greco CM. Lumbosacral plexopathy secondary to perirectal abscess in a patient with HIV infection. *Neurology.* 1989;39:1400–1401.

89. Chahin N, Temesgen Z, Kurtin PJ, Spinner RJ, Dyck PJ. HIV lumbosacral radiculoplexus neuropathy mimicking lymphoma: diffuse infiltrative lymphocytosis syndrome (DILS) restricted to nerve? *Muscle Nerve.* 2010;41:276–282.

90. Wilbourn AJ. Plexopathies. *Neurol Clin.* 2007;25:139–171.

91. Cornwall R, Radomisli TE. Nerve injury in traumatic dislocation of the hip. *Clin Orthop Relat Res.* 2000;377:84–91.

92. Stoehr M. Traumatic and postoperative lesions of the lumbosacral plexus. *Arch Neurol.* 1978;35:757–760.

93. B1 K, Wilbourn AJ, Scarberry SL, Preston DC. Intrapartum maternal lumbosacral plexopathy. *Muscle Nerve.* 2002;26:340–347.

94. You JS, Park YS, Park S, Chung SP. Lumbosacral plexopathy due to common iliac artery aneurysm misdiagnosed as intervertebral disc herniation. *J Emerg Med.* 2011;40:388–390.

95. Chhetri SK, Lekwuwa G, Seriki D, Majeed T. Acute flaccid paraparesis secondary to bilateral ischaemic lumbosacral plexopathy. *QJM*. 2013;106:463–465.

96. Bushby N, Wickramasinghe SY, Wickramasinghe DN. Lumbosacral plexopathy due to a rupture of a common iliac artery aneurysm. *Emerg Med Australas*. 2010;22:351–353.

97. Abdellaoui A, West NJ, Tomlinson MA, Thomas MH, Browning N. Lower limb paralysis from ischaemic neuropathy of the lumbosacral plexus following aorto-iliac procedures. *Interact Cardiovasc Thorac Surg*. 2007;6:501–502.

98. Melikoglu MA, Kocabas H, Sezer I, Akdag A, Gilgil E, Butun B. Internal iliac artery pseudoaneurysm: an unusual cause of sciatica and lumbosacral plexopathy. *Am J Phys Med Rehabil*. 2008;87:681–683.

99. Garland H. Diabetic amyotrophy. *Br Med J*. 1955;2:1287–1290.

100. Chokroverty S, Reyes MG, Rubino FA. Bruns-Garland syndrome of diabetic amyotrophy. *Trans Am Neurol Assoc*. 1977;102:173–177.

101. Bastron JA, Thomas JE. Diabetic polyradiculopathy: clinical and electromyographic findings in 105 patients. *Mayo Clin Proc*. 1981;56:725–732.

102. Williams IR, Mayer RF. Subacute proximal diabetic neuropathy. *Neurology*. 1976;26:108–116.

103. Dyck PJ, Norell JE, Dyck PJ. Microvasculitis and ischemia in diabetic lumbosacral radiculoplexus neuropathy. *Neurology*. 1999;53:2113–2121.

104. Garces-Sanchez M, Laughlin RS, Dyck PJ, Engelstad JK, Norell JE, Dyck PJ. Painless diabetic motor neuropathy: a variant of diabetic lumbosacral radiculoplexus neuropathy? *Ann Neurol*. 2011;69:1043–1054.

105. Dyck PJ, Engelstad J, Norell J, Dyck PJ. Microvasculitis in nondiabetic lumbosacral radiculoplexus neuropathy (LSRPN): similarity to the diabetic variety (DLSRPN). *J Neuropathol Exp Neurol*. 2000;59:525–538.

106. Dyck PJ, Norell JE, Dyck PJ. Nondiabetic lumbosacral radiculoplexus neuropathy: natural history, outcome and comparison with the diabetic variety. *Brain*. 2001;124:1197–1207.

107. Kawamura N, Dyck PJ, Schmeichel AM, Engelstad JK, Low PA, Dyck PJ. Inflammatory mediators in diabetic and nondiabetic lumbosacral radiculoplexus neuropathy. *Acta Neuropathol*. 2008;115:231–239.

108. Thaisetthawatkul P, Dyck PJ. Treatment of diabetic and nondiabetic lumbosacral radiculoplexus neuropathy. *Curr Treat Options Neurol*. 2010;12:95–99.

109. Dyck PJ, Norell JE, Dyck PJ. Methylprednisolone may improve lumbosacral radiculoplexus neuropathy. *Can J Neurol Sci*. 2001;28:224–227.

110. Dyck PJB, O'Brien P, Bosch EP, et al. The multi-centre double-blind controlled trial of IV methylprednisolone in diabetic lumbosacral radiculoplexus neuropathy. *Neurology*. 2006;66(5, Suppl 2):A191.

111. Arnason BG, Asbury AK. Idiopathic polyneuritis after surgery. *Arch Neurol*. 1968;18:500–507.

112. Laughlin RS, Dyck PJ, Watson JC, et al. Ipsilateral inflammatory neuropathy after hip surgery. *Mayo Clin Proc*. 2014;89:454–461.

113. Rattananan W, Thaisetthawatkul P, Dyck PJ. Postsurgical inflammatory neuropathy: a report of five cases. *J Neurol Sci*. 2014;337:137–140.

Chapter 10

Dysimmune small fiber neuropathies

Anne Louise Oaklander

Department of Neurology, Massachusetts General Hospital, Harvard Medical School, Boston, MA, United States; Department of Pathology (Neuropathology), Massachusetts General Hospital, Boston, MA, United States

Introduction

Among the peripheral mixed motor, sensory, and autonomic axons (aka fibers), the "small fiber" category includes the very thin (~ 1 μm) unmyelinated autonomics and C-fibers, and the thinly myelinated A-delta fibers (~ 2–5 μm). These most common peripheral neurons innervate virtually every tissue and organ.[1] Their "sensory" axonal endings (neurites) not only signal pain and itch in response to danger, but also have important efferent, paracrine, and trophic functions, including regulating immunocytes, microvessels, and osteoclasts.[2] Exteroceptive small fibers monitor our environment for external dangers and send pain and itch signals centrally to trigger conscious and involuntary evasive maneuvers while interoceptive and trophic small fibers monitor our internal environment to maintain homeostasis and marshal responses to injury and illness. The brain's insula integrates these myriad inputs to maximize our survival by triggering profoundly salient conscious and unconscious responses to these threats.[3]

Given the need to transport macromolecules long distances along axons, it is no surprise that when oxygen, nutrients, or energy supplies become chronically insufficient, the distal ends of long axons begin to malfunction, firing excessively or spontaneously, even degenerating over time. Small fibers lack of myelin precludes the use of energy-conserving saltatory conduction and requires them to synthesize, deploy, and maintain channels and other membrane structures along their entire length, rather than just at internodes. They demand more maintenance than myelinated axons. Plus, because small fibers have only miniscule quantities of axoplasm and organelles, transport and resupply are precarious. Small fibers are thus the harbingers of any type of poor internal conditions, and even motor neuropathies can include small fiber neuropathy (bystander damage).[4]

Dysimmune Neuropathies. https://doi.org/10.1016/B978-0-12-814572-2.00010-8

Epidemiology

Prevalence figures for polyneuropathy do not include small-fiber polyneuropathy (SFN), the most common neuropathy presentation, because neither surface nerve conduction study (NCS) nor electromyography, the gold-standard diagnostic tests for large-fiber polyneuropathy, capture small-fiber signaling. The only population estimate for SFN—52.95/100,000 in the Netherlands—yields a global prevalence of 4,077,150.[5] But this is the minimum prevalence as case ascertainment required specialists' report of ≥ 2 prespecified symptoms plus confirmatory skin biopsies or thermal sensory thresholds plus normal nerve conduction. If < 25% of patients are currently diagnosed by these criteria, then the global prevalence exceeds 10 million. In addition, the requirement for normal NCS excludes all others who haven't had NCS, have abnormal NCS for independent reasons, or have mixed neuropathies such as in diabetes. Also, multiple independent reports identify SFN in approximately half of patients with the fibromyalgia symptom complex.[6-9] The microneurographic recordings from C-fibers showing excess and ectopic firing in both fibromyalgia and SFN patients further unite these conditions.[10,11] With metanalysis generating a 49% prevalence of SFN in fibromyalgia (95% CI: 38%–60%),[9] and fibromyalgia reportedly affecting 2%–5% globally,[12] SFN could conceivably affect > 100 million worldwide.

Pathophysiology

Given small fibers' myriad functions, it is no surprise that SFN typically presents with diverse and varying symptoms whose unifying cause often remains unrecognized.[13] Small fibers do not control skeletal muscle, so patients lack the visible weakness and muscle atrophy that make motor neuropathies easier to diagnose. Traditional descriptions of SFN emphasize sensory symptoms such as spontaneous and stimulus-evoked distal skin pain and sensory loss, but neuropathic itch is an underappreciated somatosensory symptom. The symptoms of denervation of tissue microvessels include deep aching pains, postexertional malaise, and prolonged fatigue.[14] Postural orthostatic tachycardia syndrome (POTS) and gastrointestinal and sweating complaints reflect damage to postganglionic unmyelinated autonomic small fibers.[15,16] Sexual or urinary symptoms are less common.[17] In three-fourths of patients, sensory SFN symptoms start in the feet and spread upward, but one-fourth of patients have patchy, proximal, or total-body pain from the onset if neuronal cell bodies (ganglionopathy) are targeted.[18,19] Unexplained chronic widespread pain, particularly the classical erythromelalgia phenotype of swollen, red, and burning feet characterized by neurologist S. Weir Mitchell in 1878,[20] reflects damaged small-fiber axons firing spontaneously and transmitting unprovoked pain signals centrally while releasing vasoactive substance P and CGRP in the skin to cause redness and swelling from microvessel dilation.[21]

Other SFN symptoms are caused by neuropathic microvasculopathy that leaves tissues unable to augment perfusion during peak demand. Pathology studies clearly demonstrate impaired sympathetic motor activity causing microvascular dysregulation. In one skin biopsy study, gaping arteriovenous shunts dumped arterial blood directly into venules, bypassing tissue capillaries and reducing oxygen exchange permitting premature hypoxia, anaerobic metabolism, and hypercapnia.[22] A study of perivascular innervation in skin and muscle biopsies found denervation of the capillaries supplying primarily proximal skeletal muscles (e.g., quadriceps). This likely explains the reduced capacity for exertion and deep aching pain (from premature anaerobic metabolism and lactic acidosis) many SFN patients report.[23] SFN patients with myovascular, but not skin, perivascular denervation more often had muscle discomfort and autonomic features.[23] In another study, 60% of a cohort of patients with unexplained muscle cramps and no neuropathic complaints had skin biopsy evidence of SFN.[24] Damaged intramuscular small fibers were posited to release inflammatory mediators that excited nearby neuromuscular twigs, causing peripheral sensitization.[24]

Neurogenic vasodilation leaving blood pooled in dilated veins can also lower cardiac return (preload failure), causing orthostatic hypotension and tachycardia, further hindering the peripheral exchange of gases and nutrients. Gastrointestinal consequences are perhaps more common although less often recognized. Upper GI symptoms include nausea/vomiting from stomach dysmotility. Lower GI symptoms; constipation, diarrhea, or both (irritable bowel) appear to reflect not only misfiring and distal degeneration of enteric small fibers but dysregulation of enteric circulation that precludes normal postprandial augmentation (gastrointestinal angina).[25] Vasodysregulation in the skin causes color and temperature fluctuations and likely contributes to sensory dysfunction, rashes, and reduced hair growth and sweating. A tempting hypothesis ripe for study is that impaired cranial sympathomotor innervation contributes to the prevalent and documented cognitive dysfunction (brain fog) in SFN and fibromyalgia.[26,27] Small fibers also affect the brain directly through central synapses in the spinal cord and brain stem (central-peripheral distal axonopathy).[28] C- and A small-fiber nociceptors control the long-term potentiation-like pain amplification that can secondarily change in SFN (central sensitization). The brain effects of SFN can also be worsened by inactivity, deconditioning, depression, and medications.[26,27,29]

Clinical diagnosis

With muscle bulk, strength, and reflexes typically normal, a standard neurological examination can miss SFN, and neither surface nerve conduction study (NCS) nor electromyography, which capture large-fiber signaling, detect it. Neuropathic pain, reflecting spontaneous small-fiber firing, typically precedes the sensory loss caused by axonal degeneration, so the sensory exam can remain normal or near-normal in mild or early SFN. Recognizing SFN is straightforward when patients mention classical painful foot symptoms and they have known causes such as diabetes or chemotherapy toxicity. However, the majority of SFN patients with "initially idiopathic SFN" (iiSFN) currently remain undiagnosed for reasons including failure to conform to physician-derived textbook descriptions of symptoms and undiscovered medical causes of SFN.

Medical care and research have been throttled by the lack of a consensus case definition for SFN. Publication is anticipated in 2020 of the first consensus case definition and diagnostic criteria for research on painful iiSFN, generated by an NIH, FDA, and pharmaceutical company sponsored CONCEPPT/ ACTTION committee meeting of neuropathy experts. The new case definition will require specific pain symptoms (spontaneous or constant pain, allodynia, a nonpainful sensory symptom) plus one among the following signs: abnormal sensory perception (i.e., pinprick, light touch, vibration or position sense, allodynia, or hyperalgesia), plus objective confirmation.[30] Research case definitions prioritize specificity over sensitivity, so failure to meet the criteria does not preclude SFN, and should not justify withholding treatment or reimbursement. The impression of expert clinicians must remain the clinical diagnostic standard. The CONCEPPT criteria require skin biopsy confirmation for a "definite" research diagnosis, and biopsy confirmation is recommended before disease-modifying, costly, or risky treatments such as immunotherapies.[30]

Although there are standardized patient-reported symptom surveys for single-cause mixed neuropathies from diabetes,[31–33] sarcoidosis,[34] and specific chemotherapies,[35] and validated general questionnaires for pain and dysautonomia,[36,37] there are few comprehensive SFN-specific surveys designed to capture signs and symptoms in patients with SFN from any cause (iiSFN). For symptoms, I am aware of only the SFN-specific Rasch-built overall disability scale (SFN-RODS) and the Massachusetts General Small-Fiber Symptom Survey (SSS) as validated for SFN from all medical causes.[7,17,38] Regarding SFN exam findings, the Utah Early Neuropathy Scale was developed and validated for sensory-predominant diabetic polyneuropathy,[39] and insofar as I know only the Massachusetts General Neuropathy Exam Tool (MAGNET) is validated for SFN independent of cause.[40] Cerebrospinal fluid does not show cells or inflammatory markers in most cases, given the extradural location of the sensory and autonomic ganglia,[15] thus we no longer perform lumbar puncture.

Objective diagnostic testing

With SFN symptoms so nonspecific and exam findings often subtle or subjective, biomarker confirmation of SFN is recommended to establish the diagnosis for the estimated half of patients with iiSFN.[41,42] The shift from reliance on textbook descriptions for diagnosis (pattern recognition/circular reasoning) to unbiased biomarker confirmation can be challenging, as long-held assumptions are questioned. However, biomarker confirmation is illuminating previously unappreciated presentations and causes, including potential immune contributions. Plus, it provides a framework for medical decision-making, particularly when this involves expensive or risky treatment of uncertain efficacy, including immunotherapies. As neither surface NCS nor electromyography query small fibers, and they are invisible with conventional light microscopy, pathology remains the cornerstone of SFN confirmation.

Until recently, a sensory nerve biopsy for electron microscopy analysis was required to visualize small fibers. However, these are expensive and invasive, leaving scars, sensory deficits, and sometimes neuralgia, and they are not repeatable for tracking.[43] Hence, they have been largely replaced by minimally invasive lower-leg skin biopsies. These 2–3 mm biopsies, removed from 10 cm above the lateral malleolus, have an excellent safety profile and are more sensitive than a sural-nerve biopsy.[44] They can be removed in virtually all medical settings, then mailed in fixative to reference labs for sectioning. PGP9.5 free-floating immunohistochemical labeling then enlarges all axons coursing through the tissues to make them countable with light microscopy (Fig. 1).[45,46] They are safe enough to perform in children as well as for research and can be repeated for monitoring. The interpretation of normality is made by statistically comparing each biopsy's measured epidermal neurite density (END) to densities in a large dataset of biopsies from screened healthy volunteers.[46–49] Biopsies are considered diagnostic for SFN when the measured END is ≤ the 5th centile of the lab's predicted normal distribution for similar patients. Current limitations include the lack of standards for performance, processing, analysis, and interpretation of skin biopsies, with methods, norms, and interpretations varying considerably between labs (low inter-rater reliability). Some labs use nonrepresentative or published norms, leading to inaccurate interpretations, particularly for teens, children, or nonwhite ethnic and racial groups (Fig. 1).[47,50,51] Skin biopsies are the best test for children and applying local-anesthetic cream before intradermal lidocaine renders them painless. Age-matched norms and statistical modeling are essential for reducing the very high rates of false negative interpretations with adult norms because children have 3–4 times more epidermal neurites that are pruned during adolescence.[52] Massachusetts General has analyzed biopsies from 76 children under 21 years old, perhaps the largest pediatric normative dataset globally. Other limitations include sampling error and the fact that axons typically degenerate later than symptoms appear. Second biopsies, for example, from the thigh for nonlength-dependent neuropathies[50,53–55] or the foot,[56] add sensitivity but also cost, and there are insufficient norms for routine use. Immunofluorescent labeling visualizes twice as many fibers as bright-field microscopy, thus requiring separate, less-available norms.[57]

Among the secondary objective tests, quantitative autonomic function testing (AFT) as developed at Mayo Clinic is the best developed and most widely accepted. It includes four site comparisons of quantitative sudomotor axon reflex text (QSART) sweating to predicted norms[48] raising sensitivity to 82%, similar to a skin biopsy.[58–60] However, as few hospitals have the equipment and

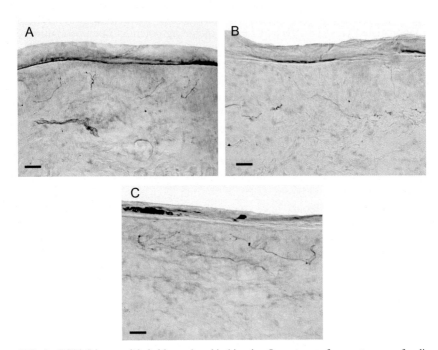

FIG. 1 PGP9.5-immunolabeled lower-leg skin biopsies: Importance of accurate norms for diagnostic interpretation. This bright-field photomicrograph illustrates standard clinical processing and morphometric evaluations used most often for clinical diagnostic confirmation of small-fiber neuropathy, and the importance of accurate norms for diagnostic interpretation. Skin biopsies are from 10 cm above the lateral malleolus in adults, or proportionally less in children. Skilled morphometrists count the number of neurites that penetrate the dermal-epidermal junction and express epidermal neurite density/mm^2 skin surface area. Each patient's END is statistically compared to the predicted normal distribution calculated from within-laboratory measurements from biopsies of screened healthy controls. Patient END ≤5th centile of predicted pathologically confirms clinical diagnoses, and predegenerative swellings, fragmentation, or inflammatory infiltrates (not shown) can be supportive. 40×. Scale bar = 100 μm. (A) Screened normal healthy control 16-year-old Caucasian male. His END (356/mm^2 skin surface area) is at the 58.0% of the age, sex, and race-matched predicted normal distribution. (B) 15.1-year-old Caucasian male patient with gastrointestinal symptoms, headache, fatigue, labile blood pressure, and POTS starting at age 3. His END of 164/mm^2 skin surface area is at the 1.3 centile of age, sex, and race-matched predicted norm, confirming the clinical diagnosis of SFN. AFT results were also abnormal, ANA was positive at 1:160, and a paraneoplastic panel identified autoantibodies against voltage-gated potassium channel. (C) Screened normal healthy Caucasian female aged 66.3 years. Her END, while only 158 epidermal/neurites/mm^2 skin surface area, is at the 37.6th centile well within the normal range although far lower than the diagnostic END in panel B. *(Reproduced with permission from Oaklander AL, Nolano M. Scientific advances in and clinical approaches to small-fiber polyneuropathy: a review. JAMA Neurol 2019;76(10):1240–51.)*

patients must stop potentially interfering medications beforehand and travel to the lab, AFT is still not regularly used or validated for trials.[48] Newer measures of sweating are insufficiently validated for routine clinical use, but the Dynamic Sweat Test assesses sweat gland density, distribution, and stimulated sweat production.[61,62] In vivo corneal confocal microscopy, which visualizes the exclusively C-fiber innervation of the cornea, is noninvasive, repeatable, and requires no preparation, but it is also not widely accessible nor sufficiently characterized for routine use.[63] Quantitative sensory testing records only patients' subjective sensations and is not an objective diagnostic test.[64]

Medical causes and contributors

Neuropathy is a cumulative result of peripheral neurons having insufficient resources to maintain their most distal regions. If the poor conditions resolve on their own, patients will note only subclinical, mild, or transient symptoms and will recover without treatment, but prolonged or serious cases require sleuthing to identify causes and alleviation of the specific impediments to neuronal health. Therefore, when SFN is suspected or confirmed, patients should be screened for potential contributors by medical history, exam, and high-value blood tests (Table 1).[13] This identifies suspects in 30%–50% of iiSFN patients.[41,42,65] Diabetes mellitus is overall the most common cause of neuropathy, but the importance of undiagnosed diabetes in iiSFN is debated. It is very rare

TABLE 1 Other medical causes to exclude in patients suspected of isolated dysimmune SFN.

Metabolic/endocrine	Diabetes, hyperthyroidism/hypothyroidism, vitamin B6 toxicity
Temporally appropriate neurotoxic exposures	Cancer chemotherapy (vinca, taxanes, platinum compounds, thalidomide, bortezomib, epothilones), antiretroviral HIV drugs, colchicine, vitamin B6, metronidazole, nitrofurantoin, fluoroquinolones, arsenic
Infectious	HIV, hepatitis B and C, leprosy
Genetic disorders	Charcot-Marie-Tooth, TTR amyloidosis, Fabry, HSAN, ion channelopathies
Hematologic	Waldenström's macroglobulinemia, multiple myeloma, monoclonal gammopathy (MGUS)
Systemic immune conditions	Sjögren's syndrome, systemic lupus erythematosus celiac, psoriatic arthritis, vasculitis
Systemic neurodegenerative conditions	Parkinson's, ALS, multisystem atrophy

in my clinic, below the US population prevalence,[41] but I test all adult iiSFN patients for it, usually with hemoglobin A1c measurement, which is inexpensive and universally available. Prediabetes conveys far less risk and I have never found it as the exclusive cause of SFN.[41,66] Nonetheless, I screen for and recommend treatment because I mitigate all conditions potentially deleterious for small fibers, including smoking, obesity, sleep apnea, and lack of aerobic exercise.[67–69] A list of evidence-based screening tests for potential contributors to SFN is available on Massachusetts General's website.[41] Regarding nutritional risks, screening for folate and vitamin B12 deficiencies is not cost-effective in countries with good nutrition and mandated supplementation. Plus, low folate causes large- rather than small-fiber sensory axonopathy.[41,65,41,65] High vitamin B_6 levels, usually from unsupervised supplementation, are a rare risk for SFN.[71]

Large-sample screening supports the hypothesis that disturbed immunity is a common contributor to iiSFN, with evaluations of children, who hardly ever have diabetes, HIV, cancer, or neurotoxic exposures, particularly illuminating. In the largest series, of 41 patients with unexplained widespread pain beginning before age 21, 76% had definite or probable early onset SFN (eoSFN) based on biomarker testing.[15] Comprehensive evaluations revealed neither familial, diabetic, nor toxic causes, but 89% had blood-test markers of dysimmunity (erythrocyte sedimentation rate, antinuclear antibody titer $\geq 1:80$, or low levels of complement components C3 or C4) and 33% had other-organ autoimmune illnesses.[15] Furthermore, immunotherapy with corticosteroids and/or intravenous immune globulins (IVIg) benefited 80% of those treated.[15] Because children and young adults are at the greatest risk of derailment yet have the greatest potential for recovery,[15,72] suspected diagnoses of eoSFN require urgent confirmation and definitive treatment. Immunotherapy should at least be considered in most cases. And all patients with nonlength-dependent iiSFN must have immune causality considered as well. Not only is immunotherapy potentially effective, but these patients may require additional treatment for conditions such as Sjogren's or paraneoplastic syndromes as iiSFN is often the initial symptom and neuromuscular evaluation brings these to light.

Links with other dysimmune conditions

Epidemiological associations with several B-cell mediated systemic immune disorders further link iiSFN to dysimmunity. This is best established for the one-fourth of SFN cases that present with nonlength-dependent or patchy presentations. This presentation suggests attack directed at the neuronal cell bodies themselves (neuronitis/ganglionitis). Many of these patients also have length-dependent symptoms, whether from attack on epitopes coexpressed along axons or because the besieged soma become unable to maintain their distal regions. Sensory cell bodies are particularly vulnerable because their ganglia migrate out from meningeal protection in utero and they develop fenestrated capillaries to survey for internal threats.[73] In ganglionitis, cerebrospinal fluid (CSF) can reveal inflammatory markers, and a ganglion biopsy can contain mononuclear infiltrates and nodules of Nageotte that mark cell-body inflammation and degeneration.[74] Sensory neuronitis often includes large-fiber neurons, also causing ataxia and reduced proprioception, hyporeflexia, and abnormal NCS or somatosensory evoked potentials.[75]

The most common and best-characterized cause of immune-mediated iiSFN is primary Sjogren's syndrome (pSS). Large screening studies of iiSFN identify varying prevalences of SS antibodies in different settings. The lowest reports of 1%–2%[42,65] are not clearly elevated, whereas my lab's report of 9.2% far exceeds population prevalence.[41] However, the actual association is even stronger, and rheumatologists report that up to 25% of pSS patients present with sensory-predominant neuropathy.[76] Although sensorimotor SS-neuropathy is marked by a high prevalence of SS autoantibodies, they are less detectable in nonataxic sensory SS-neuropathy, and 60% of SS-associated SFN is seronegative.[77,78] Perhaps this is partly because iiSFN is often an initial feature of SS. Thus, the possibility of undiagnosed SS must always be considered in iiSFN, even when patients do not have established diagnoses, and all patients should be monitored for dry eyes and dry mouth periodically, even if not present at onset. A lip biopsy to evaluate salivary gland inflammation is often the next step for iiSFN patients with Sjögren's symptoms but normal serologies. The importance of diagnosing pSS when present is that it permits comanagement with rheumatologists and ophthalmologists. In the first prospective trial of patients with SS-associated SFN, 6 months of IVIg (2 g/kg/4 weeks) was effective for improving pain and general health.[79] Other patients are managed with hydroxychloroquine, methotrexate, or rituximab.

Other systemic dysimmune conditions associated with iiSFN include celiac, lupus, and psoriatic arthritis.[41,42] Sarcoidosis is also associated with SFN. Although SFN is prevalent in sarcoidosis referral centers,[80–84] sarcoidosis is exceedingly rare in most settings, so we do not routinely screen for it, particularly given that angiotensin-converting enzyme (ACE) levels have 0% positive predictive value.[41] In a series of 115 sarcoidosis patients from Cleveland Clinic, the most common presentation was painful nonlength-dependent polyneuropathy developing in Caucasian females within 3 years of systemic sarcoidosis diagnosis. IVIg was often effective for their neuropathy and nearly two-thirds responded well to anti-TNFα treatment alone or with IVIg.[80]

A substantial proportion of patients with iiSFN and no rheumatological diagnoses still have evidence of predominantly B-cell immune dysregulation. Thirty-three percent among our 41-patient eoSFN series also had autoimmune thyroiditis, Henoch-Schönlein purpura, brachial plexitis, type 1 diabetes, postviral arthritis, immune thrombocytopenic purpura, Crohn's disease, autoimmune trochleitis, and/or Hashimoto's encephalopathy.[15] My lab has also linked SFN to other B-cell disorders, including monoclonal gammopathy (MGUS)[85] and selective immunoglobulin deficiencies. In our series of 55 IVIg-treated patients, 28% had IgG deficiency, 18% had IgG subclass deficiency, 14% had IgM deficiency, and 11% had IgA deficiency.[72]

Small-fiber-restricted dysimmunity

In 2007, I proposed that some SFN illnesses are caused by small-fiber-restricted dysimmunity and inflammation. I reported one of the first cases of an acute monophasic illness conceptually akin to GBS,[86] then I and others published many cases of apparently immune small-fiber restricted chronic courses akin to CIDP.[86] The concept of small-fiber restricted dysimmunity seemed eminently plausible given the well-documented immune-mediated neuropathies and links to systemic autoimmune disorders, plus the indirect evidence of B-cell dysregulation in many of the iiSFN patients without systemic immune diagnoses. Although the evidence is preliminary when compared to the century of data on large-fiber inflammatory neuropathy, it is summarized below.

Three types of clinical presentations of length-dependent apparently dysimmune SFN are documented so far. I and many others have reported acute severe monophasic cases.[86] These patients are often hospitalized, but for every one diagnosed and treated with immunotherapy, far more are managed undiagnosed by internists and pediatricians. Indications for hospitalization include crises of chronic pain and erythromelalgia,[86] nausea, vomiting and cachexia requiring enteral or parenteral nutrition, severe colonic dysmotility, or neurogenic syncope from POTS and resulting injuries. Reports of acute illnesses within a few weeks of infections or vaccinations, for example to the human papillomavirus vaccination,[87] suggest that molecular mimicry can be a trigger as in Campylobacter-associated acute motor axonal neuropathy (AMAN).[88] As with AMAN, most of my acute fulminant patients are children and young adults who have robust immune responsivity. Acute-onset SFN is unreported in infants and toddlers, whose immunocompetence is not yet fully established.

Less fulminant presentations of apparently immune iiSFN are far more common, but case ascertainment is poor. To facilitate diagnosis, outcome tracking, and research, my group developed, validated, and continues to improve forms to measure SFN symptoms and signs.[17,40] These permitted us to define a relapsing-remitting course by tracking a biopsy-confirmed young woman with three well-documented, stereotyped episodes of distal erythromelalgia between 2014 and 2019.[89] Each was precipitated by upper respiratory infection or immunization against influenza and courses of corticosteroids and/or IVIg returned her to full remission for months or years (Fig. 2). Far more patients have chronic subacute courses with SFN for > 6 months and gradual recovery during a few years of treatment with tapering oral prednisone and/or IVIg. Among 55 patients we tracked during IVIg administration, 16% were able to taper off IVIg and maintain sustained remission.[72] Most patients required continued IVIg tapered to the lowest effective dose, as in CIDP.

Autoantibodies and molecular pathways

Small fibers may be particularly vulnerable to immune damage given that they mediate responses to internal as well as external threats. To do so, they migrate

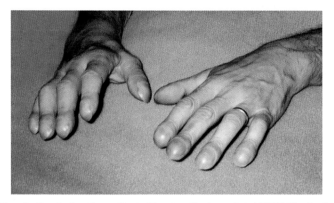

FIG. 2 Examination findings in a patient with autoantibody-mediated iiSFN. Hands of a 47-year-old man with 14 years of "total body pain" ineffectively managed with high dose opioids, gabapentin, and other treatments. A 2002 skin biopsy confirmed a clinical diagnosis of severe painful SFN, but there was no cause evident (iiSFN). However, his clubbed nicotine-stained fingers prompted immediate concern for a small-cell lung tumor with paraneoplastic SFN. A paraneoplastic panel was sent to Athena Diagnostics but testing, which then comprised only anti-MAG, antineuronal nuclear antibody, anti-CV2, sufatide, and GALOP autoantibodies, was unrevealing, and he was lost to follow-up untreated. In 2004, he died at an outside hospital of recently diagnosed lung cancer. The cause of his isolated SFN was almost certainly paraneoplastic anti-Hu autoantibodies, not yet widely recognized in 2002.[90–92] Paraneoplastic neuropathies are typically associated with small, undiagnosed cancers because the robust autoantibodies indicate good immune control of the tumor. Earlier diagnosis would have prompted a search for cancers and potentially saved his life.

from the protection of the CNS and its meninges during embryogenesis, leaving their cell bodies exposed and their distal-most neurites in intimate contact with the external and internal milieu. The dorsal root ganglia (DRG) develop fenestrated capillaries to facilitate cross-talk with infections and immunocytes as well as exposure to blood-borne infections and immune effectors. Small-fiber neurites densely innervate all mucosal barrier tissues, including in the eye, nose, and respiratory mucosa; the entire GI system; and the lower urothelium.[93] In the skin, TRPV1$^+$ nociceptive neurites initiate local axon reflexes (neurogenic inflammation) that not only cause redness and facilitate the entry of intravascular contents into threatened areas, but also initiate protective type 17 immunity that anticipates pathogen invasion.[94] A recent study shows that gastrointestinal C-fibers are not only sentinels and regulators of gut motility, circulation, and homeostasis, but they actively protect against infection in the Peyer's patches. When activated by the bacterial pathogen salmonella, sensory C-fibers regulate intestinal permeability and change the microbiome, boosting the number of protective gut organisms.[95] Sensory neurons have receptors for inflammatory mediators including histamine, cytokines, or neurotrophins, and they communicate with and help regulate mast cells, dendritic cells, eosinophils, Th2 cells, and type 2 innate lymphoid in many tissues to help mediate itch and inflammation.[96] The distal terminals of "sensory" small fibers release neuropeptides, including a calcitonin gene-related peptide, substance P, and vasoactive intestinal peptide, and the autonomics release acetylcholine and noradrenaline. Such neuro-immune signaling is increasingly recognized to be central in allergic diseases including atopic dermatitis, asthma, and food allergies. The distal small-fiber terminals are thus very visible to immune surveillance.

The identification of small-fiber epitopes and autoantibodies is in its infancy, given the limited case ascertainment. The forthcoming ACTTION/CONCEPPT consensus case definition and research diagnosis criteria will facilitate high-throughput screening.[30] In iiSFN, autoantibodies are more often reported in rapid-onset, clear-cut cases in females, and with nonlength-dependent presentations. In the Pestronk lab's study of 155 patients with iiSFN, 37% had IgM antibodies to trisulfated heparin disaccharide (TS-HDS), compared to 11% of ALS controls, and 15% had antibodies to fibroblast growth factor-3 (FGFR3) versus 3% of ALS controls.[97] In other studies, five of eight children with isolated iiSFN had IgM TS-HDS autoantibodies, as did five of 22 fibromyalgia patients among whom 86% had SFN-diagnostic skin biopsies.[55,98] Given that TS-HDS is also associated with large-fiber sensory neuropathy and other neuromuscular conditions,[99] and FGFR3 antibodies are equally prevalent in large-fiber sensory neuropathy,[97,98] specificity for SFN is uncertain, particularly for FGFR3. It is also not established whether these are pathogenic or bystander autoantibodies. Autoantibodies have been more definitively associated with dysautonomic SFN symptoms including POTS,[100,101] and immune attack on channel complexes can mimic genetic channelopathy-associated SFN.[102]

Mayo Clinic research established that paraneoplastic syndromes are rare causes of autoantibody-mediated iiSFN, with anti-Hu amphiphysin and CV2 autoantibodies well described.[103–105] Small-cell lung tumors are most common (Fig. 2), then hematological and gastrointestinal tumors, and IVIg and rituximab are reportedly effective.[106–110] However, we do not routinely send blood for paraneoplastic panels. Their far higher rate of false positive than true positive results (39% versus 20% in patients with sensory presentations) causes patient anxiety and often leads to expensive, fruitless testing.[111]

The most direct evidence of antibodies in iiSFN comes from passive transfer experiments in which animals are exposed to cell-free fluids from patients. Mice injected with sera from three patients with acute postinfectious SFN causing distal pain and dysautonomia developed SFN-like pain hypersensitivity and small-fiber-specific peripheral and spinal-cord pathology (Fig. 3).[112] The passive transfer of human autoantibodies to contactin associated protein-like 2 (CASPR2) to mice causes pain hypersensitivity and enhanced dorsal root ganglia cell excitability by reducing potassium channel Kv1 function.[102]

Given the lack of established diagnostic criteria for diagnosing autoimmune SFN, it is not yet possible to definitively identify the cellular and molecular pathways, but all evidence so far implicates not only B cells and antibody-antigen complexes, but also complement consumption. A large series reveals elevated prevalences of low levels of complement C4 and C3: Among 195 confirmed iiSFN patients, 16% had low serum C4 and 11% had low C3.[41] In our 41

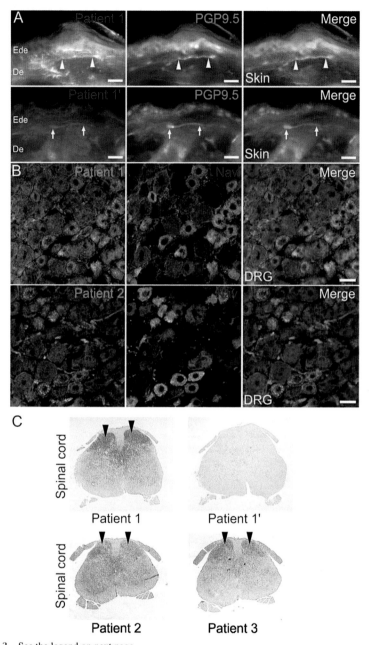

FIG. 3   See the legend on next page

patients with early onset widespread pain, 46% and 21% had low C4 and C3, respectively.[15] These findings implicate the classical and lectin pathways rather than the alternative pathway, which consumes C3 but not C4. T cells do not appear to have a prominent role, and in distinction with GBS and CIDP, cells are rare in nerve biopsies and in CSF.[15]

Considerations for immunotherapy treatment

Many patients with apparently autoimmune SFN are already recovering without treatment or have symptoms too mild to warrant immunotherapy. Unfortunately for the severely ill, nonimproving patients, there are no randomized or placebo-controlled trials or consensus guidelines to guide immunotherapy considerations. Despite this, physicians are increasingly prescribing various immunotherapies empirically, based on their clinical experience and the retrospective series published.

Corticosteroids have been rapidly effective in some but not all young patients with rapid-onset painful SFN,[86,113–115] unlike in GBS.[116] In our series of 10 clinic patients treated with oral prednisone (1 mg/kg/day for 4 weeks then rapid taper), 80% improved.[15] Among five severely ill hospitalized patients treated with intravenous methylprednisolone (1 g/day for 5 days) then prednisone taper, this was effective for only the two acute cases.[15] These results require cautious interpretation; in addition to very small samples and the lack of untreated controls, other potential confounders include nonspecific benefits for pain, activity, and mood. For clinic patients, oral prednisone, often with alternate-day dosing, is easier and cheaper than monthly pulses of intravenous methylprednisolone. Corticosteroids should particularly be considered for acute patients, young patients with minimal safety concerns, and patients without access to more expensive treatments.[86,113]

FIG. 3 Passive transfer evidence of dysimmune SFN to mice. The Nobuhiro Yuki laboratory intrathecally injected sera from three Chinese patients with new severe limb pain after shortly preceding infections. Patients' immune blood markers remained normal along with tests for other common causes and known neuropathy-associated autoantibodies. Sera from healthy volunteers or patients with CMT or CIDP provided negative controls (not shown). Serum immunoglobulin from SFN patients but not controls induced thermal hind-paw hyperalgesia (pain behaviors not shown). Panel (A) from mice's foot pads depicts strong and wide colocalization of Patient 1 sera with anti-PGP9.5 labeled small-fiber axons. Panel (B) from mouse lumbar dorsal root ganglia depicts colocalization of sera from Patients 1 and 2 with anti-Nav labeled small-fiber neuronal cell bodies. Patient sera preferentially labeled the small-diameter that express voltage-gated sodium channels. Pane 1 (C) from mouse lumbar spinal cord depicts binding of acute sera from patients 1, 2, and 3, but not convalescent sera (upper right panel) to peripheral incoming sensory axons and superficial lamina of the dorsal horn where most small fibers terminate and synapse. Scale bars = 20 μm in (A), 10 μm in (B). *(From Yuki N, Chan AC, Wong AHY, et al. Acute painful autoimmune neuropathy: a variant of Guillain-Barré syndrome. Muscle Nerve. 2018;57(2):320–324.)*

IVIg has the strongest evidence of benefit so far, further corroborating the hypothesis of B-cell mediation. Patients being considered for IVIg should have confirmed iiSFN with severe nonrecovering disability, other causes excluded (Table 1), and ideally evidence of dysimmunity, usually by medical history or test results. Sometimes I use a short trial of corticosteroids for additional evidence if unsure. In the first large series, 55 children and adults with SFN treated with ≥ 1 g/kg/4 weeks for ≥ 3 months, both primary outcomes were met. Patient pretreatment pain severity dropped ($P = .007$) and the prevalence of AFTs diagnostic for SFN dropped from 89% pretreatment to 55% ($P \leq .001$).[72] Three-quarters of patients and their neurologists reported improvement, and 16% of patients entered sustained remissions permitting IVIg withdrawal. There were no serious or unexpected adverse events, but typical infusion reactions were common.[72] All the smaller studies report positive results, including in sarcoidosis-associated SFN,[80] Sjogren's associated SFN,[79] and dysautonomia.[117] Prospective randomized controlled trials for "idiopathic SFN" are underway in the Netherlands (NCT02637700),[118] and in Boston for SFN associated with autoantibodies to TS-HDS and FGFR3 (NCT03401073).

Plasmapheresis is presumed efficacious as in GBS,[119] but it is only rarely considered because the benefit is transient and the logistics are complex. Settings in which to consider it include pregnancy, for diagnostic confirmation or next-day benefit in critically ill patients, or in selected patients with contraindications to corticosteroids and IVIg. Rituximab is increasingly supplanting plasmapheresis for depleting autoantibodies, despite no studies in SFN. It is most often used for patients with rheumatological diagnoses such as Sjogren's,[120] and B-cell associated malignancies and IgM MGUS, and efficacy is reported in seronegative autoimmune autonomic neuropathy and ganglionopathy.[121] I have found it occasionally helpful in rare patients with isolated apparently autoimmune SFN with insufficient benefit from several other immunotherapies.[122–124] Given the large number of cytokine and complement inhibitors under development, and their increasing use in neuromuscular medicine,[125] more selective inhibitors of B-cell-mediated neuroinflammation will be tried soon. Given their cost, inconvenience, and potentially serious side-effects, it is hoped that independent funding agencies will prioritize research into efficacy, safety, and indications.

Conclusions

The full range of SFN symptoms is often unappreciated even by neuromuscular specialists, leaving too many patients undiagnosed. Although many prefer to avoid patients with chronic unexplained pain, itching, or fibromyalgia diagnoses, not to mention the uncertainties about dysimmune SFN, the risks of letting severely ill and disabled patients remain untreated are underestimated. Because small-fiber axons grow throughout life, definitive diagnosis and treatment often permit axonal and functional recovery. Skin biopsy confirmation is now increasingly accepted as the small-fiber equivalent to performing nerve conduction study in large-fiber neuropathy.[30] Although diabetes is common, there is increasing evidence that B-cell mediated damage to small fibers is a significant contributor to initially idiopathic SFN, with sudden-onset monophasic GBS-like and chronic CIDP-like courses now well described. Patients with the highest probability of dysimmune causality include those with nonlength-dependent (ganglionitis) presentations, often from Sjogren's syndrome, and females and children with other evidence of disturbed immunity and immunodeficiency. All evidence so far implicates complement-mediated autoantibodies, including one small passive-transfer experiment in mice. Numerous small case-series and three unblinded studies of IVIg report similar efficacy and safety as in CIDP, with smaller case series also supporting corticosteroids. Because various factors can impede small-fiber health, all SFN patients should have potential secondary contributors (e.g., smoking and cardiovascular) addressed to maximize axon perfusion and nutrition. Finally, neuromuscular specialists need to become more familiar with clinical presentations and diagnostic and treatment options, including immunotherapies, engage in research to help discover the mechanisms, and trial existing and new therapies for apparently dysimmune small-fiber polyneuropathy.

Acknowledgments

I am grateful for years of mentorship from my fellowship supervisor John W "Jack" Griffin that began and encouraged my research on small-fiber and autoimmune neuropathy.

Financial support and sponsorship

NIH R01-NS093653 (Oaklander), US DoD GW140169 (Oaklander).

Conflict of Interest

None.

References

1. Ochoa J, Mair WG. The normal sural nerve in man. I. Ultrastructure and numbers of fibres and cells. *Acta Neuropathol.* 1969;13(3):197–216.
2. Fukuda T, Takeda S, Xu R, et al. Sema3A regulates bone-mass accrual through sensory innervations. *Nature.* 2013;497(7450):490–493.
3. Benarroch EE. Autonomic nervous system and neuroimmune interactions: new insights and clinical implications. *Neurology.* 2019;92(8):377–385.
4. Nolano M, Provitera V, Manganelli F, et al. Nonmotor involvement in amyotrophic lateral sclerosis: new insight from nerve and vessel analysis in skin biopsy. *Neuropathol Appl Neurobiol.* 2017;43(2):119–132.
5. Peters MJ, Bakkers M, Merkies IS, Hoeijmakers JG, van Raak EP, Faber CG. Incidence and prevalence of small-fiber neuropathy: a survey in the Netherlands. *Neurology.* 2013;81(15):1356–1360.

6. Boneparth A, Chen S, Horton DB, et al. *Evidence of decreased epidermal neurite density in juvenile fibromyalgia patients.* In: *Abstract Presented at Annual Meeting of the American Academy of Neurology, May 4–10, 2019, Philadelphia, PA*; 2019.

7. Lodahl M, Treister R, Oaklander AL. Specific symptoms may discriminate between fibromyalgia patients with vs without objective test evidence of small-fiber polyneuropathy. *Pain Rep.* 2018;3(1):e633.

8. Oaklander AL, Herzog ZD, Downs HM, Klein MM. Objective evidence that small-fiber polyneuropathy underlies some illnesses currently labeled as fibromyalgia. *Pain.* 2013;154:2310–2316.

9. Grayston R, Czanner G, Elhadd K, et al. A systematic review and meta-analysis of the prevalence of small fiber pathology in fibromyalgia: implications for a new paradigm in fibromyalgia etiopathogenesis. *Semin Arthritis Rheum.* 2018.

10. Evdokimov D, Frank J, Klitsch A, et al. Reduction of skin innervation is associated with a severe fibromyalgia phenotype. *Ann Neurol.* 2019;86(4):504–516.

11. Serra J, Collado A, Sola R, et al. Hyperexcitable C nociceptors in fibromyalgia. *Ann Neurol.* 2013;75(2):196–208.

12. Branco JC, Bannwarth B, Failde I, et al. Prevalence of fibromyalgia: a survey in five European countries. *Semin Arthritis Rheum.* 2010;39(6):448–453.

13. Oaklander AL, Nolano M. Scientific advances in and clinical approaches to small-fiber polyneuropathy: a review. *JAMA Neurol.* 2019;76(10):1240–1251.

14. Steinhoff M, Schmelz M, Szabo IL, Oaklander AL. Clinical presentation, management, and pathophysiology of neuropathic itch. *Lancet Neurol.* 2018;17(8):709–720.

15. Oaklander AL, Klein MM. Evidence of small-fiber polyneuropathy in unexplained, juvenile-onset, widespread pain syndromes. *Pediatrics.* 2013;131(4):e1091–e1100.

16. Thieben MJ, Sandroni P, Sletten DM, et al. Postural orthostatic tachycardia syndrome: the Mayo clinic experience. *Mayo Clin Proc.* 2007;82(3):308–313.

17. Treister R, Lodahl M, Lang M, Tworoger SS, Sawilowsky S, Oaklander AL. Initial development and validation of a patient-reported symptom survey for small-fiber polyneuropathy. *J Pain.* 2017;18(5):556–563.

18. Gwathmey KG. Sensory neuronopathies. *Muscle Nerve.* 2016;53(1):8–19.

19. Crowell A, Gwathmey KG. Sensory neuronopathies. *Curr Neurol Neurosci Rep.* 2017;17(10):79.

20. Mitchell SW. On a rare vaso-motor neurosis of the extremities, and on the maladies with which it may be confounded. *Am J Med Sci.* 1878;151:17–36.

21. Sousa-Valente J, Brain SD. A historical perspective on the role of sensory nerves in neurogenic inflammation. *Semin Immunopathol.* 2018;40(3):229–236.

22. Albrecht PJ, Hou Q, Argoff CE, Storey JR, Wymer JP, Rice FL. Excessive peptidergic sensory innervation of cutaneous arteriole-venule shunts (AVS) in the palmar glabrous skin of fibromyalgia patients: implications for widespread deep tissue pain and fatigue. *Pain Med.* 2013;14(6):895–915.

23. Dori A, Lopate G, Keeling R, Pestronk A. Myovascular innervation: axon loss in small-fiber neuropathies. *Muscle Nerve.* 2015;51(4):514–521.

24. Lopate G, Streif E, Harms M, Weihl C, Pestronk A. Cramps and small-fiber neuropathy. *Muscle Nerve.* 2013;48(2):252–255.

25. Selim MM, Wendelschafer-Crabb G, Redmon JB, et al. Gastric mucosal nerve density: a biomarker for diabetic autonomic neuropathy? *Neurology.* 2010;75(11):973–981.

26. Poda R, Guaraldi P, Solieri L, et al. Standing worsens cognitive functions in patients with neurogenic orthostatic hypotension. *Neurol Sci.* 2012;33(2):469–473.

27. Hsieh PC, Tseng MT, Chao CC, et al. Imaging signatures of altered brain responses in small-fiber neuropathy: reduced functional connectivity of the limbic system after peripheral nerve degeneration. *Pain*. 2015;156(5):904–916.

28. Briner RP, Carlton SM, Coggeshall RE, Chung KS. Evidence for unmyelinated sensory fibres in the posterior columns in man. *Brain*. 1988;111(Pt 5):999–1007.

29. Henrich F, Magerl W, Klein T, Greffrath W, Treede RD. Capsaicin-sensitive C- and A-fibre nociceptors control long-term potentiation-like pain amplification in humans. *Brain*. 2015;138(Pt 9):2505–2520.

30. Gewandter JS, Freeman R, Dworkin R, et al. *Diagnostic criteria for idiopathic distal sensory polyneuropathy and small-fiber polyneuropathy*. In: *Paper Presented at 2020 Conference of the American Academy of Neurology; Toronto, ON, Canada*; 2020.

31. Bastyr 3rd EJ, Price KL, Bril V, Group MS. Development and validity testing of the neuropathy total symptom score-6: questionnaire for the study of sensory symptoms of diabetic peripheral neuropathy. *Clin Ther*. 2005;27(8):1278–1294.

32. Zilliox L, Peltier AC, Wren PA, et al. Assessing autonomic dysfunction in early diabetic neuropathy: the Survey of Autonomic Symptoms. *Neurology*. 2011;76(12):1099–1105.

33. Meijer JW, Smit AJ, Sonderen EV, Groothoff JW, Eisma WH, Links TP. Symptom scoring systems to diagnose distal polyneuropathy in diabetes: the Diabetic Neuropathy Symptom score. *Diabet Med*. 2002;19(11):962–965.

34. Hoitsma E, De VJ, Drent M. The small fiber neuropathy screening list: construction and cross-validation in sarcoidosis. *Respir Med*. 2011;105(1):95–100.

35. Oldenburg J, Fossa SD, Dahl AA. Scale for chemotherapy-induced long-term neurotoxicity (SCIN): psychometrics, validation, and findings in a large sample of testicular cancer survivors. *Qual Life Res*. 2006;15(5):791–800.

36. Treister R, O'Neil K, Downs HM, Oaklander AL. Validation of the composite autonomic symptom scale 31 (COMPASS-31) in patients with and without small fiber polyneuropathy. *Eur J Neurol*. 2015;22(7):1124–1130.

37. Dworkin RH, Turk DC, Revicki DA, et al. Development and initial validation of an expanded and revised version of the Short-form McGill Pain Questionnaire (SF-MPQ-2). *Pain*. 2009;144(1–2):35–42.

38. Brouwer BA, Bakkers M, Hoeijmakers JG, Faber CG, Merkies IS. Improving assessment in small fiber neuropathy. *J Peripher Nerv Syst*. 2015;20(3):333–340.

39. Singleton JR, Bixby B, Russell JW, et al. The Utah Early Neuropathy Scale: a sensitive clinical scale for early sensory predominant neuropathy. *J Peripher Nerv Syst*. 2008;13(3):218–227.

40. Zirpoli G, Klein MM, Downs S, Farhad K, Oaklander AL. Validation of the Mass General Neuropathy Exam Tool (MAGNET) for initial diagnosis of length-dependent small-fiber polyneuropathy. In: *Proc. 2018 Conference of the Peripheral Nerve Society*. 2018:249–250.

41. Lang M, Treister R, Oaklander AL. Diagnostic value of blood tests for occult causes of initially idiopathic small-fiber polyneuropathy. *J Neurol*. 2016;263(12):2515–2527.

42. de Greef BTA, Hoeijmakers JGJ, Gorissen-Brouwers CML, Geerts M, Faber CG, Merkies ISJ. Associated conditions in small fiber neuropathy—a large cohort study and review of the literature. *Eur J Neurol*. 2018;25(2):348–355.

43. Dahlin LB, Eriksson KF, Sundkvist G. Persistent postoperative complaints after whole sural nerve biopsies in diabetic and nondiabetic subjects. *Diabet Med*. 1997;14(5):353–356.

44. Herrmann DN, Griffin JW, Hauer P, Cornblath DR, McArthur JC. Epidermal nerve fiber density and sural nerve morphometry in peripheral neuropathies. *Neurology*. 1999;53(8):1634–1640.

45. Wilkinson KD, Lee KM, Deshpande S, Duerksen-Hughes P, Boss JM, Pohl J. The neuron-specific protein PGP 9.5 is a ubiquitin carboxyl-terminal hydrolase. *Science*. 1989;246(4930):670–673.

46. Lauria G, Hsieh ST, Johansson O, et al. European Federation of Neurological Societies/Peripheral Nerve Society Guideline on the use of skin biopsy in the diagnosis of small fiber neuropathy. Report of a joint task force of the European Federation of Neurological Societies and the Peripheral Nerve Society. *Eur J Neurol.* 2010;17(7):903–912. e944–909.

47. Provitera V, Gibbons CH, Wendelschafer-Crabb G, et al. A multi-center, multinational age- and gender-adjusted normative dataset for immunofluorescent intraepidermal nerve fiber density at the distal leg. *Eur J Neurol.* 2016;23(2):333–338.

48. England JD, Gronseth GS, Franklin G, et al. Practice parameter: evaluation of distal symmetric polyneuropathy: role of autonomic testing, nerve biopsy, and skin biopsy (an evidence-based review). Report of the American Academy of Neurology, American Association of Neuromuscular and Electrodiagnostic Medicine, and American Academy of Physical Medicine and Rehabilitation. *Neurology.* 2009;72(2):177–184.

49. Devigili G, Tugnoli V, Penza P, et al. The diagnostic criteria for small fibre neuropathy: from symptoms to neuropathology. *Brain.* 2008;131(Pt 7):1912–1925.

50. McArthur JC, Stocks EA, Hauer P, Cornblath DR, Griffin JW. Epidermal nerve fiber density: normative reference range and diagnostic efficiency. *Arch Neurol.* 1998;55(12):1513–1520.

51. Jin P, Cheng L, Chen M, Zhou L. Low sensitivity of skin biopsy in diagnosing small fiber neuropathy in Chinese Americans. *J Clin Neuromuscul Dis.* 2018;20(1):1–6.

52. Klein MM, Downs H, O'Neil K, Oaklander AL. Skin biopsy of normal children demonstrates inverse correlation between age and epidermal nerve fiber density, meaning age-specific norms are needed. *Ann Neurol.* 2014;76(suppl 18):S69.

53. Lauria G, Holland NR, Hauer P, Cornblath DR, Griffin JW, McArthur JC. Epidermal innervation: changes with aging, topographic location, and in sensory neuropathy. *J Neurol Sci.* 1999;164(2):172–178.

54. Provitera V, Gibbons CH, Wendelschafer-Crabb G, et al. The role of skin biopsy in differentiating small-fiber neuropathy from ganglionopathy. *Eur J Neurol.* 2018;25(6):848–853.

55. Malik A, Lopate G, Hayat G, et al. Prevalence of axonal sensory neuropathy with IgM binding to trisulfated heparin disaccharide in patients with fibromyalgia. *J Clin Neuromuscul Dis.* 2019;20(3):103–110.

56. Walk D, Wendelschafer-Crabb G, Davey C, Kennedy WR. Concordance between epidermal nerve fiber density and sensory examination in patients with symptoms of idiopathic small fiber neuropathy. *J Neurol Sci.* 2007;255(1–2):23–26.

57. Nolano M, Biasiotta A, Lombardi R, et al. Epidermal innervation morphometry by immunofluorescence and bright-field microscopy. *J Peripher Nerv Syst.* 2015;20(4):387–391.

58. Low VA, Sandroni P, Fealey RD, Low PA. Detection of small-fiber neuropathy by sudomotor testing. *Muscle Nerve.* 2006;34(1):57–61.

59. Singer W, Spies JM, McArthur J, et al. Prospective evaluation of somatic and autonomic small fibers in selected autonomic neuropathies. *Neurology.* 2004;62(4):612–618.

60. Thaisetthawatkul P, Fernandes Filho JA, Herrmann DN. Contribution of QSART to the diagnosis of small fiber neuropathy. *Muscle Nerve.* 2013;48(6):883–888.

61. Duchesne M, Richard L, Vallat JM, Magy L. Assessing sudomotor impairment in patients with peripheral neuropathy: comparison between electrochemical skin conductance and skin biopsy. *Clin Neurophysiol.* 2018;129(7):1341–1348.

62. Provitera V, Nolano M, Caporaso G, Stancanelli A, Santoro L, Kennedy WR. Evaluation of sudomotor function in diabetes using the dynamic sweat test. *Neurology.* 2010;74(1):50–56.

63. Azmi S, Ferdousi M, Petropoulos IN, et al. Corneal confocal microscopy shows an improvement in small-fiber neuropathy in subjects with type 1 diabetes on continuous subcutaneous insulin infusion compared with multiple daily injection. *Diabetes Care.* 2015;38(1):e3–e4.

64. Freeman R, Chase KP, Risk MR. Quantitative sensory testing cannot differentiate simulated sensory loss from sensory neuropathy. *Neurology.* 2003;60(3):465–470.

65. Farhad K, Traub R, Ruzhansky KM, Brannagan 3rd TH. Causes of neuropathy in patients referred as "idiopathic neuropathy". *Muscle Nerve.* 2016;53(6):856–861.

66. Dyck PJ, Clark VM, Overland CJ, et al. Impaired glycemia and diabetic polyneuropathy: the OC IG Survey. *Diabetes Care.* 2012;35(3):584–591.

67. Zirpoli G, Rice MS, Huang T, Tworoger SS, Oaklander AL. Anthropometric, lifestyle, and dietary risk factors for peripheral neuropathy in the Nurses' Health Study II. In: *Proc. 2018 Conference of the Peripheral Nerve Society, Baltimore, MD.* 2018:249–250.

68. O'Brien PD, Hinder LM, Callaghan BC, Feldman EL. Neurological consequences of obesity. *Lancet Neurol.* 2017;16(6):465–477.

69. Ylitalo KR, Sowers M, Heeringa S. Peripheral vascular disease and peripheral neuropathy in individuals with cardiometabolic clustering and obesity: National Health and Nutrition Examination Survey 2001–2004. *Diabetes Care.* 2011;34(7):1642–1647.

70. Koike H, Takahashi M, Ohyama K, et al. Clinicopathologic features of folate-deficiency neuropathy. *Neurology.* 2015;84(10):1026–1033.

71. Latov N, Vo ML, Chin RL, Carey BT, Langsdorf JA, Feuer NT. Abnormal nutritional factors in patients evaluated at a neuropathy center. *J Clin Neuromuscul Dis.* 2016;17(4):212–214.

72. Liu X, Treister R, Lang M, Oaklander AL. IVIg for apparently autoimmune small-fiber polyneuropathy: first analysis of efficacy and safety. *Ther Adv Neurol Disord.* 2018;11: 1756285617744484.

73. Hsu JL, Liao MF, Hsu HC, et al. A prospective, observational study of patients with uncommon distal symmetric painful small-fiber neuropathy. *PLoS One.* 2017;12(9):e0183948.

74. Griffin JW, Cornblath DR, Alexander E, et al. Ataxic sensory neuropathy and dorsal root ganglionitis associated with Sjögren's syndrome. *Ann Neurol.* 1990;27(3):304–315.

75. Birnbaum J, Lalji A, Piccione EA, Izbudak I. Magnetic resonance imaging of the spinal cord in the evaluation of 3 patients with sensory neuronopathies: diagnostic assessment, indications of treatment response, and impact of autoimmunity: a case report. *Medicine (Baltimore).* 2017;96(49):e8483.

76. Sène D, Cacoub P, Authier FJ, et al. Sjögren syndrome-associated small fiber neuropathy: characterization from a prospective series of 40 cases. *Medicine (Baltimore).* 2013;92(5):e10–e18.

77. Lefaucheur JP, Sène D, Oaklander AL. Primary Sjögren's syndrome. *N Engl J Med.* 2018;379(1):96.

78. Sène D, Jallouli M, Lefaucheur JP, et al. Peripheral neuropathies associated with primary Sjogren syndrome: immunologic profiles of nonataxic sensory neuropathy and sensorimotor neuropathy. *Medicine (Baltimore).* 2011;90(2):133–138.

79. Gaillet A, Champion K, Lefaucheur J, Trout H, Bergmann J, Sène D. Intravenous immunoglobulin efficacy for primary Sjögren's Syndrome associated small fiber neuropathy. *Autoimmun Rev.* 2019.

80. Tavee JO, Karwa K, Ahmed Z, Thompson N, Parambil J, Culver DA. Sarcoidosis-associated small fiber neuropathy in a large cohort: clinical aspects and response to IVIG and anti-TNF alpha treatment. *Respir Med.* 2017;126:135–138.

81. Parambil JG, Tavee JO, Zhou L, Pearson KS, Culver DA. Efficacy of intravenous immunoglobulin for small fiber neuropathy associated with sarcoidosis. *Respir Med.* 2011;105(1):101–105.

82. Hoitsma E, Faber CG, van Kroonenburgh MJ, et al. Association of small fiber neuropathy with cardiac sympathetic dysfunction in sarcoidosis. *Sarcoidosis Vasc Diffuse Lung Dis.* 2005;22(1):43–50.

83. Voorter CE, Drent M, Hoitsma E, Faber KG, van den Berg-Loonen EM. Association of HLA DQB1 0602 in sarcoidosis patients with small fiber neuropathy. *Sarcoidosis Vasc Diffuse Lung Dis*. 2005;22(2):129–132.

84. Hoitsma E, Marziniak M, Faber CG, et al. Small fibre neuropathy in sarcoidosis. *Lancet*. 2002;359(9323):2085–2086.

85. Zirpoli G, Kaiser E, Yee AJ, Oaklander AL. Do conventional and light-chain MGUS increase risk for small-fiber polyneuropathy? *Ann Neurol*. 2018;84(S22).

86. Paticoff J, Valovska A, Nedeljkovic SS, Oaklander AL. Defining a treatable cause of erythromelalgia: acute adolescent autoimmune small-fiber axonopathy. *Anesth Analg*. 2007;104(2):438–441.

87. Martinez-Lavin M, Martinez-Martinez LA, Reyes-Loyola P. HPV vaccination syndrome. A questionnaire-based study. *Clin Rheumatol*. 2015;34:1981–1983.

88. McKhann GM, Cornblath DR, Griffin JW, et al. Acute motor axonal neuropathy: a frequent cause of acute flaccid paralysis in China. *Ann Neurol*. 1993;33(4):333–342.

89. Spoendlin J, Roschach B, Wilder-Smith A, Landolt M, Oaklander AL. Characterization of a relapsing/remitting, disease course for corticosteroid-responsive small-fiber polyneuropathy. In: *Paper Presented at 2019 Annual Meeting of the Peripheral Nerve Society, Genoa, Italy*; 2019.

90. Oh SJ, Gurtekin Y, Dropcho EJ, King P, Claussen GC. Anti-Hu antibody neuropathy: a clinical, electrophysiological, and pathological study. *Clin Neurophysiol*. 2005;116(1):28–34.

91. Camdessanch, JP, Antoine JC, Honnorat J, et al. Paraneoplastic peripheral neuropathy associated with anti-Hu antibodies. A clinical and electrophysiological study of 20 patients. *Brain*. 2002;125(Pt 1):166–175.

92. Oh SJ, Dropcho EJ, Claussen GC. Anti-Hu-associated paraneoplastic sensory neuropathy responding to early aggressive immunotherapy: report of two cases and review of literature. *Muscle Nerve*. 1997;20(12):1576–1582.

93. Voisin T, Bouvier A, Chiu IM. Neuro-immune interactions in allergic diseases: novel targets for therapeutics. *Int Immunol*. 2017;29(6):247–261.

94. Cohen JA, Edwards TN, Liu AW, et al. Cutaneous TRPV1(+) neurons trigger protective innate type 17 anticipatory immunity. *Cell*. 2019;178(4):919–932. e914.

95. Lai NY, Musser MA, Pinho-Ribeiro FA, et al. Gut-innervating nociceptor neurons regulate Peyer's patch microfold cells and SFB levels to mediate salmonella host defense. *Cell*. 2019;180. 33–49.e22.

96. Steinhoff M, Oaklander AL, Szabo IL, Stander S, Schmelz M. Neuropathic itch. *Pain*. 2019;160(suppl 1):S11–S16.

97. Levine TD, Kafaie J, Zeidman LA, et al. Cryptogenic small-fiber neuropathies: serum autoantibody binding to trisulfated heparan disaccharide and fibroblast growth factor receptor-3. *Muscle Nerve*. 2019. https://doi.org/10.1002/mus.26748.

98. Kafaie J, Al Balushi A, Kim M, Pestronk A. Clinical and laboratory profiles of idiopathic small fiber neuropathy in children: case series. *J Clin Neuromuscul Dis*. 2017;19(1):31–37.

99. Pestronk A, Choksi R, Logigian E, Al-Lozi MT. Sensory neuropathy with monoclonal IgM binding to a trisulfated heparin disaccharide. *Muscle Nerve*. 2003;27(2):188–195.

100. Suarez GA, Fealey RD, Camilleri M, Low PA. Idiopathic autonomic neuropathy: clinical, neurophysiologic, and follow-up studies on 27 patients. *Neurology*. 1994;44(9):1675–1682.

101. Watari M, Nakane S, Mukaino A, et al. Autoimmune postural orthostatic tachycardia syndrome. *Ann Clin Transl Neurol*. 2018;5(4):486–492.

102. Dawes JM, Weir GA, Middleton SJ, et al. Immune or genetic-mediated disruption of CASPR2 causes pain hypersensitivity due to enhanced primary afferent excitability. *Neuron*. 2018;97(4):806–822. e810.

103. Antoine JC, Camdessanche JP. Paraneoplastic neuropathies. *Curr Opin Neurol.* 2017; 30(5):513–520.
104. Oki Y, Koike H, Iijima M, et al. Ataxic vs painful form of paraneoplastic neuropathy. *Neurology.* 2007;69(6):564–572.
105. Graus F, Keime-Guibert F, Rene R, et al. Anti-Hu-associated paraneoplastic encephalomyelitis: analysis of 200 patients. *Brain.* 2001;124(6):1138–1148.
106. Zis P, Sarrigiannis PG, Rao DG, Hadjivassiliou M. Gluten neuropathy: prevalence of neuropathic pain and the role of gluten-free diet. *J Neurol.* 2018;265(10):2231–2236.
107. Honnorat J. Therapeutic approaches in antibody-associated central nervous system pathologies. *Rev Neurol (Paris).* 2014;170(10):587–594.
108. Coret F, Bosca I, Fratalia L, Perez-Griera J, Pascual A, Casanova B. Long-lasting remission after rituximab treatment in a case of anti-Hu-associated sensory neuronopathy and gastric pseudoobstruction. *J Neuro Oncol.* 2009;93(3):421–423.
109. Voltz R. Intravenous immunoglobulin therapy in paraneoplastic neurological syndromes. *J Neurol.* 2006;253(suppl 5):V33–V38.
110. Shams'ili S, de BJ, Gratama JW, et al. An uncontrolled trial of rituximab for antibody associated paraneoplastic neurological syndromes. *J Neurol.* 2006;253(1):16–20.
111. Ebright MJ, Li SH, Reynolds E, et al. Unintended consequences of Mayo paraneoplastic evaluations. *Neurology.* 2018;91(22):e2057–e2066.
112. Yuki N, Chan AC, Wong AHY, et al. Acute painful autoimmune neuropathy: a variant of Guillain-Barré syndrome. *Muscle Nerve.* 2018;57(2):320–324.
113. Dabby R, Gilad R, Sadeh M, Lampl Y, Watemberg N. Acute steroid responsive small-fiber sensory neuropathy: a new entity? *J Peripher Nerv Syst.* 2006;11(1):47–52.
114. Seneviratne U, Gunasekera S. Acute small fibre sensory neuropathy: another variant of Guillain-Barre syndrome? *J Neurol Neurosurg Psychiatry.* 2002;72(4):540–542.
115. Morales PS, Escobar RG, Lizama M, et al. Paediatric hypertension-associated erythromelalgia responds to corticosteroids and is not associated with SCN9A mutations. *Rheumatology (Oxford).* 2012;51(12):2295–2296.
116. Hughes RA, Brassington R, Gunn AA, van Doorn PA. Corticosteroids for Guillain-Barre syndrome. *Cochrane Database Syst Rev.* 2016;10:CD001446.
117. Schofield JR, Chemali KR. Intravenous immunoglobulin therapy in refractory autoimmune dysautonomias: a retrospective analysis of 38 patients. *Am J Ther.* 2018.
118. de Greef BT, Geerts M, Hoeijmakers JG, Faber CG, Merkies IS. Intravenous immunoglobulin therapy for small fiber neuropathy: study protocol for a randomized controlled trial. *Trials.* 2016;17(1):330.
119. Chevret S, Hughes RA, Annane D. Plasma exchange for Guillain-Barré syndrome. *Cochrane Database Syst Rev.* 2017;2:CD001798.
120. Mariette X, Criswell LA. Primary Sjogren's Syndrome. *N Engl J Med.* 2018;378(10): 931–939.
121. Bouxin M, Schvartz B, Mestrallet S, et al. Rituximab treatment in seronegative autoimmune autonomic neuropathy and autoimmune autonomic ganglionopathy: case-report and literature review. *J Neuroimmunol.* 2019;326:28–32.
122. Chen LY, Keddie S, Lunn MP, et al. IgM paraprotein-associated peripheral neuropathy: small CD20-positive B-cell clones may predict a monoclonal gammopathy of neurological significance and rituximab responsiveness. *Br J Haematol.* 2019. https://doi.org/10.1111/bjh.16210.
123. Huma AC, Kecskes EM, Tulba D, Balanescu P, Baicus C. Immunosuppressive treatment for peripheral neuropathies in Sjogren's syndrome—a systematic review. *Rom J Intern Med.* 2019. https://doi.org/10.2478/rjim-2019-0022.

124. Dalakas MC. Advances in the diagnosis, immunopathogenesis and therapies of IgM-anti-MAG antibody-mediated neuropathies. *Ther Adv Neurol Disord.* 2018;11. 1756285617746640.

125. Muppidi S, Utsugisawa K, Benatar M, et al. Long-term safety and efficacy of eculizumab in generalized myasthenia gravis. *Muscle Nerve.* 2019;60(1):14–24.

Index

Note: Page numbers followed by *f* indicate figures and *t* indicate tables.

Printed in the United States
By Bookmasters